Intelligent Soft Sensors

Intelligent Soft Sensors

Editor

Simon Tomažič

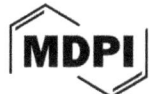

Basel • Beijing • Wuhan • Barcelona • Belgrade • Novi Sad • Cluj • Manchester

Editor
Simon Tomažič
University of Ljubljana
Ljubljana, Slovenia

Editorial Office
MDPI
St. Alban-Anlage 66
4052 Basel, Switzerland

This is a reprint of articles from the Special Issue published online in the open access journal *Sensors* (ISSN 1424-8220) (available at: https://www.mdpi.com/journal/sensors/special_issues/intelligent_soft_sensors).

For citation purposes, cite each article independently as indicated on the article page online and as indicated below:

Lastname, A.A.; Lastname, B.B. Article Title. *Journal Name* **Year**, *Volume Number*, Page Range.

ISBN 978-3-0365-8522-2 (Hbk)
ISBN 978-3-0365-8523-9 (PDF)
doi.org/10.3390/books978-3-0365-8523-9

© 2023 by the authors. Articles in this book are Open Access and distributed under the Creative Commons Attribution (CC BY) license. The book as a whole is distributed by MDPI under the terms and conditions of the Creative Commons Attribution-NonCommercial-NoDerivs (CC BY-NC-ND) license.

Contents

About the Editor vii

Simon Tomažič
Intelligent Soft Sensors
Reprinted from: *Sensors* **2023**, *23*, 6895, doi:10.3390/s23156895 1

Thijs Devos, Matteo Kirchner, Jan Croes, Wim Desmet and Frank Naets
Sensor Selection and State Estimation for Unobservable and Non-Linear System Models
Reprinted from: *Sensors* **2021**, *21*, 7492, doi:10.3390/s21227492 5

Wenjuan Mei, Zhen Liu, Lei Tang and Yuanzhang Su
Test Strategy Optimization Based on Soft Sensing and Ensemble Belief Measurement
Reprinted from: *Sensors* **2022**, *22*, 2138, doi:10.3390/s22062138 25

Katalin Mohai, Csilla Kálózi-Szabó, Zoltán Jakab, Szilárd Dávid Fecht, Márk Domonkos and János Botzheim
Development of an Adaptive Computer-Aided Soft Sensor Diagnosis System for Assessment of Executive Functions
Reprinted from: *Sensors* **2022**, *22*, 5880, doi:10.3390/s22155880 47

Alejandro Rincón, Fredy E. Hoyos and John E. Candelo-Becerra
A Simplified Algorithm for Setting the Observer Parameters for Second-Order Systems with Persistent Disturbances Using a Robust Observer
Reprinted from: *Sensors* **2022**, *22*, 6988, doi:10.3390/s22186988 63

Gorazd Karer and Igor Škrjanc
Improved Individualized Patient-Oriented Depth-of-Hypnosis Measurement Based on Bispectral Index
Reprinted from: *Sensors* **2022**, *23*, 293, doi:10.3390/s23010293 81

Shengyuan Xiao, Shuo Wang, Liang Ge, Hengxiang Weng, Xin Fang, Zhenming Peng and Wen Zeng
Hybrid Feature Fusion-Based High-Sensitivity Fire Detection and Early Warning for Intelligent Building Systems
Reprinted from: *Sensors* **2023**, *23*, 859, doi:10.3390/s23020859 99

Žiga Stržinar, Araceli Sanchis, Oscar Sipele, Boštjan Pregelj and Igor Škrjanc
Stress Detection Using Frequency Spectrum Analysis of Wrist-Measured Electrodermal Activity
Reprinted from: *Sensors* **2023**, *23*, 963, doi:10.3390/s23020963 119

Bhagoji Bapurao Sul, Dhanalakshmi Kaliaperumal and Seung-Bok Choi
Self-Sensing Variable Stiffness Actuation of Shape Memory Coil by an Inferential Soft Sensor
Reprinted from: *Sensors* **2023**, *23*, 2442, doi:10.3390/s23052442 135

Yuxuan Li, Weihao Jiang, Zhihui Shi and Chunjie Yang
A Soft Sensor Model of Sintering Process Quality Index Based on Multi-Source Data Fusion
Reprinted from: *Sensors* **2023**, *23*, 4954, doi:10.3390/s23104954 159

Bo Wang, Jun Liu, Ameng Yu and Haibo Wang
Development and Optimization of a Novel Soft Sensor Modeling Method for Fermentation Process of *Pichia pastoris*
Reprinted from: *Sensors* **2023**, *23*, 6014, doi:10.3390/s23136014 177

Simon Tomažič and Igor Škrjanc
Halfway to Automated Feeding of Chinese Hamster Ovary Cells
Reprinted from: *Sensors* **2023**, *23*, 6618, doi:10.3390/s23146618 . . . . **199**

About the Editor

Simon Tomažič

Simon Tomažič received his B.Sc. and Ph.D. degrees in electrical engineering from the Faculty of Electrical Engineering, University of Ljubljana, Slovenia, in 2012 and 2016, respectively. He is currently an Assistant Professor at the Laboratory of Control Systems and Cybernetics, University of Ljubljana. His main research interests include fuzzy model identification, mathematical and computational modelling, soft sensors, machine learning with big data, predictive control of dynamical systems and indoor positioning using computer vision and radiolocation.

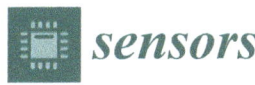

Editorial

Intelligent Soft Sensors

Simon Tomažič

Faculty of Electrical Engineering, University of Ljubljana, 1000 Ljubljana, Slovenia; simon.tomazic@fe.uni-lj.si; Tel.:+386-1-4768-760

Citation: Tomažič, S. Intelligent Soft Sensors. *Sensors* **2023**, *23*, 6895. https://doi.org/10.3390/s23156895

Received: 26 July 2023
Accepted: 2 August 2023
Published: 3 August 2023

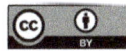

Copyright: © 2023 by the author. Licensee MDPI, Basel, Switzerland. This article is an open access article distributed under the terms and conditions of the Creative Commons Attribution (CC BY) license (https://creativecommons.org/licenses/by/4.0/).

In this Special Issue, we embark on a journey into the exciting field of intelligent soft sensors, and take a deep dive into the groundbreaking advances and potential that these software algorithms have introduced in various fields. Soft sensors, often referred to as virtual sensors, are fast becoming a cornerstone of the ever-evolving digital age. To appreciate the capabilities of soft sensors, one must acknowledge their fundamental basis. These tools are based on sophisticated mathematical models, state-of-the-art computational techniques, and rigorous algorithmic strategies. Fields as diverse as physics, electrical engineering, biology, mathematics and even economics have influenced their development, making them a true example of interdisciplinary excellence.

Because these algorithms process a large number of measurements simultaneously, insights into online estimation of complex process variables that were previously impossible have become possible. In areas such as control applications, fault detection or data fusion, the importance of soft sensors has increased. Essentially, data from numerous sources are fused to gain insights from the apparent clutter.

The broader socio-economic and environmental context must also be considered. With rising costs, increasing concerns about sustainability and the overarching need for efficiency, the importance of soft sensors is clearer than ever. They provide the adaptability necessary for optimised resources, minimised waste and improved performance, meeting the pressing needs of the 21st century. In the rapidly digitising world, the ingenuity and breakthrough capabilities of today's researchers and engineers are undeniably impressive. It is not just about finding solutions to current problems, but also about identifying opportunities that many have not yet recognized. The forward-looking nature of this field becomes even clearer in the context of soft sensors. With this technological development, it is important to also recognise the broader impacts and applications.

Among the many interesting contributions in this Special Issue, one deals with the complexity of setting observer parameters for second-order systems with constant perturbations [1]. A novel algorithm that simplifies the inherent complexity in defining the convergence rate and the range for unknown state errors is the focus of the discussion. By matching the theory with practical scenarios, its usefulness is highlighted using a microalgae bioreactor model, emphasising the effectiveness of the algorithm in ensuring an optimal convergence rate and precision. The challenges posed by unobservable and nonlinear systems are addressed in [2], which presents a unique extended Kalman filter framework. An intelligent projection onto an observable subspace is used to solve previously insurmountable instability problems. The brilliance is particularly evident in sensor selection, which helps stabilise unobservable states and optimise sensor selection without the need for actual measurements. A deeper understanding is fostered by another valuable contribution [3] that re-evaluates conventional prediction and health management techniques. In an era characterised by rapid production cycles and frequent design changes, the urgency of a more dynamic, self-contained test optimisation methodology is highlighted. By merging soft sensing, ensemble learning and extreme learning machines (ELMs), a technique is presented that excels in efficiency and adaptability to the intricacies of modern systems.

However, the applications of soft sensors are not limited to manufacturing or engineering. Their impact on the medical and psychological fields is equally significant. The research [4] presented on ToLA—a computerised adaptive testing version of the Tower of London task—is exemplary. An item response theory was combined with an adaptive algorithm. The result is a diagnostic tool with increased sensitivity that provides a deeper understanding of neurodevelopmental disorders. Similarly, a model for measuring hypnotic depth during intravenous general anaesthesia is presented [5], pointing to a future where anaesthetic treatments are perfectly individualised.

Research into electrodermal activity (EDA) for stress detection [6] highlights the importance of monitoring mental health. The application of frequency spectrum analysis in this research promises a fast, accurate and efficient assessment of stress in real time, which is particularly important given the global increase in mental health problems.

In bioprocessing, where the goal is to improve accuracy and efficiency, soft sensors are becoming increasingly useful, especially when combined with Raman spectroscopy and machine learning. A study on the automated feeding of Chinese hamster ovary cells (CHO) [7] is presented, highlighting the importance of integrating Raman spectroscopy and chemometrics to develop models for monitoring and controlling CHO bioprocesses. The profound implications of the careful preprocessing and wise selection of multivariate analysis methods to improve accuracy in the monitoring of important process variables are demonstrated.

To further explore the topic of bioprocesses, the fermentation process of Pichia pastoris is examined and the BDA-IPSO-LSSVM soft sensor modelling method is presented [8]. This model addresses the recurring problem of model errors due to discrepancies in data distribution. By leveraging the combined strengths of transfer learning, fuzzy set concepts and advanced optimisation techniques, exceptional predictive accuracy is achieved, even under changing conditions. While these advances are remarkable, the transformative impact of soft sensors extends even further in the modern technology landscape.

With the increasing integration of technologies such as artificial intelligence, machine learning and IoT (Internet of Things), the potential of soft sensors is growing exponentially. Possibilities that were once considered unattainable are now becoming tangible. It is not just about the sensors, but also about the ecosystems that enable them. Change is on the horizon as the industry is ready to adopt a proactive maintenance culture, predictive quality control and instant adaptive adjustments. In the field of soft sensor research, societal impact and directions are becoming increasingly important. Educational institutions, companies and policy makers play a crucial role in shaping this path. Their joint efforts to create an enabling environment foster innovation and drive progress in this dynamic field.

The following section looks at the versatility and scope of soft sensor applications in industry. The research on self-acting shape memory coils (SMC) with variable stiffness [9] is worth highlighting. The proposed method not only improves the performance and cost efficiency of SMA actuators, but its applicability extends across various fields from robotic grippers to biomedical devices.

The next paper [10] deals with the merging of data from different sources in sintering processes and highlights the growing importance of integrating different types of data for better predictions. By cleverly merging visual data with traditional time series process data, the method achieves significant improvements in predicting complicated quality variables such as FeO content. In the area of safety and infrastructure, research on a highly sensitive fire detection and early-warning system [11] highlights the value of fusing multiple fire indicators for timely and effective fire detection in buildings. This hybrid feature-fusion-based strategy represents potential for much safer smart building systems.

The essence of soft sensors lies in the data they interpret. These are not just any data, but a mixture of signals, inputs and variables that all help to describe the underlying processes. When these nuances are unravelled, soft sensors reveal the hidden subtleties of the world. Whether it is the microenvironment of a bioreactor, the status of a complicated machine or the subtle changes in human physiology, these virtual tools enable a comprehensive understanding.

In addition, much attention is being paid to ethics and transparency in relation to these technologies. As these sensors play an increasingly central role in determining outcomes, such as autonomous driving decisions—whether to avoid an obstacle or brake abruptly—

the need for transparency, accountability and ethical considerations in their algorithms becomes ever more important. It is our collective responsibility to ensure that the full potential of these technologies is realised while adhering to ethical principles and practices.

In summary, the articles in this Special Issue not only highlight the advancing frontiers of soft sensors in various fields, but also emphasise the importance of multidisciplinary collaboration in these developments. As technologies advance, so will the applications and opportunities for soft sensors. Challenges and opportunities await researchers and professionals in this field, as the future promises even more advanced and integrated solutions.

Funding: This research received no external funding.

Institutional Review Board Statement: Not applicable.

Informed Consent Statement: Not applicable.

Data Availability Statement: Not applicable.

Conflicts of Interest: The author declare no conflict of interest.

References

1. Rincón, A.; Hoyos, F.E.; Candelo-Becerra, J.E. A Simplified Algorithm for Setting the Observer Parameters for Second-Order Systems with Persistent Disturbances Using a Robust Observer. *Sensors* **2022**, *22*, 6988. [CrossRef] [PubMed]
2. Devos, T.; Kirchner, M.; Croes, J.; Desmet, W.; Naets, F. Sensor Selection and State Estimation for Unobservable and Non-Linear System Models. *Sensors* **2021**, *21*, 7492. [CrossRef] [PubMed]
3. Mei, W.; Liu, Z.; Tang, L.; Su, Y. Test Strategy Optimization Based on Soft Sensing and Ensemble Belief Measurement. *Sensors* **2022**, *22*, 2138. [CrossRef] [PubMed]
4. Mohai, K.; Kálózi-Szabó, C.; Jakab, Z.; Fecht, S.D.; Domonkos, M.; Botzheim, J. Development of an Adaptive Computer-Aided Soft Sensor Diagnosis System for Assessment of Executive Functions. *Sensors* **2022**, *22*, 5880. [CrossRef] [PubMed]
5. Karer, G.; Škrjanc, I. Improved Individualized Patient-Oriented Depth-of-Hypnosis Measurement Based on Bispectral Index. *Sensors* **2023**, *23*, 293. [CrossRef] [PubMed]
6. Stržinar, Ž.; Sanchis, A.; Ledezma, A.; Sipele, O.; Pregelj, B.; Škrjanc, I. Stress Detection Using Frequency Spectrum Analysis of Wrist-Measured Electrodermal Activity. *Sensors* **2023**, *23*, 963. [CrossRef] [PubMed]
7. Tomažič, S.; Škrjanc, I. Halfway to Automated Feeding of Chinese Hamster Ovary Cells. *Sensors* **2023**, *23*, 6618. [CrossRef] [PubMed]
8. Wang, B.; Liu, J.; Yu, A.; Wang, H. Development and Optimization of a Novel Soft Sensor Modeling Method for Fermentation Process of Pichia pastoris. *Sensors* **2023**, *23*, 6014. [CrossRef] [PubMed]
9. Sul, B.B.; Kaliaperumal, D.; Choi, S.B. Self-Sensing Variable Stiffness Actuation of Shape Memory Coil by an Inferential Soft Sensor. *Sensors* **2023**, *23*, 2442. [CrossRef] [PubMed]
10. Li, Y.; Jiang, W.; Shi, Z.; Yang, C. A Soft Sensor Model of Sintering Process Quality Index Based on Multi-Source Data Fusion. *Sensors* **2023**, *23*, 4954. [CrossRef] [PubMed]
11. Xiao, S.; Wang, S.; Ge, L.; Weng, H.; Fang, X.; Peng, Z.; Zeng, W. Hybrid Feature Fusion-Based High-Sensitivity Fire Detection and Early Warning for Intelligent Building Systems. *Sensors* **2023**, *23*, 859. [CrossRef]

Disclaimer/Publisher's Note: The statements, opinions and data contained in all publications are solely those of the individual author(s) and contributor(s) and not of MDPI and/or the editor(s). MDPI and/or the editor(s) disclaim responsibility for any injury to people or property resulting from any ideas, methods, instructions or products referred to in the content.

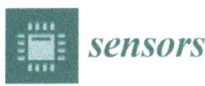

Article

Sensor Selection and State Estimation for Unobservable and Non-Linear System Models

Thijs Devos [1,2,*], Matteo Kirchner [1,2], Jan Croes [1,2], Wim Desmet [1,2] and Frank Naets [1,2]

1 LMSD Research Group, Department of Mechanical Engineering, KU Leuven, Celestijnenlaan 300, 3001 Leuven, Belgium; matteo.kirchner@kuleuven.be (M.K.); jan.croes@kuleuven.be (J.C.); wim.desmet@kuleuven.be (W.D.); frank.naets@kuleuven.be (F.N.)
2 DMMS Core Lab, Flanders Make, Gaston Geenslaan 8, 3001 Leuven, Belgium
* Correspondence: thijs.devos@kuleuven.be

Abstract: To comply with the increasing complexity of new mechatronic systems and stricter safety regulations, advanced estimation algorithms are currently undergoing a transformation towards higher model complexity. However, more complex models often face issues regarding the observability and computational effort needed. Moreover, sensor selection is often still conducted pragmatically based on experience and convenience, whereas a more cost-effective approach would be to evaluate the sensor performance based on its effective estimation performance. In this work, a novel estimation and sensor selection approach is presented that is able to stabilise the estimator Riccati equation for unobservable and non-linear system models. This is possible when estimators only target some specific quantities of interest that do not necessarily depend on all system states. An Extended Kalman Filter-based estimation framework is proposed where the Riccati equation is projected onto an observable subspace based on a Singular Value Decomposition (SVD) of the Kalman observability matrix. Furthermore, a sensor selection methodology is proposed, which ranks the possible sensors according to their estimation performance, as evaluated by the error covariance of the quantities of interest. This allows evaluating the performance of a sensor set without the need for costly test campaigns. Finally, the proposed methods are evaluated on a numerical example, as well as an automotive experimental validation case.

Keywords: extended Kalman filter; state estimation; sensor selection; observability; non-linear models

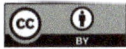

1. Introduction

Nowadays, many new mechatronic systems become available on the market, designed to perform tasks with increasing complexity while ensuring machine/operator safety. As a result of this increase in complexity, advanced controller schemes are being developed that introduce the need for accurate information on the dynamics of these systems. However, in many applications, this information cannot be directly measured because either no sensor exists that is capable of measuring the quantity of interest or the available sensors are expensive or impractical to implement [1]. This has led to the development of various virtual sensing techniques that aim at obtaining the dynamic information of a mechatronic system indirectly through estimations based on simple measurements [2]. This methodology has been investigated for use in a wide range of applications [3–6].

As a result of increased computational power, these virtual sensing schemes have gained significant traction for the analysis of structural [7] and general mechanical systems [8,9] in recent years. Driven by the need for more accurate system information, model complexity has significantly increased up to flexible multibody-related formulations [10–12]. However, this comes at the cost of increased computational effort and additional issues towards observability and thus estimator stability.

When model complexity is increased, observability requirements can become challenging as extra model degrees of freedom require additional sensor data to ensure full observability [13]. For example, in tire force estimation applications, vehicle position states are typically unobservable when no GPS measurement is present, although these measurements do not contribute significantly to the tire force estimation performance [1,14]. Furthermore, the non-linear governing equations create additional challenges to evaluate observability globally and/or locally [15,16]. Additionally, some virtual sensing applications feature models with lots of states (e.g., for meteorology or oceanography typically $> 10^6$ [6]), of which only a few significantly contribute to the estimator performance. This indicates that there is a need for an approach to deal with unobservable, and thus unstable, estimators given the interest in only a few specific quantities.

One of the approaches proposed in the literature to deal with large system models is to reduce the order of the estimator to decrease its computational efforts and set fewer constraints towards observability. Two main approaches to reduce the order of an estimator have been presented in the literature. The first approach involves reducing the model if this model can be approximated sufficiently well by a subset of modes [17–19]. However, this approach is highly model specific and is therefore not suited for all applications. The second approach involves reducing the order of the Kalman filter by transforming the Riccati equation associated with the filter [1,6]. Yonezawa et al. [20] have presented an approach for unobservable system states to be asymptotically observable, assuming that a dynamic link is present between the unobservable and the observable states. This approach has proven to be very effective when considering unknown parameters or constant bias errors. However, this approach only works when a dynamic coupling is present between unobservable and observable states, which is, in a lot of applications, rarely the case for all system states, especially when dealing with increasing model complexity.

For application cases with decoupled state dynamics, such as unknown accelerometer biases and unknown parameters, the Schmidt–Kalman filter can be deployed [21]. The covariances corresponding to the augmented states are not taken into account in the update steps as these states are typically not measurable and dynamically completely decoupled from the other states. This makes it impossible to observe these states; hence, they are simply omitted from the update step. When many of these states are present, this technique can drastically improve the computational effort as only the observable state covariances are being evaluated [22]. On the other hand, the Schmidt–Kalman filter approach can only be defined for completely decoupled augmented states.

Finally, sensor selection is a necessary step when deploying any estimation framework. A common approach is trial-and-error as sensors typically have to be bought and deployed before information can be acquired on their performance. However, previous research has already investigated some more cost-effective approaches that vary widely from equation-based modeling approaches [23] to machine learning methods [24]. Commonly proposed objective functions for model-based sensor selection algorithms are the Fisher Information Matrix (FIM) [25] or the error covariance matrix of the estimator [26], evaluated using the Riccati Equation (ARE) or the Lyapunov Equation [27]. However, all of these methods still rely heavily on sensor information being available that contains information on the sensor performance, which usually requires highly expensive test campaigns for which sensors have to be acquired.

As an alternative to the above-described schemes, this work presents a novel approach to stabilise a non-observable, non-linear estimator for both full and partially decoupled system dynamics given that only specific quantities of interests are targeted and proposes a new sensor selection strategy that is able to evaluate sensor set performances before acquiring them. Firstly, an estimator setup is proposed based on a set of non-linear governing equations for both the system model, measurements and quantities of interest, described in Section 2. Furthermore, a projection of the estimator covariance equations on an observable subspace is proposed in Section 3, which makes it possible to stabilise the estimator covariances during operation. The projection explained in Section 3.2 is based on the singular value decomposition of the linear Kalman observability matrix. Furthermore, the projected Kalman filter equations presented in Section 3.3 can stabilise the unobservable state covariances although these states remain unobservable. Hence, their resulting covariances should be interpreted with care. Additionally, a sensor selection methodology is proposed, which ranks the sensors based on their estimation performance such that the user can obtain an overview of the best sensors to choose from, as defined in Section 4. This has the great advantage that a prior analysis of the sensor performance can be carried out that eliminates the need to acquire sensors beforehand and organise costly test campaigns. Finally, the work is validated in two different cases, namely an academic example explained in Section 5.1 where the potential of the method is shown and a full experimental validation case explained in Section 5.2.

2. Model Definition and Overall Estimator Setup

In this work, a non-linear model will be considered to govern the dynamics of a physical system, the measurements and some predefined quantities of interest. These non-linear models are furthermore linearised and discretised in an Extended Kalman Filter [13] based the estimation framework. This section describes the implementation of the general estimator equations.

2.1. Definition of Model, Measurement and Quantities of Interest Equations

The non-linear equations considered in this work can be divided into system, measurements and quantities of interest equations and are introduced as:

$$\text{Model:} \quad \dot{\mathbf{x}} = \mathbf{f}(\mathbf{x}, t) \tag{1}$$

$$\text{Measurements:} \quad \mathbf{y} = \mathbf{h}(\mathbf{x}, t) \tag{2}$$

$$\text{Quantities of Interest:} \quad \mathbf{y}_{vs} = \mathbf{g}(\mathbf{x}, t) \tag{3}$$

where $\mathbf{x}$ is the state vector and t is the time. The vector $\dot{\mathbf{x}}$ describes the time derivative of the states, and the vectors $\mathbf{y}$ and $\mathbf{y}_{vs}$ are the measurements and quantities of interest, respectively.

In this work, an estimation framework is set up based on the discrete extended Kalman Filter for which an explicit relation is necessary. Therefore, these continuous non-linear equations have to be linearised and discretised. This is discussed in Section 2.2.

2.2. Linearisation and Discretisation of the Governing Equations

To obtain the linear and discrete Jacobian matrices used for the estimator evaluation, the non-linear equations are linearised and discretised. The Jacobians are obtained by performing a linearisation around the a priori estimation point $(\mathbf{x}_{k|k}, t_k)$ by:

$$\mathbf{F}_{c,k} = \left.\frac{\partial \mathbf{f}(\mathbf{x}, t)}{\partial \mathbf{x}}\right|_{\mathbf{x}_{k|k}, t_k} \tag{4}$$

Furthermore, the rest of the linearised Jacobians are calculated accordingly:

$$\mathbf{H}_k = \left.\frac{\partial \mathbf{h}(\mathbf{x}, t)}{\partial \mathbf{x}}\right|_{\mathbf{x}_{k|k+1}, t_k} \tag{5}$$

$$\mathbf{G}_{vs,k} = \left.\frac{\partial \mathbf{g}(\mathbf{x}, t)}{\partial \mathbf{x}}\right|_{\mathbf{x}_{k+1|k+1}, t_k} \tag{6}$$

Important to note is that any linearisation scheme can be deployed, which suits the application of the estimator. In this work, the linear continuous time Jacobians are obtained using forward differencing [28]:

$$\mathbf{F}_{c,k} = \frac{\partial \mathbf{f}(\mathbf{x},t)}{\partial \mathbf{x}}\bigg|_{\mathbf{x}_{k|k},t_k} \approx \frac{\mathbf{f}(\mathbf{x}_{k|k}+\epsilon,t_k) - \mathbf{f}(\mathbf{x}_{k|k},t_k)}{\epsilon} \tag{7}$$

The next step is to derive the discrete system Jacobian used for the integration of the system equations and evaluation of the Kalman filter covariance equations. Again, any type of discretisation scheme could be employed here, which best suits the application of the estimator. In this work, we chose to use a different discretisation method for the integration of the system equations and the derivation of the discretised sytem Jacobian for the Kalman covariance equations. This is conducted because it is not always practical to use the same discretisation scheme as this can lead to numerically ill-conditioned systems, for example, when dealing with a set of stiff equations [29].

For the derivation of the discretised system Jacobian used in the Kalman covariance equations, the exponential discretisation scheme [30] is used:

$$\mathbf{F}_k = e^{\mathbf{F}_{c,k}\Delta t} \tag{8}$$

where $\mathbf{F}_{c,k}$ is the continuous time system Jacobian obtained from Equation (7) and Δt is the timestep. The obtained discrete Jacobian is furthermore used in the EKF covariance equations.

For the integration of the system equations, a solver that is especially suited for stiff equations from the Matlab *ode-suite* is employed [31].

2.3. Overview of the Extended Kalman Filter Framework

In this work, the Extended Kalman Filter [13] is chosen for the estimation of the dynamic system information. This filter is an extension of the regular Kalman filter, making it applicable to non-linear equations. Using the previously calculated linearised Jacobians, the general estimator equations can be defined. In this process, the propagation of the states is conducted using the earlier defined non-linear equations, but the propagation of the covariance equations is conducted using the linearised matrices. The EKF-algorithm consists of three main steps, which are prediction, correction and update.

Prediction:

$$\mathbf{x}_{k|k+1} = \mathbf{f}(\mathbf{x}_{k|k}, t_k) \tag{9}$$
$$\mathbf{y}_{k+1} = \mathbf{h}(\mathbf{x}_{k|k+1}, t_k) \tag{10}$$
$$\mathbf{P}_{k|k+1} = \mathbf{F}_k \mathbf{P}_{k|k} \mathbf{F}_k^T + \mathbf{Q}_d \tag{11}$$

Correction:

$$\mathbf{S}_k = \mathbf{H}_k \mathbf{P}_{k|k+1} \mathbf{H}_k^T + \mathbf{R} \tag{12}$$
$$\mathbf{K}_k = \mathbf{P}_{k|k+1} \mathbf{H}_k^T \mathbf{S}_k^{-1} \tag{13}$$

Update:

$$\mathbf{x}_{k+1|k+1} = \mathbf{x}_{k|k+1} + \mathbf{K}_k(\mathbf{y}_{m,k+1} - \mathbf{y}_{k+1}) \tag{14}$$
$$\mathbf{P}_{k+1|k+1} = (\mathbb{I} - \mathbf{K}_k \mathbf{H}_k)\mathbf{P}_{k|k+1} \tag{15}$$

As the quantities of interest are governed by non-linear equations such that $\mathbf{y}_{vs} = \mathbf{g}(\mathbf{x},t)$ in this work, a first-order Taylor expansion of the quantities of interest is considered around the previously calculated state configuration $(\mathbf{x}_{k+1|k+1}, t_k)$ to derive their covariances:

$$\mathbf{y}_{vs} \approx \mathbf{g}(\mathbf{x}_{k+1|k+1}, t_k) + \mathbf{G}_{vs,k}(\mathbf{x} - \mathbf{x}_{k+1|k+1}) + \mathbf{K}_{vs,k}(t - t_k) \tag{16}$$

where $\mathbf{G}_{vs,k} = \left.\frac{\partial \mathbf{g}(\mathbf{x},t)}{\partial \mathbf{x}}\right|_{\mathbf{x}_{k+1|k+1}}$ and $\mathbf{K}_{vs,k} = \left.\frac{\partial \mathbf{g}(\mathbf{x},t)}{\partial t}\right|_{t_k}$ are the Jacobians of the quantities of interest according to Equation (6). When evaluating Equation (16) around the current configuration point $(\mathbf{x}_{k+1|k+1}, t_k)$ while assuming that the function $\mathbf{g}$ is approximately affine in this region, it can be stated that, up to a first-order approximation of the Taylor series, the quantities of interest will be a stochastic variable with the following mean and covariance [32–34]:

$$\mathbf{y}_{vs,k+1} = \mathbf{g}(\mathbf{x}_{k+1|k+1}, t_k) \tag{17}$$

$$\mathbf{P}_{vs,k+1} = \mathbf{G}_{vs,k}\mathbf{P}_{k+1|k+1}(\mathbf{G}_{vs,k})^T \tag{18}$$

Since in most applications only a selected number of quantities of interest are targeted by the estimator, this works aims at focusing the estimator performance on these specific quantities of interest while keeping the estimator stable.

In this work, only a few predefined quantities of interest are estimated, which are evaluated using their error covariance. However, the covariances of the states themselves are important for the stability of the filter as the estimator is only stable when all states are at least detectable [23]. This is unwanted when a certain sensor does not improve the estimation quality of the quantities of interest but is required to make all estimator states observable, in which case one would like to omit this sensor from the estimator. Therefore, this work aims at solving the following major difficulties:

1. Stabilisation of the EKF for non-observable system states;
2. Selection of the relevant sensors for the given quantities of interest.

Both of these approaches will be discussed in the next two sections of this work.

3. Stabilisation of the Extended Kalman Filter for Unobservable System States

When employing estimators, it is well known that observability is an important topic [1,35] as it determines the stability of the filter. Because in this work only some predefined quantities of interest are considered, it might occur that some sensors do not have any effect on the estimation performance for these specific quantities of interest. They can however cause some states to be unobservable, which can lead to stability issues of the estimator algorithm. In this work, a projection is proposed to stabilise the unobservable state covariances given that only some predefined quantities of interest are targeted. Important to note here is that only the stability issues are being tackled. The targeted states remain unobservable, but the estimator error covariances will be stable. The derivation of the observable subspace consists of three main steps:

1. Generation of the total observability matrix $\mathcal{O}_{tot}$ based on training data;
2. Calculation of the observable subspace basis $\mathbf{V}_o$;
3. Transformation of the Kalman covariance equations.

These steps are discussed in the following subsections.

3.1. Observability Analysis of the Extended Kalman Filter

The observability investigation starts with the computation of an observability criterion. In this work, the linear Kalman observability matrix [36] is used, which is based on the Jacobians $\mathbf{F}_k$ and $\mathbf{H}_k$ calculated in Equations (4) and (5):

$$\mathcal{O} = \begin{bmatrix} \mathbf{H}_k \\ \mathbf{H}_k\mathbf{F}_k \\ \mathbf{H}_k\mathbf{F}_k^2 \\ \vdots \\ \mathbf{H}_k\mathbf{F}_k^{n-1} \end{bmatrix} \tag{19}$$

If this matrix is of full rank, all states are observable. This is a sufficient condition for the estimator Riccati equation to converge to a stable solution [37]. However, this only holds for local observability, while for global observability analysis, the Lie derivatives have to be investigated [36,38]. Due to the non-linear nature of the governing equations, alternative methods need to be implemented to perform observability analysis, such as the ones in [15] or [16]. This work proposes to combine the observability matrices of different timesteps into a large observability matrix. This large observability matrix is a combination of matrices evaluated at evenly spaced timesteps of the training data:

$$\mathcal{O}_{tot} = \begin{bmatrix} \mathcal{O}_{k=1} \\ \mathcal{O}_{k=1+p} \\ \mathcal{O}_{k=1+2p} \\ \vdots \\ \mathcal{O}_{k=m} \end{bmatrix} \qquad (20)$$

where k is the timestep of evaluation, m is the total amount of timesteps in the training data and p is an integer index that defines the amount of observability matrices that are taken into account in the total observability matrix. The number p can be chosen between 1 and m depending on the wanted global observability coverage. The smaller the number p, the better global observability is analysed, but the larger the total observability matrix. Alternatively, when there are no training data available, the total observability matrix can be calculated for the first timesteps of the simulation based on which the projection can be defined.

Global observability requires the matrix from Equation (20) to be of full rank. However, to reduce costs, installing the minimum amount of sensors needed to produce good and reliable estimation results should always be the aim. Therefore, sensors that do not contribute significantly to the overall quantities of interest estimation performance but are necessary to make all system states observable are not wanted. However, they will cause the estimator to become unstable due to the unboundedness of the unobservable state covariances. This work therefore aims at tackling the stability issues related to unobservable system states. A projection of the Kalman filter Riccati equation is proposed on an observable subspace defined by the singular modes of the complete observability matrix from Equation (20). This projection will be discussed in the next subsection.

3.2. Calculation of an Observable Projection Basis

It is well known that a singular value decomposition (SVD) can be used to determine the rank of a matrix [15,39]. Furthermore, an SVD can also indicate which states are unobservable by looking into the modeset corresponding to the singular values. This modeset can also be exploited as a basis for an observable projection.

Lets consider the singular value decomposition of the complete observability matrix. As a result, the full observability matrix ($\mathcal{O}_{tot}$) can be written as a product of three matrices:

$$\mathcal{O}_{tot} = \mathbf{U\Sigma V} \qquad (21)$$

where $\mathbf{\Sigma}$ is a square matrix containing the singular values and matrices $\mathbf{U}$ and $\mathbf{V}$ contain the corresponding modes that satisfy $\mathbf{VV}^T = \mathbb{I}$ and $\mathbf{UU}^T = \mathbb{I}$. When the observability matrix is rank deficient, at least one of the calculated singular values will be close to zero and the matrix $\mathbf{\Sigma}$ will have the following structure:

$$\Sigma = \begin{bmatrix} \sigma_1 & \cdots & 0 & 0 & \cdots & 0 \\ \vdots & \ddots & \vdots & \vdots & \ddots & \vdots \\ 0 & \cdots & \sigma_m & 0 & \cdots & 0 \\ 0 & \cdots & 0 & \approx 0 & \cdots & 0 \\ \vdots & \ddots & \vdots & \vdots & \ddots & \vdots \\ 0 & \cdots & 0 & 0 & \cdots & \approx 0 \end{bmatrix} = \begin{bmatrix} \Sigma_o & 0 \\ 0 & \Sigma_u \end{bmatrix} \approx \begin{bmatrix} \Sigma_o & 0 \\ 0 & 0 \end{bmatrix} \quad (22)$$

where m is the rank of the total observability matrix $\mathcal{O}_{tot}$. To determine whether singular values are zero, a threshold value of 10^{-12} has been set by trial-and-error after investigating the singular values for the validation examples. Furthermore, the corresponding modes present in the matrix $\mathbf{V}$ can be partitioned according to the corresponding singular values in Equation (22):

$$\mathbf{V} = \begin{bmatrix} \mathbf{V}_o \\ \mathbf{V}_u \end{bmatrix} \quad (23)$$

where $\mathbf{V}_u$ are the modes that span the kernel of the observability matrix. At the same time, $\mathbf{V}_o$ is the matrix consisting of the modes corresponding to an observable subspace for this particular sensor set. Using the $\mathbf{V}\mathbf{V}^T = \mathbb{I}$ property of the SVD matrices, the following expression can be obtained:

$$\mathbf{V}\mathbf{V}^T = \begin{bmatrix} \mathbf{V}_o \\ \mathbf{V}_u \end{bmatrix} \begin{bmatrix} \mathbf{V}_o^T & \mathbf{V}_u^T \end{bmatrix} = \begin{bmatrix} \mathbf{V}_o \mathbf{V}_o^T & \mathbf{V}_o \mathbf{V}_u^T \\ \mathbf{V}_u \mathbf{V}_o^T & \mathbf{V}_u \mathbf{V}_u^T \end{bmatrix} = \begin{bmatrix} \mathbb{I} & 0 \\ 0 & \mathbb{I} \end{bmatrix} \quad (24)$$

where the $\mathbf{V}_o \mathbf{V}_o^T = \mathbb{I}$ and $\mathbf{V}_o \mathbf{V}_u^T = \mathbf{V}_u \mathbf{V}_o^T = 0$ properties can be obtained. In this work, a projection of the estimator covariance equations is proposed using the matrix $\mathbf{V}_o$ containing an observable modeset:

$$\mathbf{x} = \mathbf{V}_o^T \mathbf{q} \quad (25)$$

The aim of this transformation is to obtain new, observable estimator covariance equations such that the estimator runs stable during operation. Applying Equation (25) to Equations (4) and (5), the new linearised Jacobians can be found as:

$$\widetilde{\mathbf{F}}_k = \mathbf{V}_o \mathbf{F}_k \mathbf{V}_o^T \quad (26)$$
$$\widetilde{\mathbf{H}}_k = \mathbf{H}_k \mathbf{V}_o^T \quad (27)$$

Due to the transformation, the new estimator observability matrix will have an additional multiplication by the transformation matrix $\mathbf{V}_o^T$. Using the singular value decomposition formula from Equation (21), Equation (22) and the $\mathbf{V}_u \mathbf{V}_o^T = 0$ and $\mathbf{V}_o \mathbf{V}_o^T = \mathbb{I}$ properties, the following expression is obtained:

$$\mathcal{O}_{tot} \mathbf{V}_o^T = \mathbf{U} \Sigma \mathbf{V} \mathbf{V}_o^T = \mathbf{U} \begin{bmatrix} \Sigma_o & 0 \\ 0 & 0 \end{bmatrix} \begin{bmatrix} \mathbf{V}_o \\ \mathbf{V}_u \end{bmatrix} \mathbf{V}_o^T = \mathbf{U} \begin{bmatrix} \Sigma_o & 0 \\ 0 & 0 \end{bmatrix} \begin{bmatrix} \mathbf{V}_o \mathbf{V}_o^T \\ 0 \end{bmatrix} = \mathbf{U} \begin{bmatrix} \Sigma_o \\ 0 \end{bmatrix} \quad (28)$$

which proves that the newly obtained observability matrix will be of full rank as all singular values larger than 0 of the original total observability matrix are present in Σ_o.

The above proposed projection only works if the targeted quantities of interest, expressed in the virtual sensor equations through $\mathbf{G}_{vs,k}$, are independent of the unobservable states. Mathematically speaking, this means that the linearised Jacobian of the virtual sensors cannot be spun with any of the observability matrix kernel basis vectors $\mathbf{V}_u$. To check this, the following criterion has to be evaluated:

$$\mathbf{G}_{vs,m} \mathbf{V}_u^T = 0 \quad (29)$$

where *m* indicates that the linearised Jacobian of the quantities of interest equation is taken at the last timestep of the training data to make sure that initial transient behaviour is no longer present.

If the criterion of Equation (29) is not met, the estimator cannot be set up such that it will deliver valuable and trustworthy information on the quantities of interest. If this is the case, the sensor set connected to the Kalman filter should be changed or extended to a set that is able to capture all relevant information.

3.3. Transformation of the Estimator Covariance Equations

Now that the projection matrix $\mathbf{V}_o$ has been defined and the new Jacobians are derived, the new projected Kalman filter equations can be deduced. Using the matrices defined in Equations (9)–(13) and expressing the estimator equations in terms of the linearised Jacobians deduced from Equations (4) and (5), the following equations can be derived:

Prediction:

$$\mathbf{x}_{k|k+1} = \mathbf{f}(\mathbf{x}_k, t_k) \tag{30}$$

$$\mathbf{y}_{k+1} = \mathbf{h}(\mathbf{x}_k, t_k) \tag{31}$$

$$\mathbf{P}_{k|k+1} = (\mathbf{V}_o \mathbf{F}_k \mathbf{V}_o^T) \mathbf{P}_{k|k} (\mathbf{V}_o \mathbf{F}_k \mathbf{V}_o^T)^T + \mathbf{V}_o \mathbf{Q}_d \mathbf{V}_o^T \tag{32}$$

Correction:

$$\mathbf{S}_k = (\mathbf{H}_k \mathbf{V}_o^T) \mathbf{P}_{k|k+1} (\mathbf{H}_k \mathbf{V}_o^T)^T + \mathbf{R} \tag{33}$$

$$\mathbf{K}_k = \mathbf{P}_{k|k+1} (\mathbf{H}_k \mathbf{V}_o^T)^T \mathbf{S}_k^{-1} \tag{34}$$

Update:

$$\mathbf{x}_{k+1|k+1} = \mathbf{x}_{k|k+1} + \mathbf{V}_o^T \mathbf{K}_k (\mathbf{y}_{m,k+1} - \mathbf{y}_{k+1}) \tag{35}$$

$$\mathbf{P}_{k+1|k+1} = (\mathbb{I} - \mathbf{K}_k (\mathbf{H}_k \mathbf{V}_o^T)) \mathbf{P}_{k|k+1} \tag{36}$$

Finally, the quantities of interest and their corresponding covariances expressed by Equations (17) and (18) can be projected according to the transformation matrix $\mathbf{V}_o$:

$$\mathbf{y}_{vs,k+1} = \mathbf{g}(\mathbf{x}_{k+1|k+1}, t_k) \tag{37}$$

$$\mathbf{P}_{vs,k+1} = (\mathbf{G}_{vs,k} \mathbf{V}_o^T) \mathbf{P}_{k+1|k+1} (\mathbf{G}_{vs,k} \mathbf{V}_o^T)^T \tag{38}$$

To acquire the original state covariances, the newly acquired covariances need to be transformed back to their original values. This can be conducted by pre- and post-multiplying the covariance matrix $\mathbf{P}_{k+1|k+1}$ with the observable subspace transformation matrix $\mathbf{V}_o$:

$$\mathbf{P}_{k+1|k+1} = \mathbf{V}_o^T \mathbf{P}_{k+1|k+1} \mathbf{V}_o \tag{39}$$

As a result of the transformation, the covariance matrix $\mathbf{P}_{k+1|k+1}$ of Equation (36) is no longer of its original size any more but is of size *m* according to Equation (22). This means that, due to the negligible contribution of the unobservable states to the transformation matrix $\mathbf{V}_o$, these unobservable states will be omitted from the covariance equations, ensuring that their covariances will remain stable during the estimator operation. However, the drawback is that, when transforming the state covariances back to their original values in Equation (39), the corresponding covariances for the unobservable states are not interpretable as the transformation matrix $\mathbf{V}_o$ does not contain any contributions towards these states. However, if the defined quantities of interest are independent of the unobservable states, their corresponding covariances will be interpretable and deliver reliable results. At the same time, some measurements can be excluded from the estimator, which reduces the need to buy more sensors to solve estimator stability issues related to observability.

4. Sensor Selection Using the Stabilised EKF Estimation Framework

The second aspect that is covered in this work is the selection of the appropriate sensors. A sensor selection algorithm is proposed that ranks the sensors according to their contribution to the quantities of interest estimation performance by evaluating the covariance equations based on the training data. The mean of the covariance profile of the quantities of interest is used to evaluate the performance of a certain sensor set.

4.1. Generate Training Data by Performing a Forward Simulation

The training data are generated by performing a forward simulation and saving all relevant matrices. This allows evaluating the sensor performance beforehand, hence eliminating the need for an initial measurement campaign on a physical system and the acquisition of sensors.

During the forward simulation, the relevant information needed for further processing is stored. All sensors to be included in the sensor selection algorithm should be present in the training data, such that the generated linearised Jacobian for the measurement equation $\mathbf{H}_k^{n_s^0} \in \mathbb{R}^{(n_s^0) \times (n_{st})}$ has the correct dimensions corresponding to the total amount of sensors in the sensor space n_s^0.

4.2. Sensor Selection Algorithm

Very often in state estimation, it is not clear which sensors contribute the most towards the estimation performance. Therefore, the proposed sensor selection algorithm aims at ranking the sensors by their estimation performance, which is evaluated using the quantities of interest covariance matrices $\mathbf{P}_{vs,k}$ for each simulation timestep. During the sensor selection procedure, no state update is performed, but only the covariance propagation is evaluated. This allows the algorithm to be sped up significantly. The linearised Jacobian matrices are reused from the training data generated according to the previous subsection. The sensor selection algorithm consists of the following steps (where n_s^0 is the number of sensors in the entire sensorspace):

1. Given the measurement matrix $\mathbf{H}_k^{n_s^0 - i}$ for the entire sensor space, and previously saved matrices $\mathbf{F}_k$ from the training data, evaluate the covariance propagation $\mathbf{P}_{vs,k}$ for all simulation timesteps. The resulting mean of the quantity of interest covariance profile is the reference covariance p_0.
2. Iterate along the entire sensor space and perform during each iteration i:
   (a) remove a sensor j from the sensor space obtaining $\mathbf{H}_k^{n_s^0 - i - j}$;
   (b) calculate transformation matrix $\mathbf{V}_o$ and observability matrix kernel $\mathbf{V}_u$;
   (c) check that none of the selected sensors depend on the kernel of the observability matrix $\mathbf{G}_{vs,m} \mathbf{V}_u = 0$. If any of the selected sensors are part of the kernel, the algorithm is stopped as the sensors are incapable of accurately estimating the quantities of interest;
   (d) if the previous criterion is fulfilled, propagate Kalman covariance equations defined by Equations (32)–(38) from Section 3.3 to obtain $\mathbf{P}_{vs,i,k}$. The resulting mean of the quantity of interest is the sensor set covariance p_i.
3. Find the sensor with the lowest covariance p_i, remove it from the sensor space and restart Step 2.

The result of the algorithm is a set of sensors ranked by their respective performance contribution to the overall quantity of interest covariance. The algorithm is summarised in Algorithm 1.

Algorithm 1 Sensor selection

1: Given $\mathbf{H}_k^{n_s^0-i}$, simulate covariance propagation to obtain reference covariance p_0
2: **for** $i = 1 : n_s^0$ **do**
3:     **for** $j = 1 : n_s^0 - i + 1$ **do**
4:         Remove sensor j from sensor space to obtain $\mathbf{H}_k^{n_s^0-i-j}$
5:         Calculate transformation matrices $\mathbf{V}_o$ and $\mathbf{V}_u$ as defined in Section 3.2
6:         **if** $\mathbf{G}_{vs,m}\mathbf{V}_u = 0$ **then**
7:             Simulate covariance propagation
8:             Evaluate mean of quantity of interest covariance profile:
9:             $p_i = mean(\mathbf{P}_{vs,k} \; \forall \; k)$
10:         **else**
11:             Quantities of interest lie within the kernel of observability matrix
12:             Stop algorithm;
13:     Evaluate the sensor f with lowest covariance for the quantity of interest:
14:     $f = min(p_i)$
15:     Save sensor f and remove f from sensor space to obtain $\mathbf{H}_k^{n_s^0-j-1}$

5. Validation and Discussion

In this work, two validation cases are presented:

1. A simple, numerical example to show the potential of the proposed methods to stabilise the estimator for unobservable states;
2. An experimental validation case to show the engineering cases.

These validation cases are discussed in the next sections.

5.1. Simple Validation Case

The simple validation case presented in this work is based on a three-mass system depicted in Figure 1.

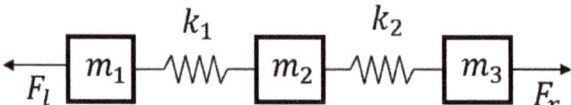

Figure 1. A visual representation of the academic validation case used consisting of three masses connected with springs.

In this case, the quantity of interest is the position of the left mass m_1, whereas the measurement used is the position of mass m_2.

5.1.1. Model Setup

For this simple example, the parameters k_1 and k_2 are chosen to be the same, such that $k_1 = k_2 = k$. The same holds for the masses $m_1 = m_2 = m_3 = m$. This is conducted to simplify the system and make the results more intuitive. All system parameters are listed in Table 1.

Table 1. Parameters of the three-mass academic example system used for validation.

Parameter	Value
m_1, m_2, m_3 (kg)	10
k_1, k_2 (N/m)	1000

Depending on variables k_1, k_2 and the masses of the blocks, three eigenmodes can be computed for this system. For this example, the three eigenfrequencies are 0, $\sqrt{k/m}$ and $\sqrt{3k/m}$. The system is excited with a sinusoidal force at the exact frequency of the second eigenmode, being $\sqrt{k/m} = 100$ Hz. Corresponding to this eigenfrequency, the eigenmode is of the form:

$$\mathbf{V}_2 = \begin{bmatrix} -1 & 0 & 1 \end{bmatrix}^T \quad (40)$$

This is the mode where both outer masses move in opposite directions, and the middle mass does not move. This means that the middle mass m_2 is located in a node of this eigenmode. Therefore, a position measurement of this mass cannot provide any information on the states of both other masses, and hence, the estimator will be unobservable. Here, the proposed projection can be executed to stabilise the Kalman filter covariances.

5.1.2. Estimator Setup

To estimate the quantities of interest, the filter has to be configured with a model noise matrix $\mathbf{Q}_d$ and a measurement noise matrix $\mathbf{R}$. For the model noise matrix $\mathbf{Q}_d$, a noise level of $(10^{-2}$ m$^2)$ has been set for the acceleration equations, whereas the noise level for the velocity equations are being set to 0. This is due to the fact that the velocity equations are a copy from the previous timestep, and therefore, no error is introduced. This means that the $\mathbf{Q}_d$-matrix is defined as follows:

$$\mathbf{Q}_d = \begin{bmatrix} 10^{-2} & 0 & 0 & 0_{1\times 3} \\ 0 & 10^{-2} & 0 & 0_{1\times 3} \\ 0 & 0 & 10^{-2} & 0_{1\times 3} \\ 0_{3\times 1} & 0_{3\times 1} & 0_{3\times 1} & 0_{3\times 3} \end{bmatrix} \quad (41)$$

The measurement noise is uncorrelated with a variance of $(2 \times 10^{-1}$ (m/s$^2)^2)$ for acceleration measurements and/or $(10^{-1}$ m$^2)$ for position measurements.

5.1.3. Discussion

This academic example allows showing that the projection onto the observable subspace can stabilise the state covariances of the Kalman filter. To show this, a special case is selected where the system is excited on exactly the second eigenmode, and a position measurement of mass m_2 is considered. The quantity of interest is the acceleration of mass m_1. Since the system is excited on an eigenfrequency, a position measurement of mass m_2 will not deliver any useful data to track the acceleration of mass m_1 as this mass lies within a node of the second eigenmode of the system. This special case is chosen to show that the proposed methodology works for any system where the unobservable modes can be isolated using a singular value decomposition.

The results of the estimation are depicted in Figure 2 and are similar to the results obtained from other simple, academic example cases [35]. One can observe that the amplitude of the oscillations raises continuously due to the system excitation on resonance frequency and the lack of damping in the model. The estimator is able to track the states of the system well, although larger variations in the position of mass m_2 can be observed where the absolute state values reach 0 m. Because this mass is not moving much, it becomes harder for the estimator to track.

For this system, a position measurement on mass m_2 will cause the states of both the outer masses m_1 and m_3 to be unobservable. This is visible in Figure 3 due to the unboundedness of the covariances of the states corresponding to masses m_1 and m_3 shown in grey as they are linked to the kernel of the observability matrix $\mathbf{V}_u$.

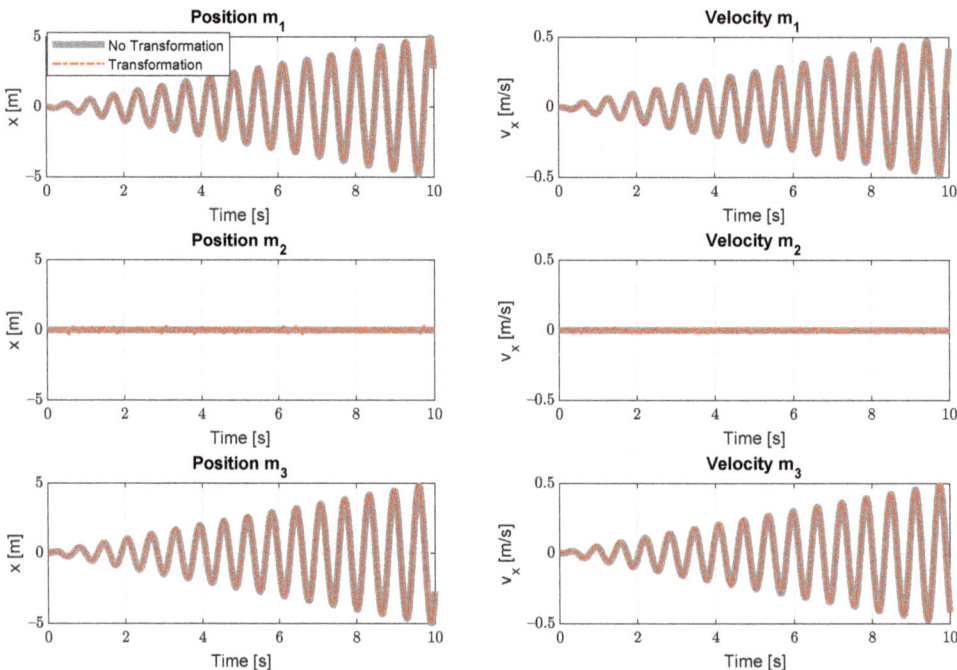

Figure 2. State estimation results for the academic model. The graphs shows the difference between the estimation results with covariance transformation versus without.

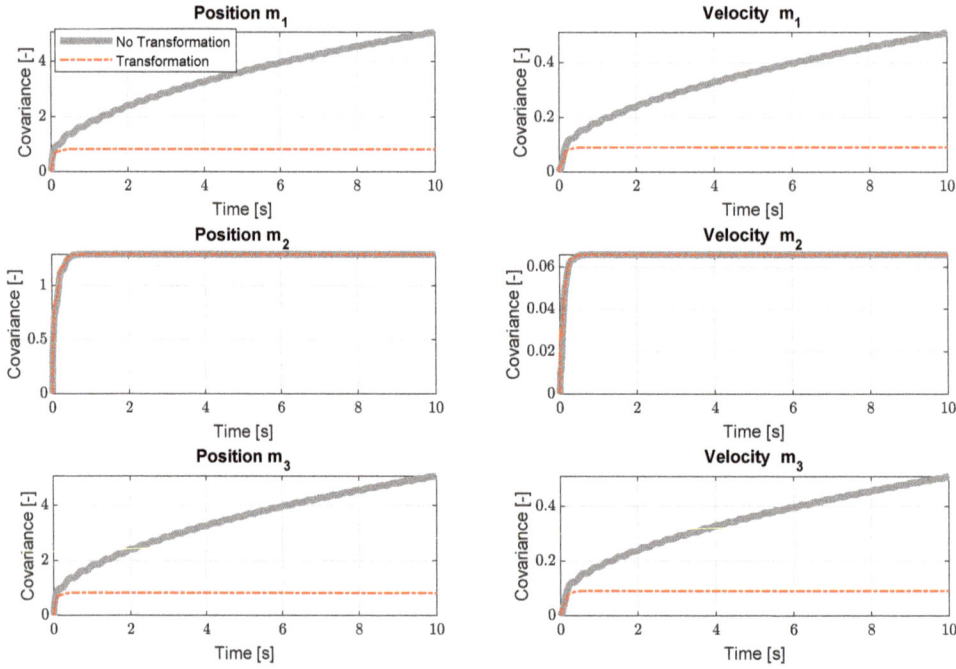

Figure 3. The resulting state covariances for the academic model using a position measurement on the middle mass m_2 and a virtual position measurement of mass m_3.

Using the projection shown in Section 3, these unstable covariances can be stabilised. When applying the projection, the resulting covariances are bounded, which is indicated by the red dashed lines in Figure 3. Figure 3 also shows that, since the states of the middle mass m_2 were already fully observable, the projection does not influence these covariances. However, one has to be careful interpreting the covariances of any quantity of interest should they be linked to an unobservable modeset $\mathbf{V}_u$, which can be investigated using Equation (29). Because the unobservable system states remain unobservable when applying the projection, the estimation results of these states should be interpreted carefully. This indicates that the transformation introduces a trade-off between the stability of the Kalman filter and the interpretability of the covariances. When this would be the case in practise, additional sensors will have to be added to the sensor set in order to comply with the observability requirements. Nevertheless, the results show that the proposed methodology is able to stabilise the unobservable covariances, hence ensuring a stable estimator containing unobservable states.

5.2. Experimental Validation Case

The second validation case for the proposed estimator approach is an experimental case performed on a vehicle. The experimental validation is conducted on a vehicle using a 10-DOF vehicle model that has been developed and validated at Flanders Make in previous work [1,40,41] and graciously provided to be used in this work.

5.2.1. Model Setup

The model used in this work is a 10-DOF freedom model is depicted in Figure 4, which is based on the Flanders Make Range Rover Evoque, visible in the same figure. The model has 16 states in total, 12 states for the body (2 for each degree of freedom) and 4 to describe the rotational degree of freedom of the wheels. Geometric parameters have been measured on the real vehicle, such as the suspension attachment points, centre of gravity location, wheel centre locations and so on. Table 2 gives an overview of the main parameters of the Range Rover Evoque, which are used by the 10-DOF vehicle model.

Table 2. Vehicle model parameters for the Range Rover Evoque [1,40].

Vehicle Property	Abbreviation	Value
Vehicle mass	m	2408 kg
Yaw moment of inertia	I_{zz}	3231 kgm^2
Distance between COG and front axle	l_f	1.4394 m
Distance between COG and rear axle	l_r	1.2356 m
Track width of front axle	t_f	1.625 m
Track width of rear axle	t_r	1.625 m
Height of COG	h_{COG}	0.65 m
Front axle cornering stiffness	$\bar{C}_{yf}$	88,500 N/rad
Rear axle cornering stiffness	$\bar{C}_{yr}$	118,200 N/rad

Next to these general body definitions, the-10 DOF vehicle models features:
- An exponential suspension spring characteristic;
- A linear suspension damper model;
- A linear tire model using cornering stiffnesses from Table 2.

The measurements were generated during a test campaign at Ford Lommel [40]. Here, the vehicle has been equipped with various sensors to measure the dynamic quantities of the system, among which a low-cost Global Navigation Satellite System receiver, an inertial measurement unit (IMU), a Corrsys Datron optical sensor and Kistler tire force transducers [1]. The IMU measured the accelerations in three directions of the centre of gravity and rotational speeds and angles (roll, pitch and yaw), defined around the axes depicted in Figure 4. The Corrsys Datron optical sensor measured the longitudinal and lateral velocity of the car, of which the slip angle could be deduced. The GPS was able to record the location of the vehicle's centre of gravity during the measurements, and the tire force transducers measured the tire forces of both rear tires.

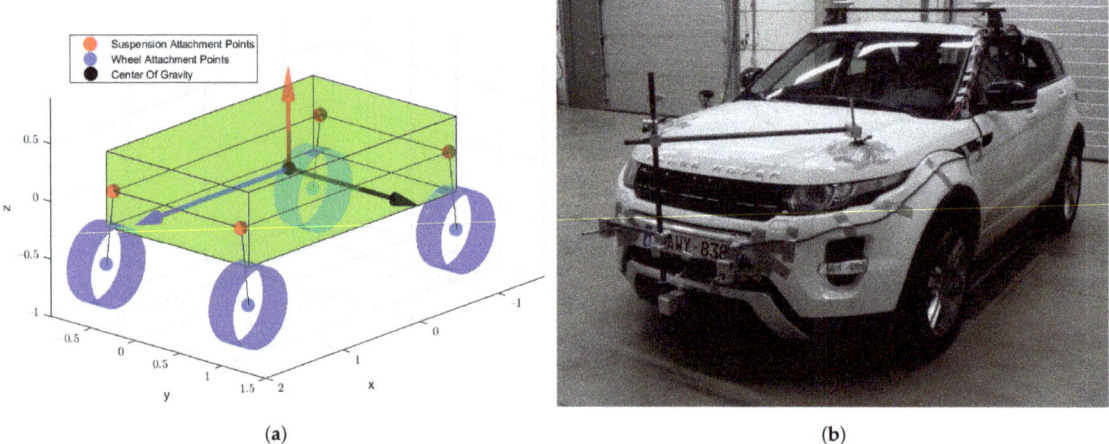

(a)   (b)

Figure 4. An overview of the vehicle application case for the validation of this work. (**a**) The 10-DOF model used for experimental validation. (**b**) The Flanders Make Range Rover Evoque represented by the 10 DOF model [1].

For this validation case, several quantities of interest have been investigated. These considered metrics are listed below:

1. Rear longitudinal tire forces;
2. Rear lateral tire forces;
3. Rear vertical tire forces;
4. Vehicle longitudinal and lateral position;
5. Vehicle side-slip angle.

The tire forces were estimated as this is commonly conducted already since tire force transducers are very expensive. The side-slip angle is also a subject of current research as this variable is hard to measure due to its dynamic nature but necessary for advanced control algorithms such as the ESP. Finally, the vehicle longitudinal and lateral position states were also included in the quantities of interest to show that the proposed projection and sensor selection methodology work for independent states.

5.2.2. Estimator Covariance Tuning

A necessary step to set up any estimator is to tune the covariance matrices. The model covariance matrix $\mathbf{Q}_d$ used for this validation case has been derived as:

$$\mathbf{Q}_d = \begin{bmatrix} 1 \times 10^{-4}\mathbb{I}_{3\times 3} & 0_{3\times 3} & 0_{3\times 3} & 0_{3\times 3} & 0_{3\times 4} \\ 0_{3\times 3} & 1 \times 10^{-3}\mathbb{I}_{3\times 3} & 0_{3\times 3} & 0_{3\times 3} & 0_{3\times 4} \\ 0_{3\times 3} & 0_{3\times 3} & 1 \times 10^{-5}\mathbb{I}_{3\times 3} & 0_{3\times 3} & 0_{3\times 4} \\ 0_{3\times 3} & 0_{3\times 3} & 0_{3\times 3} & 1 \times 10^{-1}\mathbb{I}_{3\times 3} & 0_{3\times 4} \\ 0_{4\times 3} & 0_{4\times 3} & 0_{4\times 3} & 0_{4\times 3} & 1 \times 10^{-5}\mathbb{I}_{4\times 4} \end{bmatrix} \quad (42)$$

The matrix defined above has been tuned by trial and error by means of evaluating the covariance values of the estimator.

The measurement noise matrix $\mathbf{R}$ is defined based on data sheets of the sensor manufacturer and a set of reference measurements [1]. The used noise levels are listed below:

$$R_{a_i} = 3.1 \times 10^{-3} \text{ (m/s}^2)^2, R_{gyr} = 2.491 \times 10^{-1} \text{ (m/s)}^2$$
$$R_{GPS} = 2 \text{ m}^2, R_{v_i} = 4.856 \times 10^{-2} \text{ (m/s)}^2, R_{\omega_{ij}} = 2.1 \times 10^{-1} \text{ (m/s)}^2$$

5.2.3. Discussion

Figure 5 shows the results of the estimator compared to the measurements from the Range Rover Evoque. The quantities of interest, as listed in the section above, are compared to the measurement data from the experimental campaign. The sensors used in the Kalman filter were the IMU accelerations in three directions, a gyroscope for the yaw rate measurement, the GPS (vehicle x and y) and wheel speed sensors.

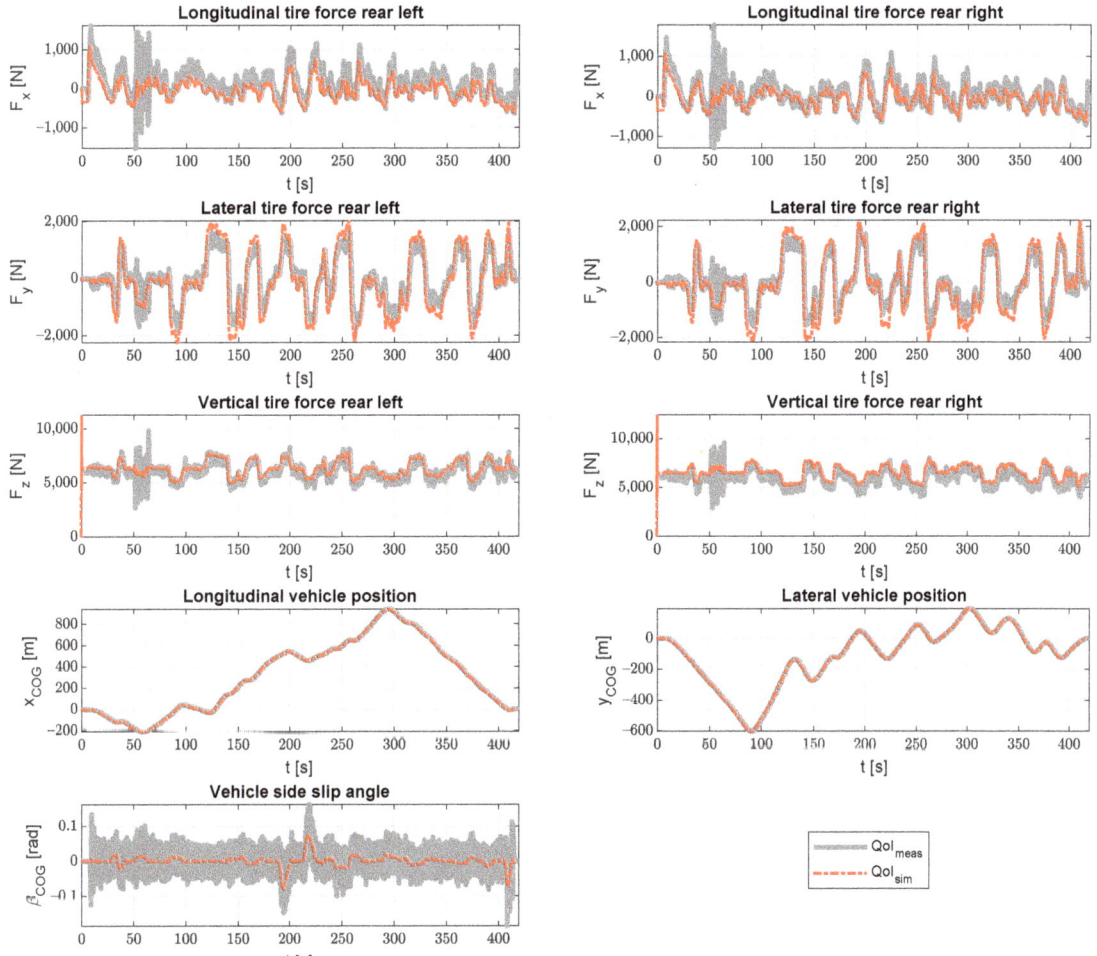

Figure 5. Validation of the quantities of interest (QoI) using real measurements from the Flanders Make Range Rover Evoque.

In general, the results match very well. One thing that can be noted is that the lateral forces are a bit over estimated in the extreme regions. Similar results were observed in [40] for the accelerations and the yaw rate when a linear tire model was used. This can be explained by the use of a linear tire model that does not take into account the saturation of the tire. This causes the forces generated by the tire to be larger than the ones actually measured. The use of a more complex, non-linear tire model that can take tire saturation into account will fix this issue and can be addressed in future work.

This validation case can show the potential of the covariance stabilisation methodology presented in this work on an engineering case as vehicle absolute position states are typically dynamically independent from the rest of the vehicle states when the road is considered flat. Therefore, if the tire forces are targeted by the estimator, the GPS measurements are less relevant for the estimator performance but will immediately cause the position states to be unobservable. This is depicted in Figure 6b where the blue covariance curve is rising continuously throughout the simulation. The green covariance curve on the same graph shows that the transformation can stabilise the covariance as it is now bounded, but orders of magnitude lower than for the observable case (red line). However, Figure 6a shows that the position is not tracked well during the simulation for all unobservable cases causing the vehicle position results to be poor. This indicates that one should be careful when interpreting the resulting covariance when using the projection for unobservable states. The proposed projecion therefore introduces a trade-off between the stability of the estimator and the interpretability of the results. However, if only interested in some specific quantities of interest, this approach can significantly reduce the cost of deploying extra sensors to obtain full observability, especially for applications with lots of states [6].

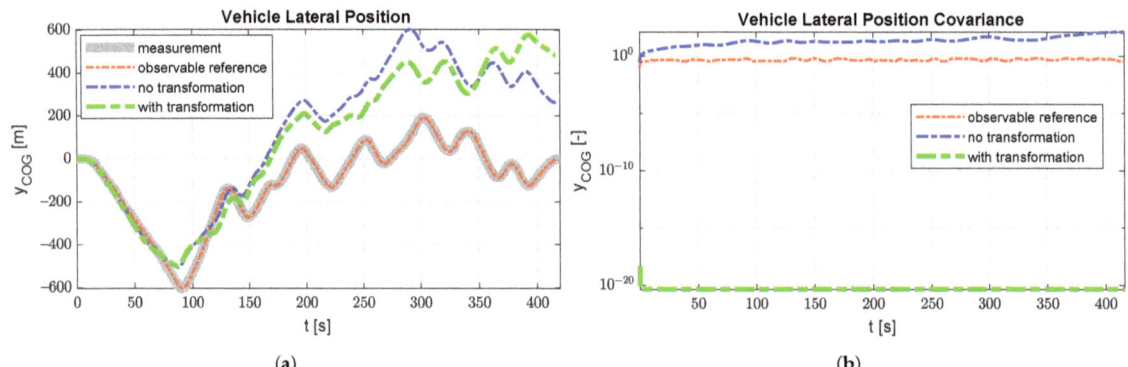

Figure 6. Comparison of the vehicle lateral position state for an observable case, an unobservable case without projection and an unobservable case with projection. (**a**) The vehicle lateral position state compared to the measured GPS Signal. (**b**) The covariance corresponding to the lateral vehicle position state.

The second part of the validation is to select the appropriate sensors for the estimation of the different quantities of interest that are considered. This is conducted by ranking the sensors based on their relative contributions to the covariance of the quantity of interest, similar to the approaches used in [26,27]. Figure 7 shows the results of the approach presented in Section 4. Figure 7 shows the contribution of each sensor to the quantities of interest covariance (p_0) relative to a simulation, including the complete sensor set (indicated by the blue line) at each iteration of Algorithm 1 where the sensor set has been reduced by exactly one sensor from left to right. Furthermore, the colour of the bars indicate information on observability. A green bar indicates that the observability is fulfilled during the entire simulation. A yellow bar indicates that the projection of Section 3 was carried out that stabilised the unobservable state covariances, and a red bar indicates that it is impossible to estimate the quantities of interest with this sensor set.

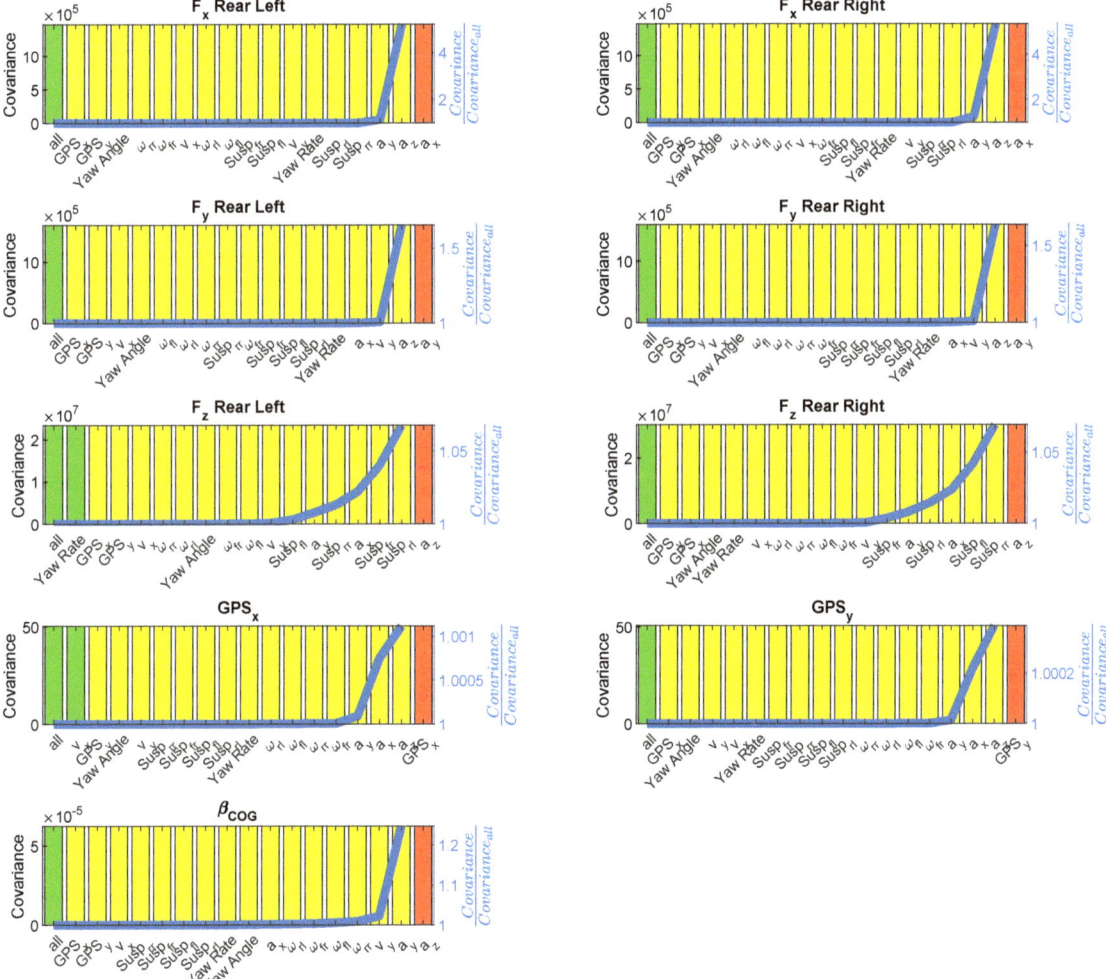

Figure 7. The sensor selection methodology results. For each quantity of interest, the sensor space has been reduced from left to right. The observability is indicated with the colour (green is fully observable, yellow is unobservable but stable and red is unobservable). The normalised metric covariance is indicated by the blue line.

In this validation case, only the last iteration is marked with a red colour, indicating that, at the least, this sensor is needed to provide the necessary data to comply with the observability requirements. Additionally, the blue line indicates that, for most quantities of interest within this validation example, only a few sensors contribute significantly to the overall quantity of interest covariance. The rest of the sensors have negligible added value relative to the quantities of interest performance.

Figure 7 shows that for the tire forces, the acceleration measurements in the respective directions are the most important sensors as they are directly related to the forces in the equations of motion. Adding these sensors can increase the estimator performance by a factor of 5, as indicated by the blue line on Figure 7. One can also observe that GPS measurements are of lesser importance here and are situated on the left side of the graph. However, omitting these GPS measurements causes the vehicle position states to be unobservable (as indicated by the yellow bar colour), which can be solved by applying the transformation proposed in Section 3.

On the other hand, when trying to evaluate the position states of the vehicle, the results depicted in Figure 7 show that not much performance can be gained by adding additional sensors as these states have no dependency to other states because they are directly obtained from integration. This means that GPS measurements are absolutely necessary to be able to track these states. The proposed approach is able to identify the situations where the estimator cannot be set up using the current sensor set by evaluating Equation (29).

In addition to the approaches presented in [25–27], the approach proposed in this work is able give a sensor performance indication for all types of sensors while also being able to handle the same type of sensors on different mounting locations as well as different sensor noise levels (cheap versus expensive sensors). Of course, the results of the sensor selection can be significantly different when considering multiple quantities of interest at the same time. This has not been investigated in this work and can be addressed in future work.

6. Conclusions

In this work, an algorithm is proposed to stabilise estimators for unobservable system states, given that only specific quantities of interest are targeted by the estimator. Through a projection of the estimator on an observable subspace, the employed Riccati equations can be stabilised, but care needs to be taken as this does not make the system inherently observable. To ensure reliable operation, the targeted quantities of interest should not rely on the non-observable omitted system subspace. This approach has been validated on a numeric academic mass-spring system, as well as an industrial automotive estimation problem. Compared to known solutions, this method is shown to consistently handle cases where decoupled states are present, strongly coupled modes are present, as well as complex non-linear behaviour.

Next to the estimation stabilisation approach, a sensor selection algorithm was proposed that ranks the sensor performance based on the expected uncertainty on the various quantities of interest. Starting form an exhaustive potential sensor set, the ranking procedure is performed by gradually removing one sensor at a time, which induces the lowest covariance rise when omitted from the estimator. On the automotive validation case, the method automatically detects that for tire forces, the acceleration measurements coming from the IMU are the most important sensors, whereas for the vehicle position states, the GPS measurements would be the most effective, which is consistent with engineering experience. Therefore, compared to known solutions, the approach is able to provide insight into the sensor set performance with respect to the predefined quantities of interest without the need for acquiring sensors and setting up costly test campaigns and is able to detect when a particular sensor set is unable to bring sufficient data in an estimator context.

Author Contributions: Conceptualisation, T.D., M.K. and J.C.; data curation, T.D., M.K. and J.C.; formal analysis, T.D.; funding acquisition, W.D. and F.N.; investigation, T.D.; methodology, T.D., M.K., J.C. and F.N.; project administration, M.K.; resources, J.C. and F.N.; software, T.D.; supervision, J.C., W.D. and F.N.; validation, T.D.; visualisation, T.D.; writing–original draft, T.D. and F.N. All authors have read and agreed to the published version of the manuscript.

Funding: This research was partially supported by Flanders Make, the strategic research centre for the manufacturing industry. The Flanders Innovation & Entrepreneurship Agency within the IMPROVED and MULTISENSOR project is also gratefully acknowledged for its support. Internal Funds KU Leuven are gratefully acknowledged for their support.

Institutional Review Board Statement: Not applicable.

Informed Consent Statement: Not applicable.

Data Availability Statement: The data presented within this study are resulting from activities within the acknowledged projects and are available therein.

Conflicts of Interest: The authors declare no conflict of interest.

Abbreviations

The following abbreviations are used in this manuscript:

GPS	Global Positioning System
SVD	Singular Value Decomposition
EKF	Extended Kalman Filter
FIM	Fisher Information Matrix
(D)ARE	(Discrete) Algebraic Riccati Equation
DOF	Degree(s) Of Freedom
IMU	Inertial Measurement Unit
ESP	Electronic Stability Program
QoI	Quantities of Interest

References

1. Naets, F.; van Aalst, S.; Boulkroune, B.; Ghouti, N.E.; Desmet, W. Design and Experimental Validation of a Stable Two-Stage Estimator for Automotive Sideslip Angle and Tire Parameters. *IEEE Trans. Veh. Technol.* **2017**, *66*, 9727–9742. [CrossRef]
2. Kullaa, J. Bayesian virtual sensing in structural dynamics. *Mech. Syst. Signal Process.* **2019**, *115*, 497–513. [CrossRef]
3. Mansouri, M.; Nounou, H.; Nounou, M. State estimation of a chemical reactor process model—A comparative study. In Proceedings of the 10th International Multi-Conferences on Systems, Signals Devices 2013 (SSD13), Hammamet, Tunisia, 18–21 March 2013; pp. 1–6. [CrossRef]
4. Langelaan, J. State Estimation for Autonomous Flight in Cluttered Environments. *J. Guidance Control Dyn.* **2007**, *30*, 1414–1426. [CrossRef]
5. Chen, B.C.; Hsieh, F.C. Sideslip angle estimation using extended Kalman filter. *Veh. Syst. Dyn.* **2008**, *46*, 353–364. [CrossRef]
6. Rozier, D.; Birol, F.; Cosme, E.; Brasseur, P.; Brankart, J.; Verron, J. A Reduced-Order Kalman Filter for Data Assimilation in Physical Oceanography. *Soc. Ind. Appl. Math.* **2007**, *49*, 449–465. [CrossRef]
7. Petersen, Ø.W.; Øiseth, O.; Nord, T.S.; Lourens, E. Estimation of the full-field dynamic response of a floating bridge using Kalman-type filtering algorithms. *Mech. Syst. Signal Process.* **2018**, *107*, 12–28. [CrossRef]
8. Ruggaber, J.; Brembeck, J. A Novel Kalman Filter Design and Analysis Method Considering Observability and Dominance Properties of Measurands Applied to Vehicle State Estimation. *Sensors* **2021**, *21*, 4750. [CrossRef]
9. Emanuele, A.; Gasparotto, F.; Guerra, G.; Zorzi, M. Robust Distributed Kalman Filtering: On the Choice of the Local Tolerance. *Sensors* **2020**, *20*, 3244. [CrossRef]
10. Rodríguez, A.J.; Sanjurjo, E.; Pastorino, R.; Ángel Naya, M. State, parameter and input observers based on multibody models and Kalman filters for vehicle dynamics. *Mech. Syst. Signal Process.* **2021**, *155*, 107544. [CrossRef]
11. Risaliti, E.; Tamarozzi, T.; Vermaut, M.; Cornelis, B.; Desmet, W. Multibody model based estimation of multiple loads and strain field on a vehicle suspension system. *Mech. Syst. Signal Process.* **2019**, *123*, 1–25. [CrossRef]
12. Adduci, R.; Vermaut, M.; Naets, F.; Croes, J.; Desmet, W. A Discrete-Time Extended Kalman Filter Approach Tailored for Multibody Models: State-Input Estimation. *Sensors* **2021**, *21*, 4495. [CrossRef]
13. Simon, D. *Optimal State Estimation: Kalman, H Infinity, and Nonlinear Approaches*; Wiley-Interscience: New York, NY, USA, 2006.
14. Hamann, H.; Hedrick, J.K.; Rhode, S.; Gauterin, F. Tire force estimation for a passenger vehicle with the Unscented Kalman Filter. In Proceedings of the 2014 IEEE Intelligent Vehicles Symposium Proceedings, Dearborn, MI, USA, 8–11 June 2014; pp. 814–819. [CrossRef]
15. Röbenack, K.; Reinschke, K.J. An efficient method to compute Lie derivatives and the observability matrix for nonlinear systems. In Proceedings of the 2000 International Symposium on Nonlinear Theory and its Applications (NOLTA'2000), Dresden, Germany, 17–21 September 2000; pp. 17–21.
16. Paradowski, T.; Lerch, S.; Damaszek, M.; Dehnert, R.; Tibken, B. Observability of Uncertain Nonlinear Systems Using Interval Analysis. *Algorithms* **2020**, *13*, 66. [CrossRef]
17. Soto, G.G.; Mendes, E.; Razek, A. Reduced-order observers for rotor flux, rotor resistance and speed estimation for vector controlled induction motor drives using the extended Kalman filter technique. *IEE Proc. Electr. Power Appl.* **1999**, *146*, 282–288. [CrossRef]
18. Aranda, J.; Cruz, J.M.D.L.; Dormido, S.; Ruipérez, P.; Hernández, R. Reduced-order Kalman filter for alignment. *Cybern. Syst.* **1994**, *25*, 1–16. [CrossRef]
19. Simon, D. Reduced Order Kalman Filtering without Model Reduction. *Control Intell. Syst.* **2007**, *35*, 169–174. [CrossRef]
20. Yonezawa, K. Reduced-Order Kalman Filtering with Incomplete Observability. *J. Guidance Control* **1980**, *3*, 280–282. [CrossRef]
21. Yang, C.; Blasch, E.; Douville, P. Design of Schmidt-Kalman filter for target tracking with navigation errors. In Proceedings of the 2010 IEEE Aerospace Conference, Big Sky, MT, USA, 6–13 March 2010; pp. 1–12.
22. Van Der Merwe, R.; Wan, E.A. Sigma-Point Kalman Filters for Probabilistic Inference in Dynamic State-Space Models. Ph.D. Thesis, Oregon Health & Science University, Portland, OR, USA, 2004.
23. Salau, N.P.; Trierweiler, J.O.; Secchi, A.R. Observability analysis and model formulation for nonlinear state estimation. *Appl. Math. Model.* **2014**, *38*, 5407–5420. [CrossRef]

24. Semaan, R. Optimal sensor placement using machine learning. *Comput. Fluids* **2016**, *159*, 167–176. [CrossRef]
25. Yamada, K.; Saito, Y.; Nankai, K.; Nonomura, T.; Asai, K.; Tsubakino, D. Fast greedy optimization of sensor selection in measurement with correlated noise. *Mech. Syst. Signal Process.* **2021**, *158*, 107619. [CrossRef]
26. Cumbo, R.; Mazzanti, L.; Tamarozzi, T.; Jiránek, P.; Desmet, W.; Naets, F. Advanced optimal sensor placement for Kalman-based multiple-input estimation. *Mech. Syst. Signal Process.* **2021**, *160*, 107830. [CrossRef]
27. Zhang, H.; Ayoub, R.; Sundaram, S. Sensor selection for optimal filtering of linear dynamical systems: Complexity and approximation. In Proceedings of the 2015 54th IEEE Conference on Decision and Control (CDC), Osaka, Japan, 15–18 December 2015; pp. 5002–5007. [CrossRef]
28. Zhou, P.B. Finite Difference Method. In *Numerical Analysis of Electromagnetic Fields*; Springer: Berlin/Heidelberg, Germany, 1993; pp. 63–94. [CrossRef]
29. Pastorino, R.; Richiedei, D.; Cuadrado, J.; Trevisani, A. State estimation using multibody models and non-linear Kalman filters. *Int. J. Non-Linear Mech.* **2013**, *53*, 83–90. [CrossRef]
30. Beylkin, G.; Keiser, J.M.; Vozovoi, L. A New Class of Time Discretization Schemes for the Solution of Nonlinear PDEs. *J. Comput. Phys.* **1998**, *147*, 362–387. [CrossRef]
31. Shampine, L.F.; Reichelt, M.W. The MATLAB ODE Suite. *SIAM J. Sci. Comput.* **1997**, *18*, 1–22. [CrossRef]
32. Gu, M.H.; Cho, C.; Chu, H.Y.; Kang, N.W.; Lee, J.G. Uncertainty propagation on a nonlinear measurement model based on Taylor expansion. *Meas. Control* **2021**, *54*, 209–215. [CrossRef]
33. Gustafsson, F.; Hendeby, G. On nonlinear transformations of stochastic variables and its application to nonlinear filtering. In Proceedings of the 2008 IEEE International Conference on Acoustics, Speech and Signal Processing, Las Vegas, NV, USA, 31 March–4 April 2008; pp. 3617–3620. [CrossRef]
34. Hartley, R.; Zisserman, A. *Multiple View Geometry in Computer Vision*, 2th ed.; Cambridge University Press: Cambridge, UK, 2003.
35. Naets, F.; Croes, J.; Desmet, W. An online coupled state/input/parameter estimation approach for structural dynamics. *Comput. Methods Appl. Mech. Eng.* **2015**, *283*, 1167–1188. [CrossRef]
36. Hermann, R.; Krener, A. Nonlinear controllability and observability. *IEEE Trans. Autom. Control* **1977**, *22*, 728–740. [CrossRef]
37. Karvonen, T.; Bonnabel, S.; Moulines, E.; Särkkä, S. On Stability of a Class of Filters for Nonlinear Stochastic Systems. *SIAM J. Control Optim.* **2020**, *58*, 2023–2049. [CrossRef]
38. Shi, X.; Williams, M.; Chatzis, M. A robust algorithm to test the observability of large linear systems with unknown parameters. *Mech. Syst. Signal Process.* **2021**, *157*, 107633. [CrossRef]
39. Banerjee, S.; Roy, A. *Linear Algebra and Matrix Analysis for Statistics*, 1st ed.; Chapman and Hall/CRC: Boca Raton, FL, USA, 6 June 2014.
40. van Aalst, S.; Naets., F.; Boulkroune, B.; Nijs, W.D.; Desmet, W. An Adaptive Vehicle Sideslip Estimator for Reliable Estimation in Low and High Excitation Driving. *IFAC-PapersOnLine* **2018**, *51*, 243–248. [CrossRef]
41. Vaseur, C.; van Aalst, S.; Desmet, W. Vehicle state and tire force estimation: Performance analysis of pre and post sensor additions. In Proceedings of the 2020 IEEE Intelligent Vehicles Symposium (IV), Las Vegas, NV, USA, 19 October–13 November 2020; pp. 1615–1620. [CrossRef]

Article

Test Strategy Optimization Based on Soft Sensing and Ensemble Belief Measurement

Wenjuan Mei [1], Zhen Liu [1,*], Lei Tang [2] and Yuanzhang Su [1,3]

[1] School of Automation Engineering, University of Electronic Science and Technology of China, Chengdu 611731, China; meiwenjuan@std.uestc.edu.cn (W.M.); syz@uestc.edu.cn (Y.S.)
[2] Southwest Institute of Technical Physics, Chengdu 611731, China; ltang20001142@163.com
[3] School of Foreign Language, University of Electronic Science and Technology of China, Chengdu 611731, China
* Correspondence: scdliu@uestc.edu.cn; Tel.: +86-028-6183-0316

Abstract: Resulting from the short production cycle and rapid design technology development, traditional prognostic and health management (PHM) approaches become impractical and fail to match the requirement of systems with structural and functional complexity. Among all PHM designs, testability design and maintainability design face critical difficulties. First, testability design requires much labor and knowledge preparation, and wastes the sensor recording information. Second, maintainability design suffers bad influences by improper testability design. We proposed a test strategy optimization based on soft-sensing and ensemble belief measurements to overcome these problems. Instead of serial PHM design, the proposed method constructs a closed loop between testability and maintenance to generate an adaptive fault diagnostic tree with soft-sensor nodes. The diagnostic tree generated ensures high efficiency and flexibility, taking advantage of extreme learning machine (ELM) and affinity propagation (AP). The experiment results show that our method receives the highest performance with state-of-art methods. Additionally, the proposed method enlarges the diagnostic flexibility and saves much human labor on testability design.

Keywords: prognostic and health management; extreme learning machine; soft sensors

1. Introduction

With the increasing use of electric devices, prognostic and health management engineering (PHM engineering) has played an extremely significant role in product lifetime management over decades [1]. PHM engineering ensures electric devices' lifetime healthy operation and provides appropriate resource assignment for product management [2]. In recent years, the production cycle has shortened because circuit technology and system design have rapidly developed [3–6]. The system structures have become more complicated, more integrated, more intelligent, and highly intensive [7]. Additionally, the potential test procedures and fault cases grow exponentially. As a result, PHM engineering has received active demand and new challenges. Practical conditional maintenance (CM) solutions become difficult to generate on modern system applications. On another hand, CM must be flexible enough to math structure complexity and system function complexity. Hence, efficient PHM engineering solutions for modern devices become an urgent problem for academic researchers and industrial engineers.

Under the CM design, testability design and maintainability design are two essential projects to determine supportability, enhance reliability, and guarantee safety during lifetime device management [8]. Testability design analyses the system's internal structures, selects test projects and arranges test procedures, estimates the system operation condition, and locates failure modes. The key difficulty for testability design is balancing the system's high structural complexity and the solution efficiency properly. Classical testability design approaches use dynamic programming (DP) to assess optimal solutions [9,10]. However, classic methods suffer from high time complexity when either the number of test projects or failures is larger than 12.

In recent years, the AO* method [11], a sequential testing generation method, balances the generation complexity of test solutions and detection performance for diagnostic procedures with heuristic searching and AND/OR graph topology. Thus, the AO* method became the most popular testability design technique. To match the growing electric system complexity, AO* has been improved to optimize searching mechanisms with information theory [12], evolution algorithms [13,14], dynamic design [15], etc. Additionally, advanced research has simplified searching procedures with rollout strategy [16] and bottom-up decision tree [17] to achieve practical large-system testability solutions. Despite good application results, these testability design approaches need to assign logic relationships between test procedures and failure modes. Hence, all these methods assume that dependent single-signal operations and sequential procedures can make all diagnostic decisions. However, modern devices contain highly complicated logistic relationships [18] between test procedures and potential failure modes under many scenarios. Consequently, the testability design consumes too much human power and affects the testability design efficiency to prepare prior knowledge, especially under short production cycles. Furthermore, the testability design wastes the entailed sensor recording information from test procedures as the existing methods rely on human-selected binary information.

The maintainability estimation model provides real-time operation condition diagnosis and realizes system health management along with testability design. In general, existing maintainability design approaches can be divided into physics-of-failure (PoF) approaches [19–22] and data-driven (DD) approaches [23–25]. PoF approaches use rules from physics or chemical dynamics to estimate electric system failure conditions [26]. With accelerated aging of experimental records and prior modeling knowledge, PoF approaches generate an accurate dynamic model under specific stress influences such as thermal, electrical, and humidity. However, most PoF approaches are only suitable under one stress function, and the methods face high limitations with real applications.

Unlike PoF methods, DD approaches rely on historical sensor information and build maps from sensor recording to failure modes. Hence, DD approaches become more flexible compared to PoF methods. Classical DD approaches use statistic methods such as stochastic methods, regression methods, distance estimation, and similarity estimation [27–30]. These methods require large samples to ensure unbiased estimation and model robustness, and are constrained in off-line modeling. Therefore, statistical approaches have limitations on maintainability design with few sampling records and short time constraints. In recent years, machine learning (ML) methods [31,32] have attracted research attention because of its high accuracy, strong adaptive ability, powerful robustness, and fast computation time. As a result, ML methods, such as neural networks (NN) [33], support vector machine (SVM) [34,35], k-nearest neighbors (KNN) [36], K-means clustering [37], and particle filters (PF) [38], have been used for maintenance design and tuned to successfully extract hidden rules from failure mode and recording information [39]. However, these methods require prior information selection and the preprocessing system degradation features. The performance of testability and maintainability may affect the preprocessing model input due to the complicated system structure and the complex recording information relationships.

We propose a test strategy optimization based on this paper's soft-sensing and ensemble belief measurement to overcome this weakness described above. We suggest a closed loop framework for PHM design to replace the sequential framework between testability and maintenance design. Instead of experienced knowledge, our method uses ensemble learning based on direct sensor recordings to gain the system state estimation. Additionally, we connect the testability and maintenance design by the minimal conditional criterion to optimize the test strategy. Consequently, the proposed method improves the flexibility of PHM design, saves labor, and enhances diagnostic efficiency. The contributions of our work follow.

- Our model builds diagnostic strategies without much prior knowledge and human-elected features. The diagnostic tree is constructed with ELM-based soft-sensor nodes. Instead of experienced features, ELM-based soft-sensor nodes provide basic probability assignment (BPA) directly from the sensor records. Hence, our methods cut the testability design human labor since the method needs no system mechanisms analysis.
- We build a closed loop between testability design and maintenance design. Thus, the maintenance design makes full use of testability design information and improves the testability design efficiency with the advantage of ELM-based construction modules.
- Our model divides the fault set adaptively into several fuzzy sets with affinity propagation and improves the diagnostic efficiency of single test procedures.

The experiment proves that our method has better diagnostic accuracy and lower false alarm ratios than other state-of-art diagnostic methods. Additionally, our diagnostic strategies take only a few tests with little test assignment consumption. For each fault state, the diagnostic procedures provide one efficient test sequence. Thus, the diagnostic procedure enjoys high efficiency for applications. Finally, affinity propagation enlarges the diagnostic flexibility and significantly reduces human labor used on testability design.

The rest of this paper is organized as follows. We introduce the PHM design problem and provide the general framework in the next section. Section 3 presents the details of the algorithms and Section 4 provides the experiment results and discussions. Finally, conclusions are drawn in Section 5.

2. Problem Formulation and General Framework

PHM engineering estimates the degradation processes and recognizes failure modes over the product's full lifetime. Based on experimental research and application surveys, PHM engineering provides fault analysis and maintenance advice to prevent failure occurrence. PHM engineering elements and the corresponding relationships are presented in Figure 1.

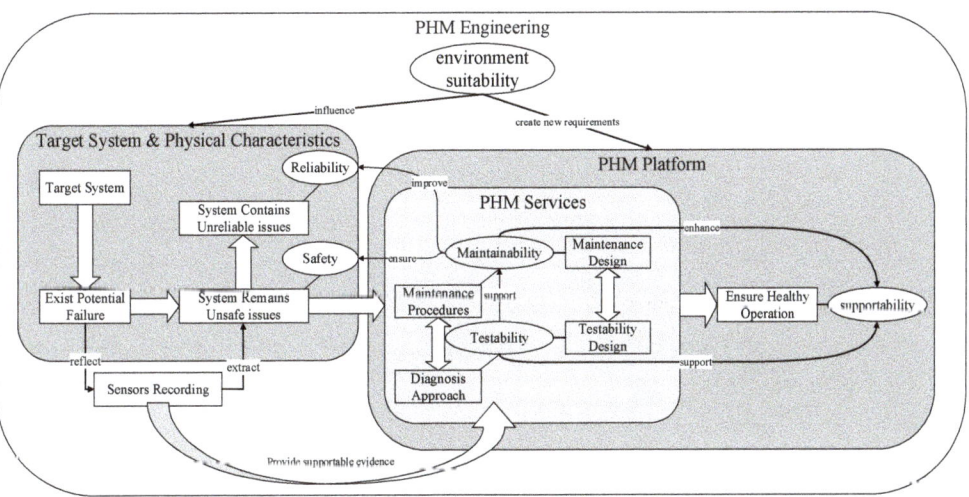

Figure 1. Element and the corresponding relationship of PHM engineering.

To study the target systems, engineers analyze potential failure modes and find unsafe and unreliable features. Thus, the target system's safety and reliability, reflected by its failure features, draw attention to system failure physical characteristics. For higher reliability and safety, the PHM platform provides maintenance procedures and diagnostic approaches for the system's supportability. The diagnostic approach depends on testability and the maintenance procedures that rely on maintainability.

Testability is the design characteristic that the health condition can be detected accurately and failure modes can be located successfully. Meanwhile, maintainability is the ability to repair and recover the system under certain conditions within a certain time. The PHM services can ensure healthy system operation and achieve the PHM engineering purpose with proper maintenance and testability design. In general, supportability is the key PHM engineering purpose influenced by testability and maintainability; thus, the PHM must meet the environmental stability needs. The physical system structure directly influences safety and reliability while system elements reflect safety and reliability critically. High testability and maintainability quality improve the system reliability and safety with good maintenance design procedures and diagnostic approaches. Hence, testability design and maintenance design are two significant PHM platform parts.

Since testability and maintenance are important, various techniques provide practical testability design and maintenance design. To our best knowledge, existing methods build a sequential approach to generate the PHM service. As Figure 2 shows, the traditional framework arranges the test procedures to assess the sensor recording and create maintenance design with the assigned sensor records. The framework is applicable for many large systems. However, the testability design uses human experience binary information such as information flow chart, dependence matrix and AND/OR graph. Therefore, the testability design suffers from extended time and the financial burden with modern complex systems, ignores the coupling effects between test procedures, and wastes valuable sensor recording information. As a result, the maintenance design receives poor performance and low efficiency because of poor information usage and low knowledge transmission efficiency from testability design and maintenance design.

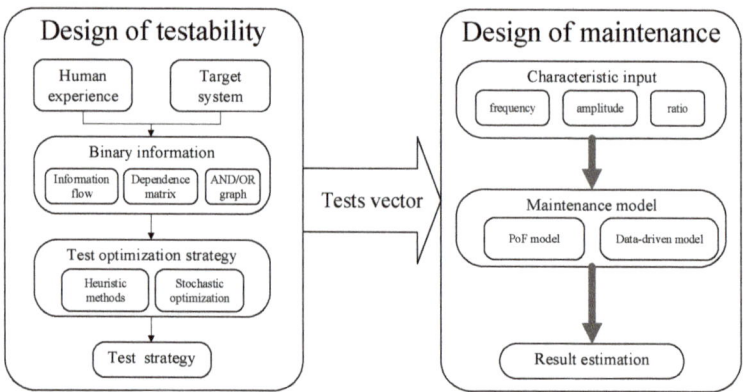

Figure 2. Traditional framework of testability and maintenance design.

We introduce a closed-loop test strategy optimization method on soft-sensor information and ensemble learning to overcome the weakness. Similar to traditional PHM design approaches, the proposed method aims to generate a fault diagnostic tree and cut the fault set with testability sensor information and maintenance signal processing. In contrast, our fault tree grows with direct sensor recording information directly along with the processing module and extends with basic probability assignments. On the other hand, the PHM design process contains a cooperative closed loop between testability and maintenance design to improve information usage and transmission efficiency during fault detection.

The general framework of the proposed method is presented in Figure 3. For maintenance design, the soft sensor integrates the recording information from assigned sensors and the processing signal, such as statistical method, support machine, and learning machine to extract suitable test features. Considering the requirement of fast diagnosis and detection, we use extreme learning machine (ELM) [34], a noniterative single-layer learning machine, to generate accurate fast processing modules of soft-sensing nodes. The details are introduced in the next section.

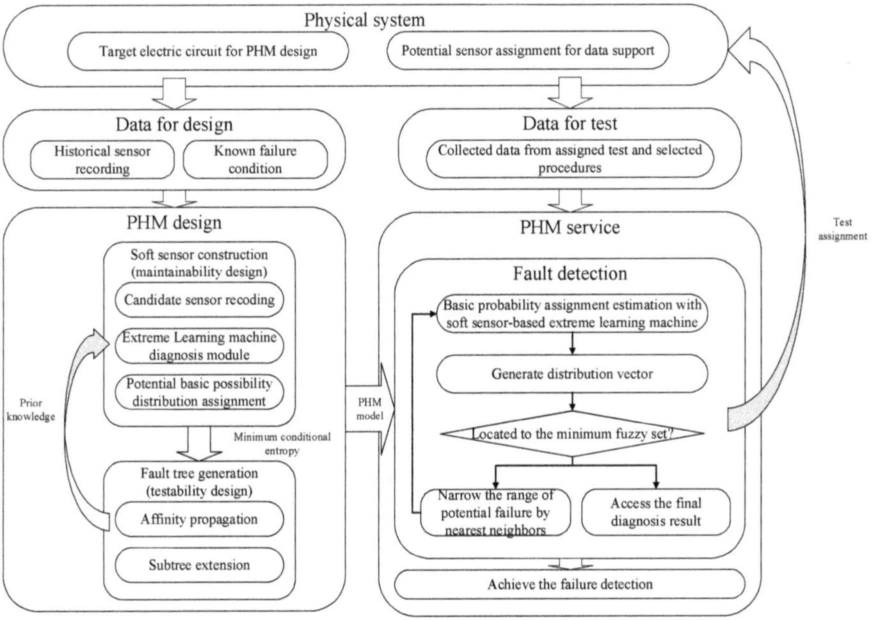

Figure 3. General framework of test strategy optimization based on soft sensing and ensemble belief measurement.

Suppose there exists N possible sensors with the PHM system design; therefore, the potential test procedures set is denoted as $T_{potential} = \{t_1, t_2, \ldots, t_i, \ldots t_{N-1}, t_N\}$, where t_i means the test procedures with i-th sensors. As each sensor contains a vector of information $x_i = \{x_{i,1}, x_{i,2}, \ldots, x_{i,K}\}, i = 1, 2, 3, \ldots, N$ with M existing samples from the targeted system, the training information is regarded as:

$$X_{train} = \begin{bmatrix} x_{1,1} & x_{1,2} & \cdots & x_{1,N} \\ x_{2,1} & x_{2,2} & \cdots & x_{2,N} \\ \vdots & \vdots & \ddots & \vdots \\ x_{M,1} & x_{M,2} & \cdots & x_{M,N} \end{bmatrix} \quad (1)$$

where x_{ij} is the recording information vector from the j-th sensor for i-th sample, $j = 1,2,3, \ldots, N$, and $i = 1,2,3, \ldots, M$.

With the sampling information, the potential fault tree soft-sensor node structure is denoted as following:

$$Node = \{S_{father}, S_{son}, T_{node}, X_{node}, Y_{node}, ELM_{node}, m_{exemplar}\} \quad (2)$$

where the T_{node} is the assigned test procedures from previous selected soft-sensor nodes and the potential selected test procedure, and X_{node} is the training sample sensor recording information to detect under the node, as follows:

$$X_{node} = \left[x_{1,T_{node}}, x_{2,T_{node}}, \ldots, x_{M_{node},T_{node}}\right]^T \quad (3)$$

$$x_{i,T_{node}} = \{x_{i,j} | t_j \in T_{node}\} \quad (4)$$

where M_{mode} is the number of the sampling data. Y_{node} provides the corresponding sample failure conditions. Suppose the whole set of failure mode is $S_{node} = \{s_1, s_2, \ldots, s_K\}$, where K is the number of fault modes considered, then Y_{node} is determined with the actual condition of training samples as follows:

$$Y_{node} = \left[y_1, y_2, \ldots, y_{M_{node}}\right]^T \tag{5}$$

$$y_i = [y_{i,1}, y_{i,2}, \ldots, y_{i,K}] \tag{6}$$

$$y_{i,j} = \begin{cases} 1 & ss_i = s_j \\ 0 & ss_i \neq s_j \end{cases} \tag{7}$$

where ss_i is the actual i-th sample fault mode. Additionally, S_{father} is the fault mode set of the soft-sensor node, represented as follows:

$$S_{father} = \{s_j | \exists x_i \in X_{node} \text{ and } s_j \in S, ss_i = s_j\} \tag{8}$$

With X_{node} and Y_{node}, the ELM serves as the soft-sensor signal processing part and aims to provide the fuzzy set of fault states as much as possible. To achieve the goal, ELM builds a map $f : R^{1 \times N} \to R^{1 \times K}$ from the training sample signals to estimate the fault states and provides the training sample prediction M_{node} as follows:

$$M_{node} = \left[f(x_{1,T_{node}} | ELM_{node}), f(x_{2,T_{node}} | ELM_{node}), \ldots, f(x_{M_{node},T_{node}} | ELM_{node})\right]^T \tag{9}$$

With M_{node}, ELM estimates the training sample failure modes. To determine the processing part performance, Y_{node} is used as the expected output marks for the fault detection process. From the view of detection process, two indexes, fault detection rate (FDR) and false alarm rate (FAR), play essential roles in evaluating the accuracy.

FDR is defined as the ratio between the failure mode probability that is successfully detected with the ELM and the total failure modes probability. Here, we assume the historical samples are subject to the general failure probability distribution of the real applications. Thus, the statistic characteristics of training samples reflect the total failure mode probability and the training sample detection performance depicts the detection probability. From above, FDR for the node is presented as follows:

$$FDR_{node} = \frac{\sum_{i=1}^{M_{node}} \sum_{j=1}^{K} P(f_j(x_{1,T_{node}} | ELM_{node}) \geq 1 - \varepsilon, y_{i,j} = 1)}{\sum_{i=1}^{M_{node}} \sum_{j=1}^{K} y_{i,j}} \tag{10}$$

where ε is the detection margin. From the generation process, $f_j(x_{1,T_{node}} | ELM_{node})$ and $y_{i,j}$ are independent of each other. Additionally, since ELM provides a continuous probability estimation, the loss function with respect to FDR_{node} is computed as follows:

$$L_{FDR_{node}} = \frac{\sum_{i=1}^{M_{node}} \sum_{j=1}^{K} \left(y_{i,j} - f_j(x_{1,T_{node}} | ELM_{node})\right) P(y_{i,j} = 1)}{\sum_{i=1}^{M_{node}} \sum_{j=1}^{K} y_{i,j}} \tag{11}$$

Along with FDR, FAR presents the ratio between false-alarm failure mode probability and the total failure detection probability. Taking consideration of $f_j(x_{1,T_{node}} | ELM_{node})$, FAR is computed as follows:

$$FAR_{node} = \frac{\sum_{i=1}^{M_{node}} \sum_{j=1}^{K} P(f_j(x_{1,T_{node}} | ELM_{node}) \geq 1 - \varepsilon, y_{i,j} = 0)}{\sum_{i=1}^{M_{node}} \sum_{j=1}^{K} P(f_j(x_{1,T_{node}} | ELM_{node}) \geq 1 - \varepsilon)} \tag{12}$$

Here, it is assumed that the model has enough accuracy so that the failure estimation and the total failure conditions have approximate values. Thus, $\sum_{i=1}^{M_{node}} \sum_{j=1}^{K} P(f_j(x_{1,T_{node}} | ELM_{node})$

$\geq 1-\varepsilon$) is able to be approximately equal to $\sum_{i=1}^{M_{node}} \sum_{j=1}^{K} y_{i,j}$. Therefore, the loss function of the FAR is denoted as:

$$L_{node} = \frac{\sum_{i=1}^{M_{node}} \sum_{j}^{K} \left(y_{i,j} - f_j\left(x_{1,T_{node}} | ELM_{node}\right)\right)^2 P(y_{i,j}=1)}{\sum_{i=1}^{M_{node}} \sum_{j}^{K} y_{i,j}}$$
$$+ \frac{\sum_{i=1}^{M_{node}} \sum_{j}^{K} \left(y_{i,j} - f_j\left(x_{1,T_{node}} | ELM_{node}\right)\right)^2 P(y_{i,j}=0)}{\sum_{i=1}^{M_{node}} \sum_{j}^{K} y_{i,j}} \qquad (13)$$
$$= \frac{\sum_{i=1}^{M_{node}} \sum_{j}^{K} \left(y_{i,j} - f_j\left(x_{1,T_{node}} | ELM_{node}\right)\right)^2}{\sum_{i=1}^{M_{node}} \sum_{j}^{K} y_{i,j}}$$

As $\sum_{i=1}^{M_{node}} \sum_{j}^{K} y_{i,j}$ is independent from the soft-sensor construction, the task of ELM is to minimize $\sum_{i=1}^{M_{node}} \sum_{j}^{K} \left(y_{i,j} - f_j(x_{1,T_{node}} | ELM_{node})\right)^2$, which is the difference between M_{node} and Y_{node}, expressed as follows:

$$ELM = argmin\left\{\sum_{i=1}^{M_{node}} ||y_i - f(x_{1,T_{node}} | ELM_{node})||^2\right\} \qquad (14)$$

Since the maintenance design of the proposed method directly relies on the recording sensor signals, the physical system knowledge is largely preserved and the information usage is highly enhanced.

Based on soft-sensor node construction, testability design process adds the soft-sensor node with best performance and builds a fault tree, taking consideration of potential soft-sensor node under the minimum conditional entropy criterion. Hence, the assigned soft-sensor nodes decrease the diagnostic uncertainty and improve the detection efficiency. Besides, affinity propagation (AP) is adapted to separate the fuzzy set of the fault modes and generate subnodes for the diagnostic model with the exemplar probability estimation $m_{exampor}$ and basic probability assignment BPA_{node}. The subnodes are denoted with the subset of failure modes $S_{son} = [S_{son,1}, S_{son,2}, \ldots, S_{son,K_{node}}]$ and satisfies the condition that $\cup_{i=1}^{K_{node}} S_{son,i} = S_{father}$.

After adding the soft-sensor nodes and extending the subset of fault modes, the information of assigned nodes T_{node} is regarded as prior knowledge, serving as feedback from testability design to maintenance design, and extending the fault tree until reaching the minimum fault condition set.

With the cooperation between testability design and maintenance design, a PHM model based on soft-senor information is generated and the sensors for PHM maintenance are assigned based on the selected test set of PHM model, as follows.

$$T_{PHM} = \{t_i : \exists T_{node}, t_i \in T_{node}\} \qquad (15)$$

To locate the fault condition when starting with the maximum set of failure modes, the corresponding sensor recording is collected and used to compute the potential basic probability assignment. Then, the subset of potential modes is determined based on existing samples with nearest neighbor strategy and the detection process is continued until finding the minimum failure sets and obtaining the failure detection. For each test sample denoted as $case_i$, the PHM detection procedures generate a test sequence corresponding to the assigned sensor recording and the estimation from the signal processing by a branch of assigned soft-sensor nodes, as follows:

$$S_{node} = \left\{Node_j : \exists m_{exemplar,k} \in m_{exemplar}, \left\|f\left(x_{case_i, T_{node,j}} | ELM_{node_j}\right) - m_{exemplar,k}\right\| = d_{node}\right\} \qquad (16)$$

where d_{Node_j} is the minimum distance from the failure condition estimation vector $f(x_{case, T_{node}} | ELM_{node_j})$ to all exemplars of soft-sensor nodes with the same father node of $Node_j$. The detection process ends when the procedures reach the terminal node of S_{node} denoted as $Node_{terminal,case}$. Then, the estimated failure condition vector is computed as:

$$\hat{y}_{case.j} = \begin{cases} 1 & s_j \in S_{node_{terminal,case}, father} \\ 0 & s_j \notin S_{node_{terminal,case}, father} \end{cases} \quad (17)$$

According to the definitions of FDR, FAR, and detection accuracy, the test performance indexes of the detection procedures are computed as follows:

$$FDR_{test} = \sum\nolimits_{X_{case}} \sum\nolimits_{j=1}^{K} P(\hat{y}_{case,j} = 1 | y_{casse,j} = 1) \quad (18)$$

$$FDR_{test} = \sum\nolimits_{X_{case}} \sum\nolimits_{j=1}^{K} P(\hat{y}_{case,j} = 0 | y_{casse,j} = 1) \quad (19)$$

$$Accuracy_{test} = \sum\nolimits_{X_{case}} \sum\nolimits_{j=1}^{K} P(\hat{y}_{case,j} = 1 | y_{casse,j} = 1) + P(\hat{y}_{case,j} = 0 | y_{casse,j} = 0) \quad (20)$$

From these, the test strategy optimization aims to select T_{PHM} from $T_{potential}$ and generate the diagnostic tree with soft sensors and AP. For each case, AP determines the next procedure and the corresponding soft sensors with previous estimations. Thus, for each case, the diagnostic tree provides an adaptive test sequence and leads to the final evaluation on the terminal node. Similar to Equation (4), the objective function is the combination of FAR loss and FDR loss, as follows:

$$L_{tree} = \frac{\sum_{i=1}^{M} \sum_{j=1}^{K} \left(y_{i,j} - F_j\left(x_{i,T_{seq,i}} \middle| T_{seq,i} \in T_{PHM}, ELM_{node} \in tree\right)\right)^2}{\sum_{i=1}^{M} \sum_{j=1}^{K} y_{i,j}} \quad (21)$$

where $T_{seq,i}$ is the required test procedure with respect to the diagnostic tree, and $F_j\left(x_{i,T_{seq,i}} \middle| T_{seq,i} \in T_{PHM}, ELM_{node} \in tree\right)$ is the state estimation from the terminal node with respect to the test procedure of the i-th case.

3. Test Strategy Optimization Based on Soft Sensing and Ensemble Belief Measurement

3.1. Construct Soft-Sensor Node with Extreme Learning Machine

As mentioned in the previous section, each soft sensor contains the recording information from the assigned sensors, the artificial intelligence signal processing modules, and probability estimation parameter for the isolation of fault states. During the construct process, maintenance design produces the soft-sensor node with candidate test procedures and candidate soft-sensor nodes with high performance, and generates the fault tree. For each candidate node, the sensor recording input is created as follows:

$$X_{candidate,\ node} = \left\{x_{s_i,T_i^*} : x_i \in X_{candidate\ node}\right\} \quad (22)$$

$$x_{s_i,T_i^*} = \{x_{s_i,t} | t \in T_i^*\} \quad (23)$$

$$T_i^* = \left\{T_{sequence}^*, t^*\right\} \text{ where } \{t^*\} \cap T_{sequence}^* = \varnothing \quad (24)$$

where $T_{sequence}^*$ integrates the previous test information of before the candidate node and makes full use of sensor recording knowledge.

At the same time, we use ELM to generate artificial intelligence signal processing modules for fast training and high generation ability. Shown in Figure 4, ELM is a noniterative three-layer neural network and contains parameters of a fully connected hidden layer and a linear-combined output layer with an activation function, as follows:

$$ELM_{candidate,node} = \{(W_{node}, b_{node}), \beta_{node}, f_h(\cdot)\} \quad (25)$$

$$W_{node} = \begin{bmatrix} w_{1,1} & \cdots & w_{1,N_T} \\ w_{2,1} & \cdots & w_{2,N_T} \\ \vdots & \ddots & \vdots \\ w_{L,1} & \cdots & w_{L,N_T} \end{bmatrix} \quad (26)$$

$$b_{node} = [b_{node.1}, b_{node.2}, \ldots, b_{node.L}] \quad (27)$$

$$\beta_{node} = \begin{bmatrix} \beta_{1,1} & \cdots & \beta_{1,N_T} \\ \beta_{2,1} & \cdots & \beta_{2,N_T} \\ \vdots & \ddots & \vdots \\ \beta_{L,1} & \cdots & \beta_{L,N_T} \end{bmatrix} \quad (28)$$

where W_{node} is denoted as the weights matrix of the hidden layer while b_{node} is the hidden layer bias, and L is the number of hidden nodes. β_{node} is the output layer weight and $f_h(.)$ determines the activation function from the sensor input and hidden output. Here, the sigmoid function is taken as the activation functions for all soft-sensor nodes. Relative to $X_{candidate\ node}$, the hidden outputs of training samples are produced as follows:

$$H_{node} = \begin{bmatrix} f_h(w_1 x_{1,T^*} + b_{node,1}) & \cdots & f_h(w_L x_{1,T^*} + b_{node,L}) \\ f_h(w_1 x_{2,T^*} + b_{node,L}) & \cdots & f_h(w_L x_{2,T^*} + b_{node,L}) \\ \vdots & \ddots & \vdots \\ f_h(w_1 x_{M_{node},T^*} + b_{node,1}) & \cdots & f_h(w_L x_{M_{node},T^*} + b_{node,L}) \end{bmatrix} \quad (29)$$

As ELM is a noniterative learning machine, W_{node} and b_{node} can be assigned randomly with respect to arbitrary probability distribution, and the output of the model is computed as a linear combination of the hidden output with trained β_{node}, as follows:

$$\dot{Y}_{candidate\ node} = \beta_{node} H_{node} \quad (30)$$

To estimate the failure situation as accurately as possible, $\dot{Y}_{candidate\ node}$ is supposed to be consistent with actual failure states Y_{node} defined based on Equations (5)–(7). According to Equation (14), the loss function of the candidate node is computed as follows:

$$Loss_{candidate\ node} = ||Y_{node} - \dot{Y}_{candidate\ node}||^2 = ||Y_{node} - \beta_{node} H_{node}||^2 \quad (31)$$

Taking differential of $Loss_{candidate\ node}$ with respect to β_{node}, the trained output weight is accessed as follows:

$$\beta_{node} = \left(H_{node} H_{node}^T + \lambda I \right)^{-1} H_{node} Y_{node} \quad (32)$$

Based on the proper assignment of ELM parameters, the soft-sensor nodes gain knowledge from the training samples and obtain accurate condition estimation with the test samples.

From above, considering the candidate node with sensor recording inputs $X_{candidate,\ node}$, the previous test sequence $T^*_{sequence}$, and candidate test point t^*, the procedure to generate the ELM_{node} follows:

Step 1: Assign the candidate node with Equation (2), where $S_{father} = \{s_i | s_{candidate\ node} = s_i, s_i \in S\}$. Meanwhile, T_{node} is generated as Equation (24), Y_{node} is assigned with Equations (5)–(7);
Step 2: Initialize ELM parameters (W_{node}, b_{node}) randomly in $[-1,1]$;
Step 3: Calculate the hidden output with respect to $X_{candidate,\ node}$ as in Equation (29);
Step 4: Train the output weights β_{node} with Equation (32);
Step 5: Obtain the estimation of candidate set $\dot{Y}_{candidate\ node}$ with Equation (30).

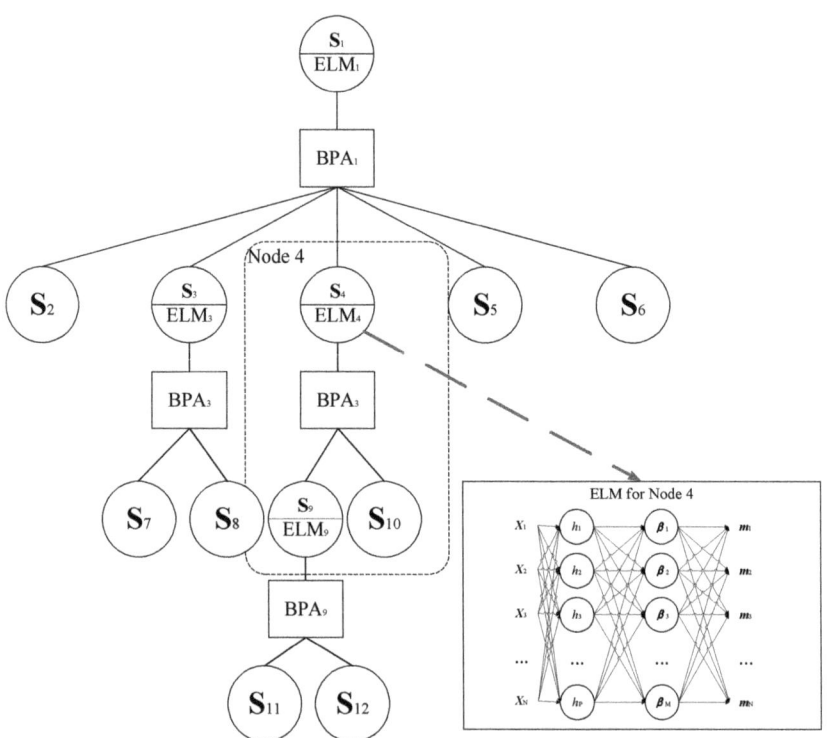

Figure 4. Fault tree of test strategy optimization based on soft sensing and ensemble belief measurement.

3.2. Separate the Fault Set Based on Affinity Propagation

With ELM-based soft-sensor nodes, the condition of trained samples and test samples can be estimated with high efficiency. Meanwhile, owing to the individual sensor recording knowledge limitation, the ELM condition evaluation has a vague part with unrelated failure modes. Thus, the fault set of corresponding nodes S_{father} is divided into several fuzzy sets $S_{son} = [S_{son,1}, S_{son,2}, \ldots, S_{son,K_{node}}]$ based on the fault state evaluation value $\dot{Y}_{candidate\ node}$. When constructing traditional diagnostic tree and fault analysis processes, the failure mode subset is divided by comparing the fault state evaluation and reference value of the failure mode or the failure mode calibration value. However, these strategies are only applicable to systems with small structures or systems with known mechanisms and a historical sample may ignore the diversity and validity. Hence, in the proposed method, we introduce a new dividing strategy based on affinity propagation (AP) to cut the fuzzy set and samples with evaluation similarity measurement between pairs of data points. With AP, S_{son} it is constituted based on the similarity between condition estimates and the fault tree generation flexibility is enhanced.

Instead of assigning engineering-experience reference information, AP generates clusters based on all training set evaluation values $\dot{Y}_{candidate\ node} = \{y_1, y_2, \ldots, y_{M_{node}}\}$. The clustering method treats each training sample as one data edge point and transmits two real-valued messages: the responsibility value $r(y_i, y_j)$ and the availability value $a(y_i, y_j)$, to realize communication between edge nodes until a good set of exemplars and corresponding clusters emerges. The responsibility value $r(y_i, y_j)$ indicates the accumulated evidence for how well suited a historical data point y_j is to serve as the exemplar for the historical data point y_i. In addition, the availability value $a(y_i, y_j)$ represents how appropriate it would be for a historical data point y_i to choose a historical data point y_j

as its exemplar. For initialization, the similarity between the historical points (y_i, y_j) is calculated based on Euclidean distance, as follows:

$$d(y_i, y_j) = -\left\Vert y_i - y_j \right\Vert^2 \tag{33}$$

where $d(y_i, y_j)$ reflects how well the historical data point y_j is suited to be the exemplar for historical data point y_i. AP aims to provide a clustering solution that satisfies the historical data points with larger values of distance estimation, which are more likely to serve as exemplars. To achieve this purpose, the clustering method recursively conducts the following updating process, sending the responsibility message from each data point to the corresponding data point.

First, the responsibility value $r(y_i, y_j)$ is computed based on the following data driven approach:

$$r(y_i, y_j) = d(y_i, y_j) - \max_{k, s.t. k \neq j} \{a(y_i, y_k) + d(y_i, y_k)\} \tag{34}$$

As the availability value $a(y_i, y_j)$ is set to 0, the responsibility value $r(y_i, y_j)$ is initialized as the input similarity $d(y_i, y_j)$ minus the largest similarity value between y_i and other exemplars. Hence, the updating process does not consider how many other points favor each candidate exemplar. In later process, if some point is efficient to assign with other exemplars, the corresponding availability value will drop to less than 0 with the updating of $a(y_i, y_j)$. Then, negative $a(y_i, y_j)$ will decrease the effective value of the similarities value $d(y_i, y_j)$ by Equation (34) and removes the corresponding candidate exemplars from competition. Especially, the self-responsibility value $r(y_i, y_j)$ is set to the input preference that the training data point y_i becomes one of the exemplars of clusters and reflects accumulated evidence that y_i is an exemplar based on its input preference tempered by how ill-suited it is for assignment to another exemplar.

After calculating the responsibility value, the availability value is updated to gather evidence from the training data point as to whether each candidate exemplar makes a good exemplar, as follows:

$$a(y_i, y_j) = min\{0, d(y_i, y_j) + \max_{k, s.t. k \neq j} \{a(y_i, y_k) + d(y_i, y_k)\}\} \tag{35}$$

In addition, the self-availability value $a(y_i, y_j)$ is updated as follows:

$$a(y_i, y_j) = \sum_{k, s.t. k \neq j, k \neq i} max\{0, r(y_i, y_k)\} \tag{36}$$

where $a(y_i, y_j)$ reflects accumulated evidence that the training data point y_i becomes an exemplar. For data point y_i, the data point y_j that maximizes $a(y_i, y_j) + r(y_i, y_j)$ is chosen to be the exemplar. Additionally, it $i = j$, then it is necessary to identify the data point y_i as the exemplar and assign its estimation value y_i as the exemplar value $m_{exemplar}$. The set of all the $m_{exemplar}$ is denoted as $M_{exemplar}$. Based on each exemplar, one subset of S_{father} satisfies.

$$\forall m_{exemplar} \in M_{exemplar}, \exists S_{son,k} \subset S_{son,k} \ s.t. \ S_{son,k}$$
$$= \{s_i : \exists x_j \in X_{node}, a(y_i, m_{exemplar}) + r(y_i, m_{exemplar}) \tag{37}$$
$$= argmax\{a(y_i, y_j) + r(y_i, y_j)\}\}.$$

From above, the AP process with respect to the candidate node is conducted as follows:

Step 1: For $\dot{y}_i, \dot{y}_j \in \dot{Y}_{candidate\ node}$, initialize the responsibility value $r(\dot{y}_i, \dot{y}_j)$ as the Euclidean distance $d(\dot{y}_i, \dot{y}_j)$ with Equation (33), and set the availability value $a(\dot{y}_i, \dot{y}_j)$ to zero;

Step 2: Update the responsibility value $r(\dot{y}_i, \dot{y}_j)$ with Equation (34);

Step 3: Update the availability value $a(\dot{y}_i, \dot{y}_j)$ with Equations (35) and (36);

Step 4: If $r(\dot{y}_i, \dot{y}_j)$ and $a(\dot{y}_i, \dot{y}_j)$ become stable, conduct Step 5, otherwise return to Step 2;

Step 5: For each sample $\dot{y}_i \in \dot{Y}_{candidate\ node}$, assign the sample data corresponding to $a(y_i, y_j) + r(y_i, y_j)$ as exemplar node $m_{exemplar}$ and then generate the exemplar set $M_{exemplar}$;

Step 6: Separate S_{father} with Equation (37).

3.3. Generate the Fault Diagnostic Tree under Minimum Conditional Criterion

Based on soft-sensor construction and subset division, the fault states of the target system can be located by cutting the set of potential failure sets with the function of sequences of soft-sensor nodes. In this section, we introduce how to generate the fault tree using a potential soft-sensor node under heuristic strategy based on the minimum conditional criterion. For the assigned failure set S_{father}, the contains numbers of potential sensor nodes corresponding to the candidate procedures. To choose the soft sensor for fault tree construction, the condition entropy $H(Y_{node}|\dot{Y}_{node}, ELM_{candidate})$ is introduced as follows:

$$H(Y_{node}|\dot{Y}_{node}, ELM_{candidate}) = -\sum_{y \in Y_{node}} p(y, \dot{y}|ELM_{candidate}) \log(y|\dot{y}, ELM_{candidate}) \tag{38}$$

Since the soft-sensor model is data-driven, the estimation value of the conditional entropy is computed as follows:

$$H(Y_{node}|\dot{Y}_{node}, ELM_{candidate}) = \sum_{y \in Y_{node}} \log p(y|\dot{y}, ELM_{candidate}) \tag{39}$$

Assuming the data information $(Y_{node}, \dot{Y}_{node})$ is subject to Gaussian distribution, then $\dot{H}(Y_{node}|\dot{Y}_{node}, ELM_{candidate})$ is simplified as follows:

$$\dot{H}(Y_{node}|\dot{Y}_{node}, ELM_{candidate}) = \sum_{y \in Y_{node}} \|Y_{node} - \dot{Y}_{node}\|^2 \tag{40}$$

For all candidate soft-sensor nodes, the node with the lowest conditional entropy is selected to build the fault diagnostic tree. From above, the process to construct the fault diagnostic tree follows:

Step 1. Initialize the root node $Node_{root}$ of the decision tree. Assign the father fault set S_{father} as the total fault set S_{total} and set the data set X_{node} as the whole training data set. Take all the test procedures as the potential test set $T_{potential}$ for $Node_{root}$. Set $T^*_{sequence}$ to $\varnothing$.

Step 2. Generate the potential soft-sensor node $Node_{candi, t_{potential}}$ for each test procedure $t_{potential} \in T_{potential}$ based on Equations (24), (28) and (31).

Step 3. Evaluate with Equation (39) the condition entropy $\dot{H}(Y_{node}|\dot{Y}_{node}, ELM_{candidate})$ for the entire potential soft-sensor node. Select the corresponding soft-sensor node $Node_{candi, t_{potential}}$ with the lowest condition entropy as the target node to the diagnostic tree, and update the $T^*_{sequence}$ as $\{T^*_{sequence}, t_{opt}\}$. Additionally, remove t_{opt} from $T_{potential}$.

Step 4. Apply AP to separate the fault set S_{father} based on $\dot{Y}_{node}$ and assign the exemplar reference $M_{exemplar}$ with Equation (36).

Step 5. For each subset S_i in S_{son}, construct the extending node $Node_{S_i}$. For each extending node $Node_{S_i}$, the father set is assigned as S_i and the data set is constructed based on AP result. $T^*_{sequence}$ is initialized as $\left\{ T^*_{sequence}, t_{opt} \right\}$.

Step 6. Generate the subset node by repeating **Steps 2** to **5** until reaching the minimal subset of failure mode. The construction process is completed when all the subnodes of the failure tree are constructed.

With the minimum conditional criterion, the fault diagnostic tree is generated with data-driven mechanisms and requires few engineering experiences. Thus, the generating process is applicable to complex systems with insufficient knowledge about structures, functions, and mechanisms.

With the diagnostic tree generated, the diagnostic process of the target system is implemented as follows:

Step 1. Initialize the target node $Node_{target}$ with the root node $Node_{root}$ of the diagnostic tree. Assign the potential fault set $S_{potential}$ to the total fault set S_{total}. Set the target sensor recording x_{target} as $\varnothing$ and set the test sequence $T_{sequence}$ to $\varnothing$.

Step 2. Conduct the new test procedure t^* in the $Node_{target}$ and obtain the sensor recording x_{target,t^*}. Add t^* into $T_{sequence}$ and merge x_{target,t^*} into x_{target}. Compute the estimation of the target system $\hat{y}_{target}$ with ELM_{node} in $Node_{target}$ by Equations (29) and (30).

Step 3. Find the optimal $m_{exemplar}$ in $M_{exemplar}$ of $Node_{target}$ with smallest distance. Locate the subfault set S^* as the updated $S_{potential}$ with Equation (37).

Step 4. Search the soft-sensor node in the diagnostic tree with $S_{father} = S_{potential}$ and assign the corresponding node as the new target node $Node_{target}$.

Step 5. Continue the diagnostic procedure by steps 2 to 4 until reaching the minimal subset of the failure set. After the diagnosis is finished, achieve the final estimation by using Equation (17).

4. Experiment

In this section, we use the analog circuit in [40] to evaluate the detection performance of the proposed method with state-of-art methods. As Figure 5 shows, the target system contains four second-order filters and one adding device. The detail of the system is presented in Table 1. The tolerance of R_1, R_2, R_3, R_4, R_5, R_6, R_7, and R_8 is $\pm 10\%$ while the tolerance of R_9, R_{10}, and R_{11} is $\pm 1\%$. For capacitances, the tolerance is set to $\pm 5\%$. Under healthy operation, the transmission gain of Av_1, Av_2, Av_3, and Av_4 is within a range of $\pm 1\%$.

Here, the failures caused by different changes of amplifiers are taken into failure detection. The failure modes are defined based on the range of transmission gain for Av_1, Av_2, Av_3, and Av_4, as shown in Table 2. Since 80% of failures in real applications have a single-failure mode, we only consider failure detection of single failure modes. For example, the failure condition of Av1 is divided into five phases with different ranges of transmission gain while the transmission gain of Av_2, Av_3, and Av_4, are collected with four different frequencies (10 Hz, 100 Hz, 10 kHz, and 100 kHz) of input signals. The details are shown in Table 3. These voltage outputs from Av_1, Av_2, Av_3, and Av_4 are regarded as the potential test points for failure detection. In total, there are 16 candidate test points and 17 potential fault states that consider the health state.

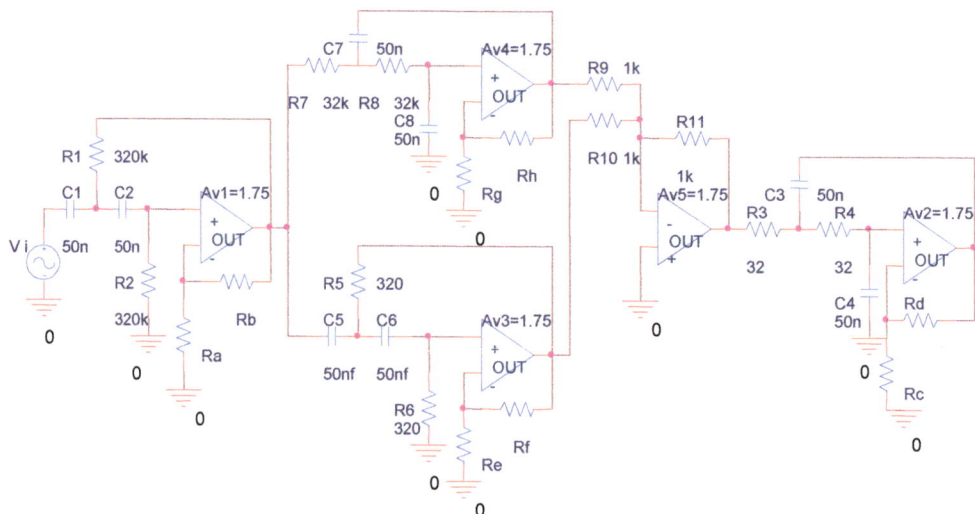

Figure 5. Target analog circuit.

Table 1. Details for the components of the circuit.

Components	Nominal Value	Tolerance	Subsystem
R_1	320 kΩ	10%	
R_2	320 kΩ	10%	
C_1	50 nF	5%	High-Pass Filter 1 F_1 = 10 Hz
C_2	50 nF	5%	
Av_1	1.75	1%	
R_3	32 Ω	10%	
R_4	32 Ω	10%	
C_3	50 nF	5%	Low-Pass Filter 1 F_2 = 100 kHz
C_4	50 nF	5%	
Av_2	1.75	1%	
R_5	320 Ω	10%	
R_6	320 Ω	10%	
C_5	50 nF	5%	High-Pass Filter 2 F_3 = 10 kHz
C_6	50 nF	5%	
Av_3	1.75	1%	
R_7	32 kΩ	10%	
R_8	32 kΩ	10%	
C_7	50 nF	5%	Low-Pass Filter 2 F_4 = 100 Hz
C_8	50 nF	5%	
Av_4	1.75	1%	
R_9	1 kΩ	1%	
R_{10}	1 kΩ	1%	Adder
R_{11}	1 kΩ	1%	

Table 2. Denotation of fault states.

Fault Index	Av_1 Value Range	Av_2 Value Range	Av_3 Value Range	Av_4 Value Range
S_0(normal)	(1.70,1.80)	(1.70,1.80)	(1.70,1.80)	(1.70,1.80)
S_1	(1.60,1.70)	(1.70,1.80)	(1.70,1.80)	(1.70,1.80)
S_2	(1.80,1.90)	(1.70,1.80)	(1.70,1.80)	(1.70,1.80)
S_3	(1.50,1.60)	(1.70,1.80)	(1.70,1.80)	(1.70,1.80)
S_4	(1.90,2.00)	(1.70,1.80)	(1.70,1.80)	(1.70,1.80)
S_5	(1.70,1.80)	(1.60,1.70)	(1.70,1.80)	(1.70,1.80)
S_6	(1.70,1.80)	**(1.80,1.90)**	(1.70,1.80)	(1.70,1.80)
S_7	(1.70,1.80)	(1.50,1.60)	(1.70,1.80)	(1.70,1.80)
S_8	(1.70,1.80)	(1.90,2.00)	**(1.70,1.80)**	(1.70,1.80)
S_9	(1.70,1.80)	(1.70,1.80)	(1.60,1.70)	(1.70,1.80)
S_{10}	(1.70,1.80)	(1.70,1.80)	(1.80,1.90)	(1.70,1.80)
S_{11}	(1.70,1.80)	(1.70,1.80)	(1.50,1.60)	(1.70,1.80)
S_{12}	(1.70,1.80)	(1.70,1.80)	(1.90,2.00)	(1.70,1.80)
S_{13}	(1.70,1.80)	(1.70,1.80)	(1.70,1.80)	(1.60,1.70)
S_{14}	(1.70,1.80)	(1.70,1.80)	(1.70,1.80)	(1.80,1.90)
S_{15}	(1.70,1.80)	(1.70,1.80)	(1.70,1.80)	(1.50,1.60)
S_{16}	(1.70,1.80)	(1.70,1.80)	(1.70,1.80)	**(1.90,2.00)**

We apply Monte Carlo simulation to generate 20 samples for each failure mode by using Pspice software to access data.

According to the traditional PHM framework shown in Figure 3, the optimization process requires binary fault marks based on human experience and design detection circuits for each fault state. Since there are four fault states for each second-order filter, the detection is a large burden on circuit design. Testability design may also fail to relate the relationship between binary estimations of different test procedures. On the other hand, the maintenance design suffers low estimation efficiency as the testability does not consider the detailed information of sensor recordings.

Unlike the sequential framework, the proposed method considers the direct sensor information under testability and maintenance design. With cooperative procedures in Figure 4, the proposed method generates the candidate soft-sensor nodes for maintenance. At the same time, the testability design uses the minimal conditional criterion to generate the optimized diagnostic strategy. The minimal conditional criterion enhances the flexibility of testability design by considering the soft-sensor estimation in maintenance phases. On the other hand, the maintenance performance with full sensor recording increases information usage efficiency. Instead of human-experience processing, the proposed method saves many costs during the PHM design. To evaluate diagnostic performance, we compared our method with the hidden Markov method (HMM), support learning machine (SVM), and radial basis function (RBF) by using all recordings of 16 test points as input information. To estimate the feature extraction performance and learning machine function, we also took HMM and SVM with principal component analysis (PCA) and extreme learning machine (ELM) into comparison. For each method, we used 70% of the samples in each fault state as the training samples to construct the model and the other 30% as the sensor information of target systems. We assigned 100 kernels or hidden nodes for our soft-sensor nodes for the SVM, RBF, and ELM models. Each method was conducted 30 times to obtain the average performance.

Table 3. Performance comparison.

Method	Performance	S0	S1	S2	S3	S4	S5	S6	S7	S8	S9	S10	S11	S12	S13	S14	S15	S16
HMM	FAR	25.0	0.00	0.00	0.00	0.00	0.00	0.00	20.00	33.3	0.00	20.0	0.00	0.00	0.00	52.6	33.3	16.7
	FDR	96.3	100	100	100	100	98.8	96.3	100	100	100	100	100	100	98.7	98.7	100	98.7
	accuracy	95.3	100	100	100	100	97.7	95.3	100	98.9	100	100	100	100	95.3	96.5	98.8	98.8
SVM	FAR	0.00	0.00	0.00	0.00	0.00	0.00	0.00	0.00	0.00	0.00	0.00	0.00	0.00	0.00	0.00	0.00	0.00
	FDR	92.3	94.1	94.1	98.8	96.4	94.1	94.1	97.6	100	94.1	94.1	94.1	94.1	94.1	94.1	96.4	97.6
	accuracy	92.9	94.1	94.1	98.9	96.5	94.1	94.1	97.7	100	94.1	94.1	94.1	94.1	94.1	94.1	96.5	97.7
RBF	FAR	33.3	66.7	33.3	33.2	36.5	0.00	0.00	37.5	0.00	0.00	0.00	50.0	60.0	33.3	60.0	54.4	28.6
	FDR	92.9	95.1	93.9	98.7	100	96.4	100	100	100	95.2	94.1	100	98.7	96.3	96.3	100	100
	accuracy	91.7	93.0	95.1	96.5	90.6	96.5	96.5	96.5	100	96.5	100	95.3	94.1	94.1	95.3	93.0	97.7
PCA HMM	FAR	25.0	0.00	0.00	0.00	0.00	0.00	20.0	0.00	0.00	0.00	0.00	0.00	0.00	0.00	28.6	0.00	0.00
	FDR	96.3	100	100	100	100	100	98.8	100	100	100	100	100	100	100	100	100	100
	accuracy	95.3	100	100	100	100	100	97.7	100	100	100	100	100	100	100	97.7	100	100
PCA SVM	FAR	0.00	0.00	0.00	0.00	0.00	0.00	2.30	0.00	0.00	0.00	0.00	0.00	0.00	0.00	0.00	0.00	0.00
	FDR	93.0	94.1	94.1	98.8	96.4	94.1	94.1	97.6	100	94.1	94.1	94.1	94.1	94.1	94.1	96.4	97.6
	accuracy	93.0	94.1	94.1	98.9	96.5	94.1	97.7	100	94.1	94.1	94.1	94.1	94.1	94.1	94.1	96.5	97.7
ELM	FAR	0.00	0.00	0.00	0.00	0.00	0.00	2.30	0.00	0.00	0.00	0.00	0.00	0.00	0.00	0.00	0.00	0.00
	FDR	91.4	100	100	100	100	100	100	100	100	100	100	100	100	100	100	96.4	97.6
	accuracy	92.3	100	100	100	100	100	100	100	100	100	100	100	100	100	100	96.4	97.6
OURS	FAR	0.00	0.00	0.00	0.00	0.00	0.00	0.00	0.00	0.00	0.00	0.00	0.00	0.00	0.00	0.00	0.00	0.00
	FDR	99.7	100	100	100	100	100	100	100	100	100	100	100	100	100	100	100	100
	accuracy	100	100	100	100	100	100	100	100	100	100	100	100	100	100	100	100	100

Table 3 shows the FAR, FDR, and accuracy of each method. HMM has high diagnostic accuracy without feature extraction, especially for S_0. This is because HMM has a higher statistical analysis ability than SVM and RBF. However, HMM gives poorer FAR than the other methods. Unlike HMM and RBF, SVM and ELM have lower FAR and become more sensitive to false-negative samples by the advantage of the learning machine. Comparing HMM, SVM, PCA–HMM, and PCA–SVM, PCA improves HMM diagnosis for S5 and S8 and proves that proper feature extractions can benefit from the diagnostic performance. Our method has the lowest FAR, the highest FDR, and the highest accuracy compared with the other methods. Based on the same sensor recordings or even less information, the generated strategy provides an accurate location for all test samples for all 16 fault states. Hence, with ensemble learning based on soft sensors, the functions of sensor recording are largely improved.

Figure 6 shows the diagnostic tree of our method. All fault conditions are separated and recognized with 13 individual testing sequences with the tree structure. Each testing sequence takes less than 5 test procedures and the whole diagnostic tree contains only 9 testing points out of 16 potential test points. In other words, the fault state of the target systems is located within 2–5 test procedures instead of collecting all 16 sensor recordings. From above, the diagnostic tree has higher efficiency and lower cost testing consumptions than diagnostic strategies that require full-tests built by SVM, HMM, and ELM, as well as the constrained diagnostic tests strategies that require PCA-based methods. Additionally, unlike traditional diagnostic trees with binary structures, our method separates the fuzzy set with the evaluation results from constructing and dividing modules. As a result, our testability design extends the diagnostic flexibility and improves the diagnostic accuracies of each fault mode.

Based on soft-sensor construction, the potential test accuracies of the diagnostic tree root node are compared based on different test procedures. As shown in Figure 7, different test procedures differ on diagnostic accuracies, especially for S_0–S_5. Therefore, the minimum conditional criterion-based fault tree constructions can efficiently select proper soft-sensor nodes into the diagnostic tree and ensure that the diagnostic FAR and FDR and their accuracies receive high improvement under the constructing process.

The affinity propagation result from the diagnostic-tree-root node is presented in Figure 8. As the root nodes evaluate all samples, the affinity results are generated with fault mode evaluations of all 17 fault conditions (from S_0 to S_{16}). Here, we depict the affinity propagation result from three fault states, which occur at the same space, such as Av_1 failures (S_0, S_1, and S_2), Av_2 failures (S_5, S_7, and S_{14}), and Av_4 failures (S_{12}, S_{13}, and S_{15}). Additionally, we present the affinity propagation results with three failure modes in different places: S_2 in Av_1, S_7 in Av_2, and S_{14} in Av_4.

From Figure 8, the soft-sensor nodes provide distinguishable BPA evaluations for each data point. The affinity propagation generates sample clusters from different dimensions adaptively with the data point similarity measurements. Most data points are clustered with topological closer clusters; others may differ on other dimensions. Compared with traditional clustering strategies for diagnosis, affinity propagation provides practical, automatic fault-state divisions and saves much human labor on engineering applications.

Finally, the sequence testing performance for fault states is shown in Figure 9. Here, we present the test sequence of S_0, S_3, S_8, and S_{15}. These four test sequences achieve their best diagnostic accuracy within three to five test procedures, and the test efficiency is much higher than traditional maintenance methods. Test accuracy grows increasingly for all test sequences as test nodes are added into the test procedures. Especially for the test sequence of S_0, the diagnostic accuracy is less than 60% in the first test procedures as the corresponding fuzzy state set contains many members. However, the accuracy grows fast as more nodes are added into the sequences and the potential states become smaller. Thus, the ensemble function of soft-sensor nodes improved the diagnostic performance with high efficiency.

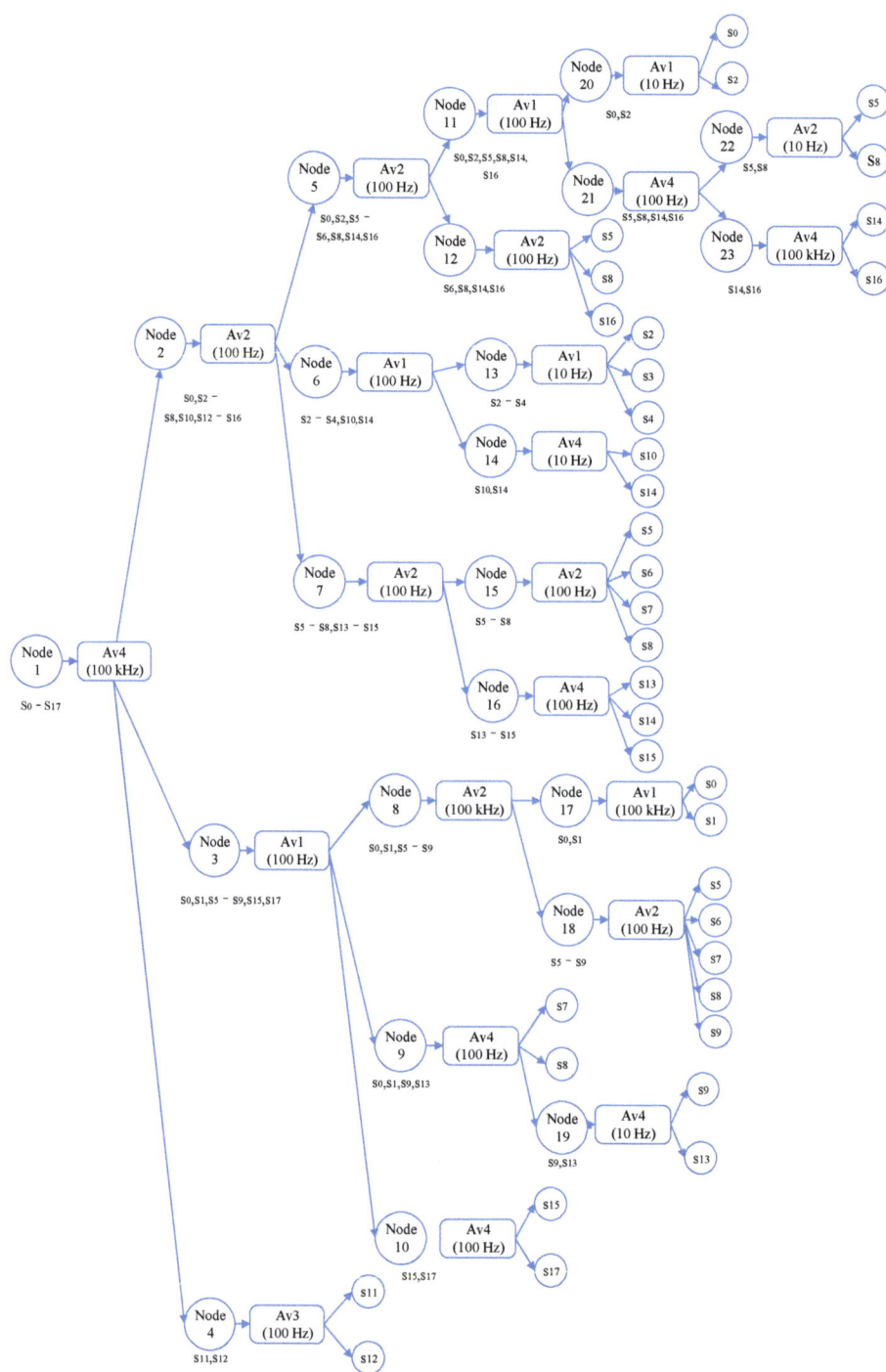

Figure 6. Analog circuit diagnostic tree.

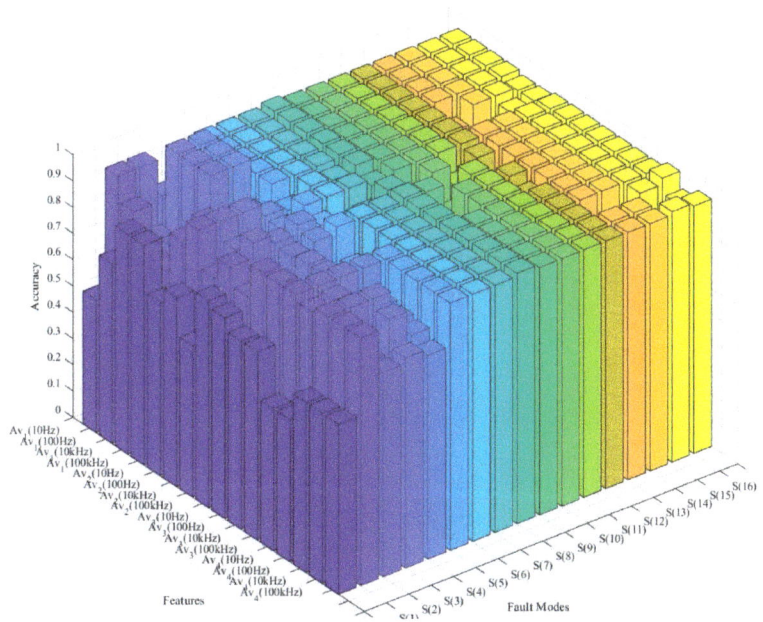

Figure 7. Analog circuit diagnostic tree potential ELM model accuracy comparison.

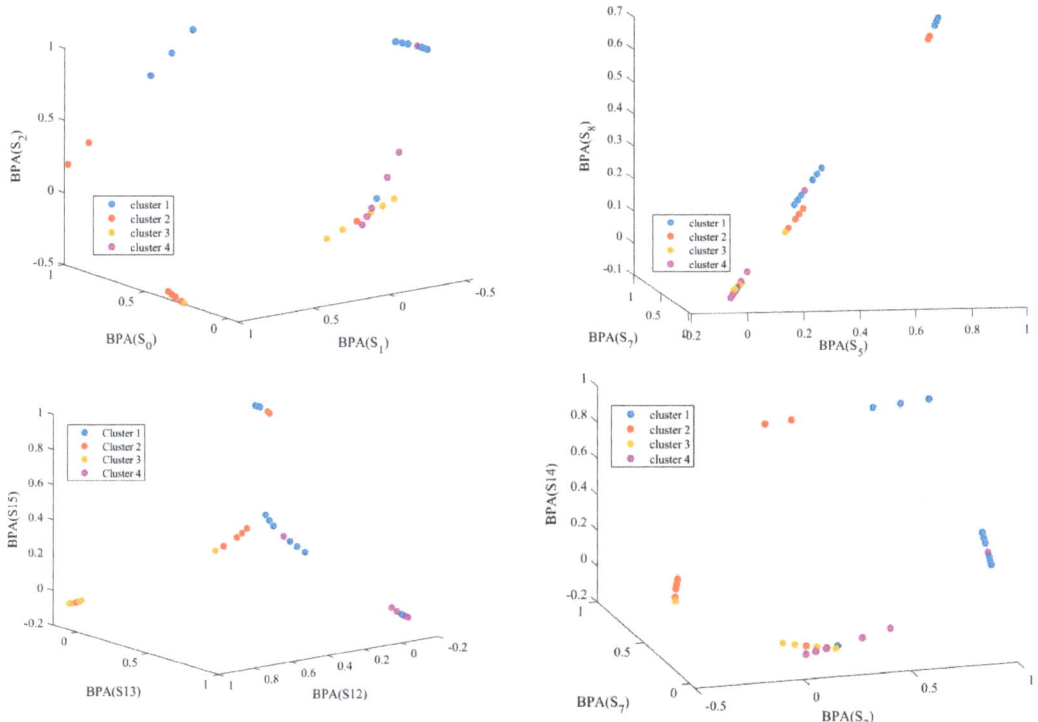

Figure 8. Potential ELM model accuracy comparison.

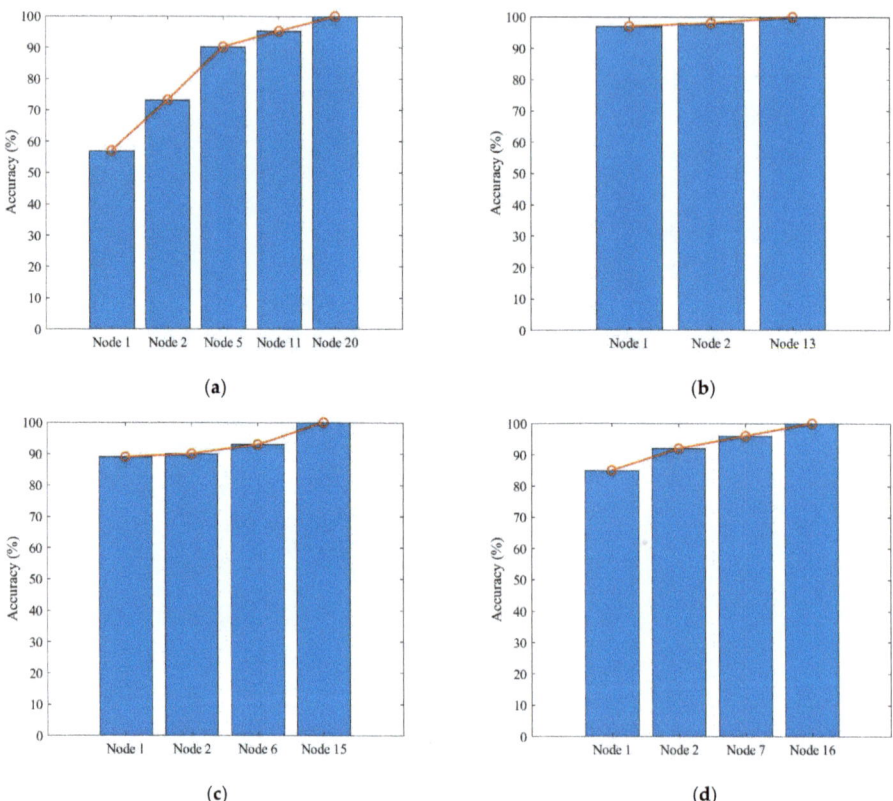

Figure 9. Test sequence accuracy comparison: (**a**) S_0 test sequence, (**b**) S_3 test sequence, (**c**) S_8 test sequence, and (**d**) S_{15} test sequence.

From above, our method has better diagnostic accuracies and lower FARs compared with other state-of-art diagnostic methods. Additionally, our diagnostic strategies take only 9 out of 16 tests points and save much test assignment consumption. For each fault state, the diagnostic procedures provide 1 test sequence within 5 test procedures. Thus, the diagnostic procedure enjoys high efficiency for applications. Finally, the affinity propagation enlarges the diagnostic flexibility and saves much human labor on testability design.

5. Conclusions

Along with a short production cycle and rapid development of design technology, existing PHM techniques have become impractical and fail to match the structural and functional complexity. Prior knowledge preparation costs too much in human labor and binary decision-making strategies waste the entailed sensor recording, especially for large complicated systems.

We propose a test strategy optimization based on soft sensing and ensemble belief measurement to overcome these weaknesses. The proposed method constructs a closed loop between testability design and maintenance design, generating an efficient fault diagnostic tree with ELM-based soft-sensor nodes. Unlike traditional diagnostic approaches, our diagnostic tree adaptively separates the fault sets by affinity propagation, and the soft-sensor nodes are assigned with the minimum conditional criterion. Thus, our methods can achieve high efficiency and flexibility for diagnostic processes.

The experiment results prove that our methods have minimum FAR and maximum accuracies on fault diagnosis among state-of-art methods. Additionally, our methods require fewer test procedures and increase the test efficiency compared with other methods. Because the construction processes are based on ELM and AP, the PHM design saves much human labor and becomes more flexible compared to traditional PHM approaches. Hence, the proposed method has good performance on test strategy design. However, the proposed method uses an offline construction technique for the diagnostic tree. As a result, the diagnostic performance only depends on the assigned fault set, and the recordings of online operations do not work on the PHM design. Therefore, the online updating of the diagnostic strategy should be further investigated.

Author Contributions: Conceptualization, W.M. and Y.S.; methodology, W.M.; software, W.M.; validation, Y.S., L.T. and Z.L.; formal analysis, L.T.; investigation, Z.L.; resources, Z.L.; data curation, W.M.; writing—original draft preparation, W.M.; writing—review and editing, W.M.; visualization, W.M.; supervision, Y.S.; project administration, L.T.; funding acquisition, Z.L. All authors have read and agreed to the published version of the manuscript.

Funding: This work was supported by the National Natural Science Foundation of China under Grant No. U1830133(NSFC) and the Project of Sichuan Youth Science and Technology Innovation Team, China (Grant No. 2020 JDTD0008).

Institutional Review Board Statement: Not applicable.

Informed Consent Statement: Not applicable.

Data Availability Statement: The data that support the findings of this study are available on request from the authors.

Conflicts of Interest: The authors declare no conflict of interest.

References

1. Braunfelds, J.; Senkans, U.; Skels, P.; Janeliukstis, R.; Salgals, T.; Redka, D.; Lyashuk, I.; Porins, J.; Spolitis, S.; Haritonovs, V.; et al. FBG-based sensing for structural health monitoring of road infrastructure. *J. Sens.* **2021**, *2021*, 8850368. [CrossRef]
2. Suryasarman, V.M.; Biswas, S.; Sahu, A. Automation of test program synthesis for processor post-silicon validation. *J. Electron. Test.* **2018**, *34*, 83–103. [CrossRef]
3. Liu, H.; Chen, X.; Duan, C.; Wang, Y. Failure mode and effect analysis using multi-criteria decision-making methods: A systematic literature review. *Comput. Indust. Eng.* **2019**, *135*, 881–897. [CrossRef]
4. Yin, T.; Huang, D.; Fu, S. Intrinsic determinants and harmonic measure of flight safety. *IEEE Tans. Ind. Electron.* **2019**, *67*, 881–897. [CrossRef]
5. Zhu, Z.; Pan, Y.; Zhou, Q.; Lu, C. Event-Triggered adaptive fuzzy control for stochastic nonlinear systems with unmeasured states and unknown Backlash-like hysteresis. *IEEE Trans. Fuzzy Syst.* **2020**, *19*, 1273–1283. [CrossRef]
6. Roman, R.C.; Precup, R.E.; Petriu, E.M. Hybrid data-driven fuzzy active disturbance rejection control for tower crane systems. *Eur. J. Control* **2021**, *58*, 373–387. [CrossRef]
7. Li, S.; Yu, G.; Tang, D.; Li, M.; Han, H. Vibration diagnosis and treatment for a crubber system connected to a reciprocating compressor. *J. Sens.* **2020**, *2020*, 6697295. [CrossRef]
8. Boumen, R.R.; Ruan, S.; De Jong, I.S.M.; Van De Mortel-Fronczak, J.A.; Rooda, J.K.; Pattipati, K.R. Hierarchical testing sequencing for complex systems. *IEEE Trans. Syst. Man Cybern. Part A Syst. Hum.* **2009**, *39*, 640–649. [CrossRef]
9. Garey, M.R. Optimal binary identification procedures. *SIAM J. Appl. Math.* **1972**, *23*, 173–186. [CrossRef]
10. Unler, A.; Murat, A. A discrete particle optimization method for feature selection in binary classification problem. *Eur. J. Oper. Res.* **2010**, *206*, 528–539. [CrossRef]
11. Pattipati, K.R.; Alexandrid, M.G. Application of heuristic search and information theory to sequential fault diagnosis. *IEEE Trans. Syst. Man Cybern.* **1990**, *20*, 872–887. [CrossRef]
12. Xu, S.; Bi, W.; Zhang, A.; Mao, Z. Optimization of flight test tasks allocation and sequencing using genetic algorithm. *Appl. Soft Comput.* **2022**, *115*, 108241. [CrossRef]
13. Sun, L.; Zhang, X.; Qian, Y.; Xu, J.; Zhang, S. Feature selection using neighborhood entropy-based uncertainty measures for gene expression data classification. *Inf. Sci.* **2019**, *502*, 18–41. [CrossRef]
14. Zhang, S.; Song, L.; Zhang, W.; Hu, Z.; Yang, Y. Optimal sequential diagnostic strategy generation considering test placement cost for multi-mode systems. *Sensors* **2015**, *15*, 25592–25606. [CrossRef] [PubMed]
15. Yang, C.; Liu, Z.; Cong, H. Fault diagnosis of analog filter circuit based on genetic algorithm. *IEEE Access* **2019**, *7*, 54969–54980. [CrossRef]
16. Fang, T.U.; Pattipati, K.R. Rollout strategies for sequential fault diagnosis. *IEEE Trans. Syst. Man Cybern.* **2003**, *33*, 86–99. [CrossRef]

17. Kundakcioly, O.E.; Unluyurt, T. Bottom-up construction of minimum cost AND/OR trees for sequential fault diagnosis. *IEEE Trans. Syst. Man Cybern.* **2007**, *37*, 621–629. [CrossRef]
18. Roy, S.; Rashid, A.U.; Abbasi, A.; Murphree, R.C.; Hossain, M.M.; Faruque, A.; Metreveli, A.; Zetterling, C.-M.; Fraley, J.; Sparkman, B.; et al. Silicon carbide bipolar analog circuits for extreme temperature signal conditioning. *IEEE Trans. Electron. Dev.* **2019**, *66*, 3764–3770. [CrossRef]
19. Yao, F.; Ma, J.; Tang, S.H. IGBT module bonding demage mechanism, evolution law and condition monitoring. *Chin. J. Sci. Instrum.* **2019**, *40*, 88–99.
20. Shi, Y.; Li, Q.; Meng, X.; Zhang, T.; Shi, J. On time-series InSAR by SA-SVR algorithm: Prediction and analysis of mining subsidence. *J. Sens.* **2020**, *2020*, 8860225. [CrossRef]
21. Liang, Y.; Yang, S.; Wen, X.; Yin, H.; Huang, L. Research on defect quantification technology in pulsed eddy current non-destructive testing. *Chin. J. Sci. Instrum.* **2018**, *39*, 70–78.
22. Samie, M.; Perinpanayagam, S.; Alghassi, A.; Motlagh, A.M.; Kapetanios, E. Developing prognostic models using duality principles for DC-DC converters. *IEEE Trans. Power Electron.* **2015**, *30*, 2872–2884. [CrossRef]
23. Seixas, A.; Cesar, R.; Flesch, C.A. Data-driven soft sensor for the estimation of sound power levels of refrigeration compressors through vibration measurements. *IEEE Trans. Ind. Electron.* **2020**, *67*, 7065–7120.
24. Senguta, E.; Jain, N.; Garg, D.; Choudhury, T. A review of payment card fraud detection methods using artificial intelligence. In Proceedings of the International Conference on Computational Techniques, Electronics and Mechanical Systems (CTEMS), Belagavi, India, 21–23 December 2018; pp. 494–499.
25. Ampatzidis, Y.; Partel, V.; Meyering, B.; Alberecht, U. Citrus rootstock evaluation utilizing UAV-based remote sensing and artificial intelligence. *Comput. Electron. Agric.* **2019**, *164*, 104900. [CrossRef]
26. Yue, D.; Han, Q. Guest editorial special issue on new trends in energy internet: Artificial intelligence-based control, network security and management. *IEEE Trans. Syst. Man Cybern. Syst.* **2019**, *49*, 1551–1553. [CrossRef]
27. Gupta, P.; Batra, S.S. Sparse short-term time series forecasting models via minimum model complexity. *Neurocomputing* **2017**, *243*, 1–11. [CrossRef]
28. Jia, L.; Tao, R.; Wang, Y.; Wada, K. Forward prediction solution for adaptive noisy FIR filtering. *Sci. China Inf. Sci.* **2001**, *52*, 10071014. [CrossRef]
29. Zhang, J.S.; Xiao, X.C. A reduced parameter second-order volterra filter with application to nonlinear adaptive prediction of chaotic time series. *Acta Phys. Sin.* **2001**, *50*, 1248–1254. [CrossRef]
30. Liu, C.; Dong, J. Simultaneous fault detection and containment control design for multi-agent systems with multi-leaders. *J. Frankl. Inst.* **2020**, *357*, 9063–9082. [CrossRef]
31. Yin, L.; He, Y.; Dong, X.; Lu, Z. Muti-step prediction of volterra neural network for traffic flow based on chaos algorithm. In Proceedings of the 3rd International Conference on Information Computing and Applications, Chengde, China, 14–16 September 2012; pp. 232–241.
32. Ge, Z. Mixture Bayesian regularization of PCR model and soft-sensing application. *IEEE Trans. Ind. Electron.* **2015**, *62*, 4336–4343. [CrossRef]
33. Geng, H.; Liang, Y.; Liu, Y.; Alsaadi, F.E. Bias estimation for asynchronous multi-rate multi-sensor fusion with unknown inputs. *Inf. Fusion* **2018**, *39*, 15–139. [CrossRef]
34. Hong, W.-C. Chaotic particle swarm optimization algorithm in a support vector regression electric load forecasting model. *Energ. Convers. Manag.* **2009**, *50*, 105–117. [CrossRef]
35. Liang, Z.; Zhang, L. Intuitionistic fuzzy twin support vector machines with the insensitive pinball loss. *Appl. Soft Comput.* **2022**, *15*, 108231. [CrossRef]
36. Cai, H.S.; Feng, J.S.; Yang, Q.B.; Li, W.Z.; Li, X. A virtual metrology method with prediction uncertainty based on Gaussian process for chemical mechanical planarization. *Comput. Ind.* **2020**, *119*, 103228. [CrossRef]
37. Singh, J.; Darpe, A.K.; Singh, S.P. Bearing remaining useful life estimation using an adaptive data-driven model based on health state change point identification and K-means clusterin. *Meas. Sci. Technol.* **2020**, *31*, 085601. [CrossRef]
38. Deng, Y.F.; Du, S.C.; Jai, S.Y.; Zhao, C.; Xie, Z.Y. Prognostic study of ball screws by ensemble data-driven particle filter. *J. Manuf. Syst.* **2020**, *56*, 359–372. [CrossRef]
39. Huang, Y.-W.; Lai, D.-H. Hidden node optimization for extreme learning machine. *AASRI Procedia* **2012**, *3*, 375–380. [CrossRef]
40. Catelani, M.; Fort, A. Soft sensor detection and isolation in analog circuits: Some results and a comparison between a fuzzy approach and radial basis function networks. *IEEE Trans. Instrum. Meas.* **2002**, *51*, 196–202. [CrossRef]

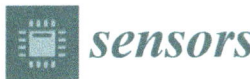

Article

Development of an Adaptive Computer-Aided Soft Sensor Diagnosis System for Assessment of Executive Functions

Katalin Mohai [1], Csilla Kálózi-Szabó [1], Zoltán Jakab [1], Szilárd Dávid Fecht [2], Márk Domonkos [2] and János Botzheim [2,*]

[1] Bárczi Gusztáv Faculty of Special Needs Education, Institute for the Psychology of Special Needs, Eötvös Loránd University, Ecseri út 3, 1097 Budapest, Hungary

[2] Department of Artificial Intelligence, Faculty of Informatics, Eötvös Loránd University, Pázmány P. Sétány 1/A, 1117 Budapest, Hungary

* Correspondence: botzheim@inf.elte.hu

Abstract: The main objective of the present study is to highlight the role of technological (soft sensor) methodologies in the assessment of the neurocognitive dysfunctions specific to neurodevelopmental disorders (for example, autism spectrum disorder (ASD), attention deficit hyperactivity disorder (ADHD), and specific learning disorder). In many cases neurocognitive dysfunctions can be detected in neurodevelopmental disorders, some of them having a well-defined syndrome-specific clinical pattern. A number of evidence-based neuropsychological batteries are available for identifying these domain-specific functions. Atypical patterns of cognitive functions such as executive functions are present in almost all developmental disorders. In this paper, we present a novel adaptation of the Tower of London Test, a widely used neuropsychological test for assessing executive functions (in particular planning and problem-solving). Our version, the Tower of London Adaptive Test, is based on computer adaptive test theory (CAT). Adaptive testing using novel algorithms and parameterized task banks allows the immediate evaluation of the participant's response which in turn determines the next task's difficulty level. In this manner, the subsequent item is adjusted to the participant's estimated capability. The adaptive procedure enhances the original test's diagnostic power and sensitivity. By measuring the targeted cognitive capacity and its limitations more precisely, it leads to more accurate diagnoses. In some developmental disorders (e.g., ADHD, ASD) it could be very useful in improving the diagnosis, planning the right interventions, and choosing the most suitable assistive digital technological service.

Keywords: computerized adaptive testing (CAT); soft-sensor based diagnosis; executive functions; neurodevelopmental disorders

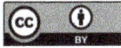

1. Introduction

Technological development from the second half of the 20th century on has contributed to the development of the sciences of the mind in at least two ways. First, the advent of computers gave rise to a theoretical breakthrough in understanding cognition as fundamentally information processing. This insight was reinforced, from the very beginning (e.g., [1,2]) by various approaches to computational modeling of cognitive functions. Second, a great number of tools and applications such as brain imaging, data processing, and other computerized and soft-sensor-based forms of data collection came in to support empirical studies and hypothesis testing. One part of this development was that of cognitive neuropsychology, which has, among other things, led to a deeper understanding of neurodevelopmental disorders [3,4]. The rapid progression of infocommunication technology has contributed to the process of fine-tuning psychometric tools based on neuropsychology [5,6]. At present, traditional paper-and-pencil tests are giving way to their computerized counterparts in neuropsychological practice, just like they do in many other areas.

Paper-and-pencil tests are the name given to the various measurement procedures developed to assess psychological functioning, despite the fact that only some of the tests currently in use require the use of paper and pencil. The paper-and-pencil tests are designed to explore objective performances and usually have a fixed formed, linear arrangement, i.e., each assessment follows the same strict procedure ([7]).

2. Classical or Technology-Based Testing

Technology-based assessment (TBA) can involve the use of any information and communication technology (ICT) device, such as a laptop or desktop computer, smartphone, tablet, and various applications running on these devices. Thus technology-based testing includes computer-based assessment as well as e-testing (for review see [8]). TBA simplifies the test assessment and administration and results in more valid and reliable measurement data. It is also more time- and cost-efficient, provides immediate assessment and feedback, eliminates data loss, and allows the development of interactive exercises, multimedia elements, and simulations [7,9,10].

The computer implementation of paper-and-pencil tests can take place at several levels, exploiting different potentials. On the one hand, existing paper-and-pencil tests can be converted into digital form without virtually any change [11]. Using the technology of soft sensors at this level offers a number of benefits, such as immediate scoring and feedback, and even higher motivational power. On the other hand, traditional tests can also be implemented in such a way that meanwhile the assessment tool is extended (e.g., by including multimedia tools, by collecting additional information such as reaction time, eye movement tracking, etc.), which allows the simultaneous handling of stimuli of multiple modalities from both the input and the output side. Thirdly, a well-developed task bank can be created, which can be the basis for automatic item generation. This creates an opportunity to give participants different tasks of the same difficulty. In assessing individual variations in cognitive and emotional development, a much more specific and fine-tuned diagnosis can be made at this level [6,12]. At the highest level, a so-called adaptive testing procedure can be implemented by introducing novel test algorithms using fully parameterized task banks. This allows the creation of tasks that match the participants' abilities so that they receive tasks with the greatest diagnostic power in their case. All of this would be unachievable in linear paper-and-pencil testing. So adaptive testing exceeds the functionality of the original test and significantly increases the diagnostic sensitivity of a given test [10,13–16]. For example, dimensions of cognitive capacity and their limits can be measured more accurately, allowing more sensitive testing procedures to be developed. This may help to clarify the diagnosis of certain disorders (e.g., Parkinson's disease or developmental disorders such as ADHD or dyslexia) [5,17–19]. This last level is known in the literature as computerized adaptive testing (CAT), and it has the greatest potential [14,20,21]. In our interpretation, CAT and computer-based testing (CBT) are not two dichotomous measurement systems, but there are different levels of CBT. In our opinion, CAT is the highest form of CBT with the most potential and diagnostic power. The essence of CAT is to create an individualized test situation. The software immediately evaluates the person's answer, which determines the difficulty of the next task, and the participant is given items from the task bank that match their estimated ability level. To achieve this, two key components are needed: (1) a precisely calibrated item bank, and (2) a suitable algorithm that can estimate the participant's ability level during testing. For the first, that is, calibrating item difficulty, we used item response theory (IRT). For the second component we constructed an algorithm to choose the subsequent item based on the participant's performance on earlier items (see below for details) [13,22,23]. In addition to its many advantages, CAT has some disadvantages as well. It can aggravate unequal opportunities, as the lack of experience and the unfamiliarity with technology can have a negative impact on results. Using technology-based assessment care must be taken to avoid the disadvantage of certain groups. At the same time, it is worth considering whether the lack of experience can be eliminated by the widespread use of technology [9].

Another disadvantage is the high start-up costs. Developing a calibrated task bank of hundreds of items is time-consuming and costly [24]. In the long run, however, the benefits listed above will offset the significant initial resource inputs, so that significant savings can be made later.

Technology-based testing also raises a number of psychometric questions: although technology-based procedures are more and more widespread, before they replace traditional paper-and-pencil tests, it is necessary to examine whether the two different methods measure the same construct in psychological terms, i.e., whether they produce equivalent results to traditional tests. Therefore, similar results are expected for paper-and-pencil and technology-based tests, unbiased by any medium effect. (The type of the test used in the study—paper-pencil vs. technology-based procedure—should not result in significant variance.) However, this also raises the question of whether it is necessary for the results to be equivalent at all. Future research and impact studies will provide the answers to these questions [8,11].

3. Technology and Neurodevelopmental Disorders

Using tests for assessing the characteristics of atypical development is common practice in almost all developed (OECD) countries, but the purpose and method of assessment and the range of people assessed varies considerably [25,26]. There is a general trend for digital test developments to appear primarily in the assessment of a wider student population for screening and measuring more generalized knowledge (e.g., classroom participant tests, knowledge level, and academic performance). In the case of children and learners with special educational needs, digital test development efforts tend to focus on specific, more delimited functional areas (e.g., attentional and executive skills). Technology-based measurement and assessment offer a number of opportunities for the identification of developmental disorders. The technology enables the specialist—educator, teacher, psychologist, doctor—to make a more efficient (e.g., less time-consuming, more valid, more reliable) diagnostic decision, to determine whether a particular disorder can be diagnosed in a certain participant, and makes it possible to assess personality, reveal knowledge or ability profile. For the person concerned, the indirect benefit is that the diagnosis is made more quickly, the results of the diagnosis or assessment are more precise and reliable, so the person can have the most suitable support and education adjusted to his/her personal and ability profile [27].

Overall, the countless possibilities of the digital interface (tablet, smartphone, laptop, etc.) enable an optimal, cost-effective, and more precise investigation of atypical patterns in the cognitive architecture [6]. It is also important to stress that digital assessment of atypical development takes into account well-known standards regarding service and development [26,28]. One of these standards is not to develop separate assessment tools for the typical and for the atypical development, but to create "design for all", so the main universal concept is to ensure equal access and use [29,30], which of course includes needs-based design.

4. The assessment of Executive Functions (EF) in Neuropsychology

In many cases, neurocognitive dysfunctions can be detected in neurodevelopmental disorders (ASD, ADHD, specific learning disorder), some of them having well-defined syndrome-specific clinical pattern [31,32]. Many evidence-based neuropsychological batteries are available for identifying these domain-specific functions. Some of these atypical cognitive functions, although in different patterns, are present in all developmental disorders, such as the executive functions [33–35]. Executive functioning is an umbrella term for the general component of all complex cognitive processes that play a key role in solving novel, difficult and goal-oriented tasks, and in flexibly adapting to environmental changes [36,37]. In fact, the function of executive processes is the differential coordination of mental functioning, the coordination of psychological processes along the lines of perception, emotion, cognition, and execution [37]. It can be defined as a set of capabilities that allows you to represent distant goals, develop plans for achieving the goals, organize and control the cognitive and psychological functioning and behavior, monitor the environment, and, if it is necessary, do flexible modification on the developed plans [38]. This ensures the regulation of behavior, including self-regulation [39] and, as the authors of [38] point out, this is what distinguishes humans from the instinctive and reflexive responses of animals. Although there is no consensus on the precise definition of executive functions, most authors state the multidimensional nature of EF, differed by the number of components, processes, and complexity. Among the components of executive function can be mentioned the inhibitory control or response inhibition, working memory, updating, and shifting [40,41].

5. Goal of the Present Study

The aim of this paper is to present CAT-based procedures of a well-known and widely used neuropsychological test assessing executive functions as a soft sensor.

Although most neuropsychological tests of executive functions are already computer based, our search did not reveal any studies presenting CAT-based versions of these tools. To understand why, we need to know that the development of psychometric tests used in the assessment of neurodevelopmental disorders is based mostly on classical test theory. Classical test theory (CTT) focuses on total test score; it characterizes item difficulty as the relative frequency of examinees who answer an item correctly and derives item discriminability from item-total correlations. Item response theory, on the other hand, focuses on individual items characterizing item difficulty and examinee ability on the same scale whose units are logits (log odds of the probability of correct response). An important advantage of IRT over CTT is that the former assures that the joint difficulty–ability scale is at interval level [13].

In general, most neuropsychological tests are based on classical test theory. At the same time, the development of item banks at considerable financial cost seems unnecessary, as the main function of the tests is to help the diagnosis and differential diagnosis, which can be achieved best by increasing the sensitivity of the items rather than by creating a large item bank.

Based on adaptive test theory, we developed the Tower of London Adaptive Test and the Corsi Adaptive Test, measuring different aspects of executive functions, the former is used for assessing planning and problem-solving ability, while the latter is used for assessing visual working memory. In this paper, we present the Tower of London Adaptive Test (ToLA). Our aim was to assess the level of ability as sensitively as possible and do so in a relatively short time. This helps us, for example, eliminate the effect of attention disorder (i.e., by abolishing the need to maintain attention for an extended time) from planning and strategy-making ability, thereby enabling a more accurate differential diagnosis. In order to achieve this, the focus was not only on creating an item bank but on the analysis of the characteristics (e.g., solution time, number of steps required to solve a given item) of initially well-thought-out items and the use of these results.

In addition to the above-mentioned benefits, the synergy of this kind of adaptive solution with the soft sensor system also has a higher added value, hence a very precise measurement is enabled this way in terms of the interactions which is often time and effort-demanding from the specialist's side during or after the tests. Additionally, the evaluation phase is made less burdensome for the specialist by only presenting the (often calculated) measures necessary during a diagnosis. In this respect, this study has a significant added value and innovative power in the assessment of neurodevelopmental disorders with soft sensors.

6. Administering the Tower of London Adaptive Test
6.1. Background

The Tower tasks constitute a widely used method for examining planning and strategic thinking as subcomponents of executive functions. Based on the earlier Hanoi Tower task, the London Tower task was developed by [42], for studying the planning processes of patients with frontal lesions. Attaining the goal state using the smallest number of moves often involves a bypass strategy whereby initially the distance from the goal state needs to increase in order for the key moves to become feasible (according to some metrics at least, e.g., how many of the discs are currently located in the stack where they should be in the end state).

In the Tower of Hanoi task, discs of different sizes piled up on a peg from largest at the bottom to smallest on top have to be transferred to one of two similar pegs in such a way that only one disc is moved at a time, and bigger discs must never be placed on smaller ones. The minimum number of moves needed is $2^n - 1$ for n discs in the initial pile.

In the Tower of London task, there are four discs that are the same size but all are differently colored; they are located in stacks of different heights—typically one stack can hold three discs, whereas two others can hold two discs each. The discs are arranged in a starting configuration, and the required goal configuration is also shown; the task is to reproduce the goal configuration from the starting one while never placing more discs in a stack than what it can hold.

The development of the tests in their current form was preceded by a pilot study; the results of which can be found in [43].

The current study is based on the results of an earlier pilot study. In 2015 we had an opportunity to develop computer-based tests for education centers involved in special-needs diagnoses. Since up to that point digital testing had not been applied in Hungary in any systematic way, in developing tests and their framework we had to build on the limited available means at the time. (The pilot study was supported by EU funds, in particular the Social Renewal Operation Programme—project number TÁMOP-3.4.2.B-12-2012-0001.) In this pilot project, we developed reading and language tests along with a few digitalized procedures to measure neurocognitive functions. The software was developed for touch screen tablets and optimized for the Windows 8.1 operation system. The tests were validated on a large sample of atypically developing children in 2014–2015 (please see the Results for detail). The American Psychological Association's (APA) ethical standards were followed to conduct this study. Written informed consent was obtained from the parents of all participating children. The participants were informed about their anonymity protection as well as about the possibility to withdraw from the study at any point during the process. Every participant was given a code for research purposes. The most important result of this pilot study was a clinical trial, and the development of corresponding test norms (see [43] and Appendix of [43]). Within a few years, however, the instruments and operation system for which these tests were developed became outdated, therefore their regular use grew more and more difficult, even though the need for their application persisted. In the present study, we substantially reworked our earlier computerized tests of executive functions including the Tower of London (TOL) Test. This new version has not been subjected to clinical trial yet, however, here we offer a reanalysis of the TOL data collected by the first version and published earlier. Our purpose in the present study is to create a web-based soft sensor for multiple users which suits the needs of both the users and clinical experts and can be developed further whenever the need arises.

6.2. The Framework

As a first step toward transforming classical neuropsychological tests into an adaptive form, we developed a framework that can be applied to several instruments. The framework comprises three major phases. The first is Familiarization, which allows the participant to become familiar with the interface and understand the task, followed by the Assessment level, which aims to assess the capabilities of the participant and is the starting point for the Testing level. Finally, during the Testing phase, the computer generates tasks of different difficulty levels based on the score obtained at the Assessment level (this is the adaptive feature of our algorithm). An overview of the described system can be seen in Figure 1.

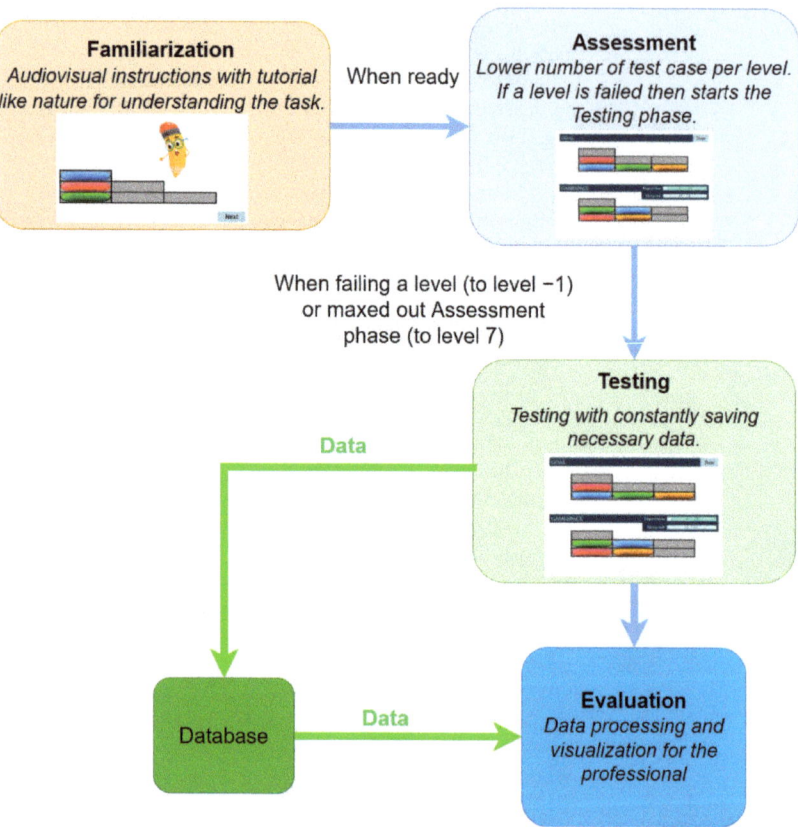

Figure 1. Overview of the system with the three phases described.

This framework provides an opportunity for the participants to familiarize themselves with the test situation before the actual testing, and to train themselves in the way of responding. All of these stages are supported by multimedia elements (including sound files and animation). In the so-called verification phase belonging to the Familiarization phase, the participant receives corrective feedback on the solution of the task, while the examiners can verify the correct understanding of the task. The standardized structure of the test helps the participant in adapting to the tasks. The evaluation is also automated; the different test parameters and scores are displayed in an output file.

6.3. Software

The developed software application was optimized for web-based usage for Chromium-based browsers. This ensures great flexibility and the test is not restricted to running on personal computers, it also has the ability to be used with smartphones or tablets, merely an internet connection and a browser are needed.

During the development, an important factor was that the system needs to be designed for usage by professionals as they can properly interpret the test results. Therefore, a Laravel 8 framework-based portal was created around the test that handles the access to the test and its results. When choosing the framework of the portal, it was considered that it should be a stable technology that is widely used this way during further development it is not tied to a specific developer in the future, and due to its widespread use, fewer bugs or vulnerabilities can be expected.

Registered professionals can enroll participants for testing. Participants must be of sufficient age to be allowed by the framework to complete the test. The data of the professionals and the participants can both be modified anytime. The participants are in 1-N relation to the tests that can be completed. The usage of this relation was necessary in order to enable the tracking of the participant's development. Sensitive data are stored through a cryptographic hash function, which prevents them from being extracted from the database in an event of unauthorized access.

The test itself is a JavaScript-based game with a logger of events. Its framework is based on Phaser 3, which greatly facilitates easy implementation. The essentially open source HTML5 framework, as a built-in functionality, handles various web browsers, while providing sufficient flexibility and not limiting the development. In Phaser, the test's levels of difficulty are built upon so-called "Scenes" in Phaser. These scenes are accessed by the test via the system's automation according to the predefined conditions (i.e., whether the participant gave a good or bad answer). At the end of a test, the data is sent to the server at the touch of a specific button by the specialist.

According to the current implementation, the test consists of the following three phases as mentioned in Section 6.2:

- During the Familiarization phase, an animated tutorial is performed, which is designed to get high attention from the participants' age group (see Figure 2). At the end of the Familiarization, there are two test cases with feedback. There is no measurement during the Familiarization phase test cases.
- The Assessment phase has a maximum of four test cases. The four assessment phase tests have different levels of difficulty. Here the predefined stopping condition is a bad answer, the assessment phase ends and the Testing phase begins.
- Finally, according to the participant's results, the Testing phase is started at a level defined by the results from the Assessment phase. The number of all test cases is 10×3, there are 3 test cases per level.

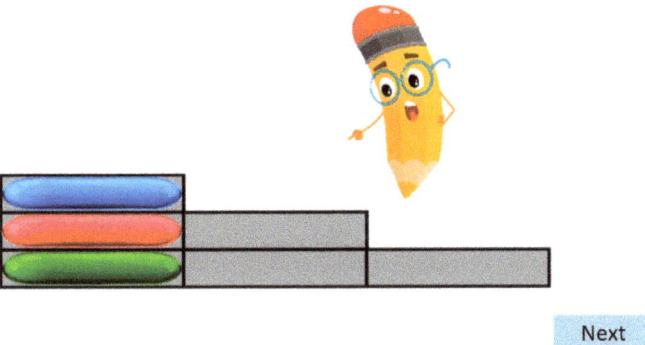

Figure 2. Tutorial with animation during the Familiarization phase.

During the game, it is considered a wrong solution if the participant does not reach the specified layout or the allowed time expires or the participant runs out of the allowed number of moves. In this case, the program sets an error flag but lets the participant keep on working, does not advance the tests, and does not indicate the failure despite that the test's answer is already recorded as an incorrect one.

If the participant has solved all the assessment tests then he/she starts the Testing phase from level 7. Otherwise, he/she has to start the level prior to the unsolved level. There must be at least two correctly completed test cases from the three for the participant to pass a level.

Only discs under the inscription "GameSpace" and discs on the top of the stack can be moved. They are moved by dragging them and dropping them to the desired place. The game saves the number of the given level and the flags of the errors. From the start of the test case, all the events are logged in milliseconds (i.e., when a disc is grabbed or is dropped, and when the participant pressed the "Done" button). The program then determines, based on the disc coordinates, whether the layout of the discs is the same as the target layout. The system checks whether there were any error flags. After the evaluation, the system chooses the new level of difficulty according to the algorithm and the participant automatically enters the next test case or the testing is stopped.

The saved data is stored on a server categorized by participant ID. By clicking on the participant's data sheet, the system returns the results of the completed tests ordered by date and in tabular form. In this case, it is checked whether the requester has the right to access the given data or not: so the participant belongs to the given user, otherwise, the request is refused and data is not sent from the server to the client.

6.4. Test Administration

The development of the Tower of London Adaptive Test required the determination of difficulty levels, the assignment of the optimal duration, and the number of steps required to solve the problems, as well as the development of the algorithm. Difficulty levels were determined by the number of steps needed to solve certain tasks. For selecting the most appropriate items for each difficulty level we used computer simulation. Based on simulation it became clear that upwards of the eight-step task, the three-disc space is no longer sufficient. Therefore, from level 1 onwards, we introduced not only the three-disc but also the four-disc task, so that children could get familiarized with both arrangements (see Figure 3).

During the task, the participant had to arrange the discs according to the configuration shown on the top of the screen. Only one disc was allowed to be moved at a time, and the number of discs piled up in a stack could not exceed stack height (see Figure 3). There were ten difficulty levels in total (corresponding to the number of moves necessary to reach the goal configuration) with three different tasks at each level. If the participant successfully solved two out of the three tasks, he/she passed the level and proceeded to the next difficulty level. If the level was not passed, a task from a lower difficulty level followed. Figure 4 summarizes the adaptive testing algorithm that was used for data collection in our earlier study [43].

The duration and number of steps for solving a given problem were limited, and both of them could be monitored on the screen. The test was interrupted if two consecutive levels were not passed.

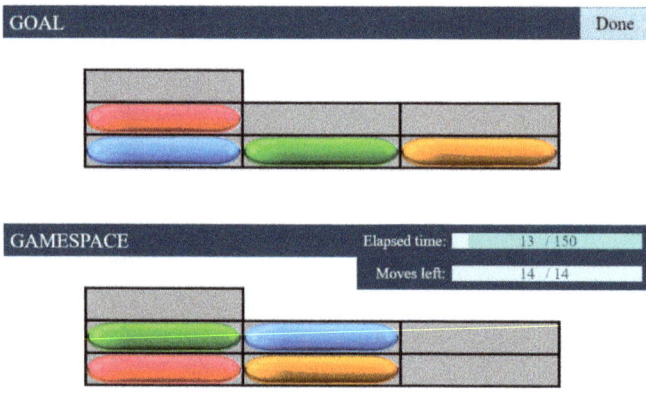

Figure 3. Screenshot of the gamespace during the Tower of London Test.

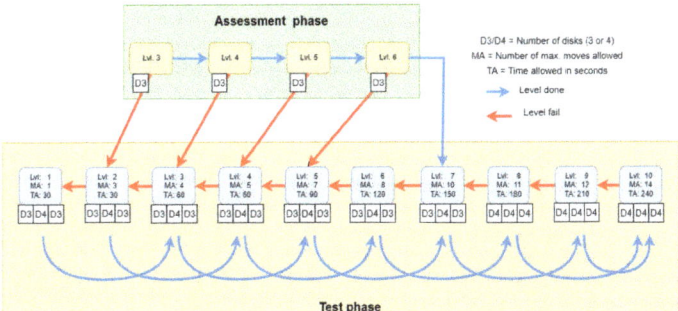

Figure 4. The algorithm of Tower of London Adaptive Test. Blue arrows represent the step if a test level is done, and red arrows the failing of a test. D3 and D4 represent the number of discs in the test case (three discs and four discs respectively). MA denotes the allowed maximum moves, and TA stands for the allowed maximum time.

However, in the original study, we set high limits for both time and number of steps. In particular, at each difficulty level the number of allowed moves was twice that of minimally necessary moves (e.g., 20 for problems that can be solved in ten moves). Evaluating the collected data using these high limits resulted in a ceiling effect (that is, high success probabilities for even the most difficult items). Therefore, in the current reanalysis we set lower maxima on the moves allowed, at each difficulty level. That is, some responses that were eventually successful, but used many more moves than necessary were now not accepted as correct. Put another way, if the required strategic planning was diluted by too much trial and error on the part of the participant, we did not score the performance. Figure 4 shows the new parameter values (see the upper values in the small red rectangles attached to ovals representing difficulty levels).

6.5. Analysis and Results

As mentioned above, the development of our present test was preceded by a pilot study [43]. In this study, the data were collected by our adaptive algorithm, and the results were analyzed by classical test theory. In what follows we reassess these data, and analyze them using item response theory.

The original sample consisted of 302 children of whom 214 were typically developing, and 84 had a learning disorder (dyslexia and/or attention deficit). All children were native Hungarians from different settlement types in Hungary. Although the sample was not representative (i.e., not compiled with the assistance of the Central Statistical Office), care was taken for the sample to approximate the characteristics of the population of same-aged children in Hungary, as well as possible. Type of residence, parents' level of education, and gender ratios were taken into account to this end. The mean age was 9.1 years (sd: 1.0 yr); the youngest participant was 7 years old, whereas the oldest one was 12 years. There were 102 second graders, 91 third graders, and 105 fourth graders in the sample; two participants were in grade 5, and two were in grade 6. Exclusion criteria for the neurotypical sample were premature birth; sensory impairment; any extant neurological syndrome (e.g., epilepsy); taking any medicine affecting the nervous system; non-promotion (repeating a school year); diagnosed need for special education (dyslexia, dyscalculia, ADHD, intellectual disability). Inclusion criteria for the clinical sample were a diagnosed disorder of reading, writing/orthography, or arithmetic ability; a diagnosis of ADHD; taking corresponding medications was not a reason for exclusion. Diagnosis took place according to the Hungarian psychological and special education protocol: assessment was conducted in psychodiagnostic centers based on teamwork.

Data used in this study was collected from 214 typically developing children (age range: from 7.08 years to 11.92 years; mean: 9.00 years, sd: 1 year; 99 females, 115 males).

Each participant completed an adaptive testing procedure involving 30 TOL problems as items. The items were divided into ten broader levels of difficulty according to the minimal number of moves necessary to reach the solution (1 to 10; three items at each level). The probability of a correct response was readjusted by lowering limits on the maximum number of moves at each level; the new limits are summarized in Table 1.

Table 1. Difficulty adjustment by setting maxima on the number of moves allowed in the Tower of London Test. Exceeding the number of allowed moves for an item resulted in a score of 0 for that item regardless of whether the participant eventually reached the required configuration or not. As a result of this adjustment, the probability of correct response to the easiest item was 0.991, whereas that to the most difficult one was 0.271.

Level (number of minimally necessary moves)	1	2	3	4	5	6	7	8	9	10
Moves allowed	1	3	4	5	7	8	10	11	12	14

Theoretically, there is no guarantee that two problems with the same number of minimally necessary moves are equally difficult from a psychological point of view. Therefore there is no reason to expect batches of three items to have identical (or nearly identical) difficulty indices (theta values in item response theory used below), and for this reason, initially, each item was entered in the analysis. However, five of the items were so easy as to produce extreme, and in one case, obviously incorrect difficulty estimates. (The item with a grossly incorrect theta estimate was one with 100% correct responses. This item was subsequently omitted from the analysis along with four others which resulted in 212 or 213 correct responses out of 214).

Note also that the guessing parameter can be reasonably ignored in our case as there is a vanishingly small chance for a participant to come up with the correct solution to a TOL problem by randomly moving discs. (In fact, for the simplest problems that require only one move, the probability of a random correct response may be up to 1/3, but as the number of necessary moves increases, the probability of correct guessing rapidly falls off. Thus there is no stable level for the probability of correct guessing. Moreover, due to the adaptive procedure used, most correct responses to the simplest problems were granted to participants without actually administering the items to them, so correct guessing did not seem to have played an important role in these cases. In further studies, however, an option is to omit extremely simple problems altogether from the analysis.) Therefore a 2PL, dichotomous items model was suitable for our purposes. We used the Latent Trait Models (ltm) package in R to conduct the analysis [23,44]. (Latent trait models assume that all test items measure the same underlying ability relying on largely the same mental processes. Given that the TOL test comprises tasks of one type, this assumption is reasonable in the present case. Each such model uses at least one parameter, namely item difficulty, which is calculated from the probability of correct response for an item using the sigmoid—or logistic—function. 1PL—that is, one-parameter logistic—models are built on the difficulty parameter alone, 2PL models introduce, in addition, an item discriminability parameter, whereas 3PL models include a third parameter which is the probability of correct guessing [45]). Table 2 shows the model summary.

Table 2. Summary of the 2PL model parameters.

	Difficulty			Discrimination		
	Value	std.err	z.vals	Value	std.err	z.vals
Item_1_2	−4.8904	1.9344	−2.5281	0.9907	0.4987	1.9866
Item_3_1	−4.9173	2.006	−2.4513	1.1036	0.6024	1.8318
Item_3_2	−4.3959	1.4469	−3.0382	1.0487	0.4528	2.316
Item_3_3	−2.957	0.8585	−3.4443	0.6356	0.1981	3.2088
Item_4_1	−2.5104	0.5025	−4.9956	1.0311	0.2511	4.1064
Item_4_2	−2.0959	0.3384	−6.1936	1.3667	0.294	4.649
Item_4_3	−2.1625	0.3542	−6.1046	1.3482	0.2946	4.5768
Item_5_1	−1.4868	0.2948	−5.0429	1.0414	0.2134	4.8809
Item_5_2	−1.1268	0.347	−3.2473	0.6743	0.1731	3.8946
Item_5_3	−0.7598	0.2605	−2.9172	0.7722	0.1812	4.2625
Item_6_1	−0.6452	0.1684	−3.8325	1.3412	0.2423	5.5359
Item_6_2	−0.8772	0.1888	−4.6455	1.3214	0.2396	5.5148
Item_6_3	−0.504	0.1139	−4.4251	2.7899	0.491	5.6826
Item_7_1	0.1914	0.2075	0.9228	0.7322	1855	3.9468
Item_7_2	−0.7521	0.1988	−3.7842	1.0973	0.2121	5.1743
Item_7_3	−0.1788	0.1442	−1.2404	1.2702	0.237	5.3586
Item_8_1	0.2875	0.126	2.2826	1.4433	0.2802	5.1509
Item_8_2	0.2639	0.0895	2.9476	2.9337	0.5436	5.397
Item_8_3	0.1208	0.0788	1.5325	5.3265	1.434	3.7145
Item_9_1	0.5437	0.1192	4.5604	1.7809	0.3563	4.9981
Item_9_2	0.9257	0.1589	5.824	1.7362	0.3887	4.4662
Item_9_3	0.7767	0.1279	6.0739	1.9745	0.4043	4.8842
Item_10_1	0.7677	0.1262	6.0855	1.9243	0.397	4.8475
Item_10_2	0.6361	0.0872	7.2932	3.4896	0.8635	4.0411
Item_10_3	0.8017	0.12	6.6781	2.1448	0.4535	4.7295

Item difficulty ranges from −4.89 (Item_1_2) to 0.8017 (Item_10_3), which is not symmetrical around 0, therefore further, more difficult items should be introduced later. Item discrimination is generally good, as 21 out of 25 items have discrimination parameters above or very close to 1; four items are at the margin of acceptability (Item_3_3; Item_5_2; Item_5_3; Item_7_1), and none are very poor. Figure 5 shows the test information function which again indicates that the introduction of further, more difficult items are needed—as the curve is asymmetrical; the present set of items gives us somewhat less information about participants with high ability, although it is good in the range from moderately low through average to moderately high range.

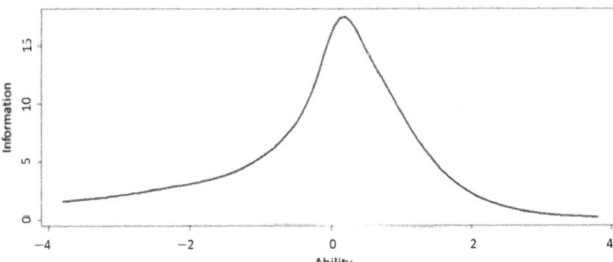

Figure 5. Test information function for the 25 Tower of London items.

Item fit is also acceptable; 9 out of 25 items had significant Chi-square values (Table 3).

Table 3. Item fit for the 25 Tower of London tasks. Significant *p*-values are marked with bold.

	χ^2	sig.
Item_1_2	8.4019	0.3952
Item_3_1	14.8232	0.0627
Item_3_2	7.9789	0.4355
Item_3_3	13.322	0.1012
Item_4_1	4.9713	0.7606
Item_4_2	3.9275	0.8636
Item_4_3	7.2758	0.5072
Item_5_1	9.1146	0.3327
Item_5_2	23.0207	**0.0033**
Item_5_3	29.703	**0.0002**
Item_6_1	18.1583	**0.0201**
Item_6_2	17.2215	**0.0279**
Item_6_3	10.4865	0.2325
Item_7_1	26.7456	**0.0008**
Item_7_2	19.8636	**0.0109**
Item_7_3	24.3304	**0.002**
Item_8_1	16.5941	**0.0346**
Item_8_2	3.5923	0.8919
Item_8_3	7.1894	0.5163
Item_9_1	9.9894	0.2658
Item_9_2	17.9461	**0.0216**
Item_9_3	8.5134	0.385
Item_10_1	11.2503	0.1879
Item_10_2	7.5525	0.4784
Item_10_3	9.3497	0.3137

Next, we compared this 2PL model with the 3PL alternative including a guessing parameter expressing the probability that a low-ability participant solves the item correctly. The highest value of the guessing parameter was 0.0024 (Item_3_2), and the lowest one was 10^{-301} (Item_10_3), that is, introducing this parameter indeed made no difference. This is also confirmed by the summary of the ANOVA comparing the two models (Table 4). In Table 4, three indicators are reported to compare the two models in terms of how well they fit to the data. Aikake's information criterion (AIC), and the Bayesian information criterion (BIC) can generally be interpreted only via using pairs of their values; of two models the one with better fit is the one with a smaller AIC or BIC. As can be seen in Table 4, the 3PL model actually exhibits a poorer fit than the 2PL one, however, the difference between them is not significant. The log-likelihood statistic is more stable in this case, corresponding to the absence of a significant difference between these two models.

Table 4. Model comparison: 2PL and 3PL.

Model	AIC	BIC	log.Lik	LRT	df	sig.
2PL	4766.76	4935.06	−2333.38			
3PL	4816.76	5069.21	−2333.38	0	25	1

Although the variability of the item discrimination values (Table 2) indicates that a one-parameter Rasch (or 1PL) model would introduce an undesirable constraint, the comparison between the Rasch model and the 2PL model was also made (Table 5). As the results show these two models do differ substantially, to the advantage of the 2PL model. AIC, BIC, and log-likelihood are all higher for the one-parameter model, indicating poorer fit, and the difference in the goodness of fit between the two models is highly significant.

Table 5. Model comparison: Rasch and 2PL.

Model	AIC	BIC	log.Lik	LRT	df	p Value
Rasch	4890.91	4975.06	−2420.46			
2PL	4766.76	4935.06	−2333.38	174.15	25	<0.001

7. Summary

Present technological development can be harnessed to assess the individual needs of children in different areas, including developmental diagnosis and support [46]. To this end, we need up-to-date instruments based on soft sensors to measure individual differences and pair them with suitable interventions when necessary. In the diagnosis of persons with disability, the involvement of technological innovations has become a subject of systematic study. Digital testing is a key component of this process whereby individualized training regimes, as well as population-level monitoring of performance, can be implemented. The soft sensor we developed serves the purpose of educational diagnosis, that is, it helps pedagogues, special education experts, psychologists, and doctors to establish faster and more efficiently whether a certain developmental status obtains for an individual being examined. As part of this, our system measures certain aspects of personality, ability profile, and knowledge. For the examined individual the benefit is that they can have a diagnosis faster, and the results are more reliable than with traditional testing procedures. As a result, the ensuing support and education will be better tailored to personal needs [27]. We need to emphasize, however, that involving technology in diagnosis, and tailoring it to special needs support is a preliminary stage to application in learning environments [6,47]. In maximizing the benefit of using technology we need also to pay attention to minimizing possible risks. Limitations—and future perspectives—of our study are the following. First, with the present version of our test software, we have not collected data yet—this is a task for a future study. Instead, we reanalyzed data collected by an earlier version of our TOL test program. Our results showed that TOL data are amenable to IRT analysis, and the results obtained are satisfactory, indeed, promising. In this respect, our expectations are fulfilled. A second limitation is that so far we have used a fixed adaptive algorithm that did not include a machine learning component. Another objective for further research is to include machine learning in our adaptive algorithm, with the aim of measuring participants' potential for relatively short-term improvement, not just performance at a given point in time. What a participant can achieve with modest support, as opposed to completely autonomously, is called the zone of proximal development [48]. Using machine learning, it becomes possible to conduct dynamic measurement which, unlike static measurement, supplies information about changes in individual learning strategies, or individual learning potential [49,50]. This information can in turn be utilized in adjusting education to individual needs. This information can be fed back into improving educational effectiveness adapted to the needs. A third limitation, or plan, is to extend our item bank, especially by constructing more difficult items (with more than 10 moves necessary to succeed) as this would tap better into the high ability range of planning and executive functions. Taking the present line of research further, we plan to conduct a systematic comparison of non-adaptive paper-and-pencil tests with their CAT versions to contribute to such benefit-and-risk analyses. We think that info-communication technology-based procedures need to be supplemented by empirical studies of application and effectiveness to become reliable and trustworthy methodologies.

Author Contributions: Conceptualization, K.M., C.K.-S. and Z.J.; data curation, Z.J.; formal analysis, Z.J.; funding acquisition, K.M.; investigation, K.M., C.K.-S., Z.J., S.D.F., M.D. and J.B.; methodology, K.M., C.K.-S. and Z.J.; project administration, K.M.; resources, K.M., C.K.-S., Z.J., S.D.F., M.D. and J.B.; software, S.D.F., M.D. and J.B.; supervision, K.M. and J.B.; validation, K.M., C.K.-S. and Z.J.; visualization, Z.J., S.D.F. and M.D.; writing—original draft, K.M., C.K.-S., Z.J., S.D.F., M.D. and J.B.; writing—review and editing, K.M. and J.B. All authors have read and agreed to the published version of the manuscript.

Funding: This research was supported by the Research Programme for Public Education Development, Hungarian Academy of Sciences, and the National Laboratory for Social Innovation.

Institutional Review Board Statement: As the present study did not involve data collection from participants, but rather, a reanalysis of data collected in an earlier, published study [43], the present study did not require ethical approval.

Informed Consent Statement: Informed consent was obtained from all subjects involved in the study.

Data Availability Statement: Enquiries concerning data generated or analyzed during this study can be directed to the corresponding author.

Conflicts of Interest: The authors declare no conflict of interest.

References

1. Ernst, G.W.; Newell, A. *GPS: A Case Study in Generality and Problem Solving*; Academic Press: New York, NY, USA, 1969.
2. Newell, A.; Simon, H.A. *Human Problem Solving*; Prentice-hall Englewood Cliffs: Hoboken, NJ, USA, 1972; Volume 104.
3. Tager-Flusberg, H. Chapter: Introduction to Research on Neurodevelopmental Disorders from a Cognitive Neuroscience Perspective. In *Neurodevelopmental Disorders*; MIT Press: Cambridge, MA, USA, 1999.
4. Denckla, M.B. Neurodevelopmental disorders from a cognitive neurosciences perspective. *Marian. Found. Paediatr. Neurol. Ser.* **2005**, *13*, 1.
5. Parsey, C.M.; Schmitter-Edgecombe, M. Applications of technology in neuropsychological assessment. *Clin. Neuropsychol.* **2013**, *27*, 1328–1361. [CrossRef] [PubMed]
6. Hakkinen, M. Assistive technologies for computer-based assessments. *R&D Connect.* **2015**, *24*, 1–9.
7. Csapó, B.; Ainley, J.; Bennett, R.E.; Latour, T.; Law, N. Technological issues for computer-based assessment. In *Assessment and Teaching of 21st Century Skills*; Springer: New York, NY, USA, 2012; pp. 143–230.
8. Alrababah, S.A.; Molnár, G. The evolution of technology-based assessment: Past, present, and future. *Int. J. Learn. Technol.* **2021**, *16*, 134–157. [CrossRef]
9. Csapó, B.; Molnár, G. Online diagnostic assessment in support of personalized teaching and learning: The eDia system. *Front. Psychol.* **2019**, *10*, 1522. [CrossRef]
10. Rezaie, M.; Golshan, M. Computer adaptive test (CAT): Advantages and limitations. *Int. J. Educ. Investig.* **2015**, *2*, 128–137.
11. Wang, T.; Kolen, M.J. Evaluating comparability in computerized adaptive testing: Issues, criteria and an example. *J. Educ. Meas.* **2001**, *38*, 19–49. [CrossRef]
12. Singleton, C. Using Computer-Based Assessment to Identify Learning Problems. In *ICT and Special Educational Needs: A Tool for Inclusion*; McGraw-Hill Education: London, UK, 2004; pp. 46–63.
13. Istiyono, E. Computer adaptive test as the appropriate model to assess physics achievement in 21st century. In Proceedings of the 1st International Conference on Innovation in Education (ICoIE 2018), Padang, Indonesia, 6–7 September 2019; pp. 304–309.
14. Sands, W.A.; Waters, B.K.; McBride, J.R. *Computerized Adaptive Testing: From Inquiry to Operation*; American Psychological Association: Washington, DC, USA, 1997.
15. Sorrel, M.A.; Barrada, J.R.; de la Torre, J.; Abad, F.J. Adapting cognitive diagnosis computerized adaptive testing item selection rules to traditional item response theory. *PLoS ONE* **2020**, *15*, e0227196. [CrossRef]
16. Khoshsima, H.; Toroujeni, S.M.H. Computer Adaptive Testing (CAT) Design; Testing Algorithm and Administration Mode Investigation. *Eur. J. Educ. Stud.* **2017**, *3*, 764–795.
17. Moore, T.M.; Calkins, M.E.; Satterthwaite, T.D.; Roalf, D.R.; Rosen, A.F.; Gur, R.C.; Gur, R.E. Development of a computerized adaptive screening tool for overall psychopathology ("p"). *J. Psychiatr. Res.* **2019**, *116*, 26–33. [CrossRef]
18. Redecker, C.; Johannessen, Ø. Changing assessment—Towards a new assessment paradigm using ICT. *Eur. J. Educ.* **2013**, *48*, 79–96. [CrossRef]
19. Singleton, C.; Thomas, K.; Horne, J. Computer-based cognitive assessment and the development of reading. *J. Res. Read.* **2000**, *23*, 158–180. [CrossRef]
20. Madsen, H.S. Chapter: Computer-Adaptive Testing of Listening and Reading Comprehension. In *Computer-Assisted Language Learning and Testing: Research Issues and Practice*; Newbury House: New York, NY, USA, 1991.
21. Weiss, D.J. Computerized adaptive testing for effective and efficient measurement in counseling and education. *Meas. Eval. Couns. Dev.* **2004**, *37*, 70–84. [CrossRef]
22. Kingsbury, G.G. Adaptive Item Calibration: A Process for Estimating Item Parameters within a Computerized Adaptive Test. In Proceedings of the 2009 GMAC Conference on Computerized Adaptive Testing, 2 June 2009. Available online: www.psych.umn.edu/psylabs/CATCentral/ (accessed on 10 July 2022).
23. Rizopoulos, D. ltm: An R package for latent variable modeling and item response analysis. *J. Stat. Softw.* **2007**, *17*, 1–25.
24. Thompson, N.A.; Weiss, D.A. A framework for the development of computerized adaptive tests. *Pract. Assess. Res. Eval.* **2011**, *16*, 1.
25. Desforges, M.; Lindsay, G. *Procedures Used to Diagnose a Disability and to Assess Special Educational Needs: An International Review*; National Council for Special Education: Trim, Ireland, 2010.

26. Phelps, R.P. Synergies for better learning: An international perspective on evaluation and assessment. *Assess. Educ. Princ. Policy Pract.* **2014**, *21*, 481–493. [CrossRef]
27. Györi, M.; Mohai, K. A diagnosztikus, támogató és edukációs technológiák pszichológiája. In *A Humán Fogyatékosságok Pszichológiája—A Gyógypedagógiai Pszichológia Alapjai*; ELTE Eötvös Kiadó: Budapest, Hungary, in press.
28. Abbott, C.; Brown, D.; Evett, L.; Standen, P.; Wright, J. *Learning Difference and Digital Technologies: A Literature Review of Research Involving Children and Young People Using Assistive Technologies 2007–2010*; King's College London: London, UK, 2011.
29. Whitney, G.; Keith, S.; Bühler, C.; Hewer, S.; Lhotska, L.; Miesenberger, K.; Sandnes, F.E.; Stephanidis, C.; Velasco, C.A. Twenty five years of training and education in ICT Design for All and Assistive Technology. *Technol. Disabil.* **2011**, *23*, 163–170. [CrossRef]
30. Williams, P.; Jamali, H.R.; Nicholas, D. Using ICT with people with special education needs: What the literature tells us. *Aslib Proc. New Inf. Perspect.* **2006**, *58*, 330–345. [CrossRef]
31. Tistarelli, N.; Fagnani, C.; Troianiello, M.; Stazi, M.A.; Adriani, W. The nature and nurture of ADHD and its comorbidities: A narrative review on twin studies. *Neurosci. Biobehav. Rev.* **2020**, *109*, 63–77. [CrossRef]
32. Morris-Rosendahl, D.J.; Crocq, M.A. Neurodevelopmental disorders—The history and future of a diagnostic concept. *Dialogues Clin. Neurosci.* **2022**, *22*. [CrossRef]
33. Zelazo, P.D. Executive function and psychopathology: A neurodevelopmental perspective. *Annu. Rev. Clin. Psychol.* **2020**, *16*, 431–454. [CrossRef] [PubMed]
34. Crisci, G.; Caviola, S.; Cardillo, R.; Mammarella, I.C. Executive functions in neurodevelopmental disorders: Comorbidity overlaps between attention deficit and hyperactivity disorder and specific learning disorders. *Front. Hum. Neurosci.* **2021**, *15*, 594234. [CrossRef]
35. Corbett, B.A.; Constantine, L.J.; Hendren, R.; Rocke, D.; Ozonoff, S. Examining executive functioning in children with autism spectrum disorder, attention deficit hyperactivity disorder and typical development. *Psychiatry Res.* **2009**, *166*, 210–222. [CrossRef]
36. Hughes, C.; Ensor, R. Does executive function matter for preschoolers' problem behaviors? *J. Abnorm. Child Psychol.* **2008**, *36*, 1–14. [CrossRef]
37. McCloskey, G.; Perkins, L.A.; Van Divner, B. *Assessment and Intervention for Executive Function Difficulties*; Routledge Taylor & Francis Group: New York, NY, USA, 2008.
38. Skoff, B. Executive functions in developmental disabilities. *Insights Learn. Disabil.* **2004**, *15*, 4–10.
39. Barkley, R. *Executive Functions: What They Are, How They Work, and Why They Evolved*; The Guilford Press: New York, NY, USA, 2012.
40. Miyake, A.; Friedman, N.P.; Emerson, M.J.; Witzki, A.H.; Howerter, A.; Wager, T.D. The unity and diversity of executive functions and their contributions to complex "frontal lobe" tasks: A latent variable analysis. *Cogn. Psychol.* **2000**, *41*, 49–100. [CrossRef] [PubMed]
41. Baggetta, P.; Alexander, P.A. Conceptualization and Operationalization of Executive Function. *Mind Brain Educ.* **2016**, *10*, 10–33. [CrossRef]
42. Shallice, T. Specific impairments of planning. *Philos. Trans. R. Soc. London. Biol. Sci.* **1982**, *298*, 199–209.
43. Mohai, K.; Kalózi-Szabó, C.; Rózsa, S. A végrehajtó funkciók adaptív mérésének lehetőségei. *Psychol. Hung. Caroliensis* **2016**, *4*, 40–85.
44. Rizopoulos, D. Package 'ltm'. 2022. Available online: https://cran.r-project.org/web/packages/ltm/ltm.pdf (accessed on 10 July 2022).
45. DeMars, C. *Item Response Theory*; Oxford University Press: Oxford, UK, 2010.
46. Pennington, B.F.; McGrath, L.M.; Peterson, R.L. *Diagnosing Learning Disorders: From Science to Practice*; Guilford Publications: New York, NY, USA, 2019.
47. Florian, L. Uses of Technology that Support Pupils with Special Educational Needs. In *ICT and Special Educational Needs: A Tool for Inclusion*; McGraw-Hill Education: London, UK, 2004; pp. 7–20.
48. Vygotsky, L. Thinking and speech. In *The Collected Works of LS Vygotsky*; Rieber, R.W., Carton, A.S., Eds.; Plenum Press: New York, NY, USA, 1987.
49. Lebeer, J. Shifting perspective: Dynamic assessment of learning processes in children with developmental disturbances. *Transylv. J. Psychol. Spec. Issue* **2005**, *1*, 57–85.
50. Grigorenko, E.L. Dynamic assessment and response to intervention: Two sides of one coin. *J. Learn. Disabil.* **2009**, *42*, 111–132. [CrossRef] [PubMed]

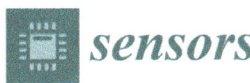

Article

A Simplified Algorithm for Setting the Observer Parameters for Second-Order Systems with Persistent Disturbances Using a Robust Observer

Alejandro Rincón [1,2,*], Fredy E. Hoyos [3] and John E. Candelo-Becerra [3]

1. Grupo de Investigación en Desarrollos Tecnológicos y Ambientales—GIDTA, Facultad de Ingeniería y Arquitectura, Universidad Católica de Manizales, Carrera 23 No. 60-63, Manizales 170002, Colombia
2. Grupo de Investigación en Microbiología y Biotecnología Agroindustrial—GIMIBAG, Instituto de Investigación en Microbiología y Biotecnología Agroindustrial, Universidad Católica de Manizales, Carrera 23 No. 60-63, Manizales 170002, Colombia
3. Departamento de Energía Eléctrica y Automática, Facultad de Minas, Universidad Nacional de Colombia, Sede Medellín, Carrera 80 No. 65-223, Robledo, Medellín 050041, Colombia
* Correspondence: arincons@ucm.edu.co; Tel.: +57-(604)-42055000

Abstract: The properties of the convergence region of the estimation error of a robust observer for second-order systems are determined, and a new algorithm is proposed for setting the observer parameters, considering persistent but bounded disturbances in the two observation error dynamics. The main contributions over closely related studies of the stability of state observers are: (i) the width of the convergence region of the observer error for the unknown state is expressed in terms of the interaction between the observer parameters and the disturbance terms of the observer error dynamics; (ii) it was found that this width has a minimum point and a vertical asymptote with respect to one of the observer parameters, and their coordinates were determined. In addition, the main advantages of the proposed algorithm over closely related algorithms are: (i) the definition of observer parameters is significantly simpler, as the fulfillment of Riccati equation conditions, solution of LMI constraints, and fulfillment of eigenvalue conditions are not required; (ii) unknown bounded terms are considered in the dynamics of the observer error for the known state. Finally, the algorithm is applied to a model of microalgae culture in a photobioreactor for the estimation of biomass growth rate and substrate uptake rate based on known concentrations of biomass and substrate.

Keywords: state estimation; robust observer; bioprocess monitoring; nonlinear systems

1. Introduction

In the monitoring and control of biological and biochemical processes, it is crucial to have real-time knowledge of variables such as the concentrations of biomass, products or reactants; the growth rate of microorganisms; and the substrate consumption rate [1–4]. Online knowledge of the substrate uptake rate is needed for the application of automatic control [4], whereas online knowledge of the specific growth rate (μ) is usually required in the following cases: (i) in automatic control with the biomass concentration as the output [5]; (ii) in automatic control with μ as the output (see [6,7]); (iii) in the maximization of growth rate via an extremum seeking controller [8]; (iv) in the maximization of the gaseous outflow rate via an extremum seeking controller [9]. The concentrations and reaction rates can be estimated by using state observers combined with the measurement of some state variables, and a known mass balance model for the measured states [1,10–12]. Control design for multi-agent systems is another active area of observer design. In these systems, observers are designed to estimate the unmeasured states of adjacent agents [13–15].

Robust observer designs have been developed for tackling uncertainty in the dynamics of observation errors. Common designs consider: (i) a lack of knowledge in the dynamics of the observation error for the unknown state; (ii) an unknown term of the unknown state

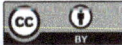

in the dynamics of the observation error for the known state [10,16–22]. In the case that the dynamics of the observation error for the known state involves an additional additive uncertain term and it is persistent but bounded, the steady state estimation involves error, even if a discontinuous observer is used. However, the estimation error depends on the observer parameters, so it can be reduced to a certain extent, provided that the known limits of the uncertainty [23,24].

In [25], a tuning procedure is proposed for setting the parameters of an extended state observer (ESO) for a closed loop second-order system with measurement noise and bounded external disturbance. The used observer is a Luenberger-like extended state, which is intended to estimate the external disturbance. The stability of the resulting estimation error dynamics is determined based on the state matrix, and two choices are proposed for setting the observer gains that lead to the real negative eigenvalues of the state matrix. Furthermore, the time-dependent bound of the transient behavior of the observation errors is determined, which gives the exponential convergence rate and the width of the convergence region in terms of observer parameters and some disturbances of the dynamics of the observation errors. However, the time derivative of the external disturbance is required to be bounded, and the input gain is required to be locally Lipschitz continuous.

In [21], an observer is designed to estimate the parameters of the tunneling current in a Scanning Tunneling Microscope (STM). The measurement of the tunneling current (i_t) is described by additive noise and first-order sensor dynamics, with the current i_t as its input. The observer is used for estimating the tunneling current i_t. The estimate is expressed in terms of Laplace transforms of the actual current and additive noise. The observer parameters must be chosen to have poles with strictly negative real parts in the transfer functions. A simple choice is proposed, which yields a second-order characteristic polynomial with a damping coefficient of one. However, no external disturbance is considered in the first-order sensor dynamics.

In [10], a filtered high gain observer is designed for a class of non-uniformly observable systems, and then it is applied to a phytoplanktonic growth model. Bounded disturbances and noisy measurements are considered, although bounded disturbances are not considered in the dynamics of the known state. The observation errors exponentially converge to a compact set whose width is a function of the observer parameters and bounds of the disturbances and measurement noise. Thus, the boundary of the transient behavior of the observation errors is determined. Furthermore, an improved observer is formulated for the case of sampled outputs, and the transient boundary of the observation errors is determined. Finally, the observer is applied to a model of continuous culture of phytoplankton, with an estimation of the substrate and cell quota concentrations based on biomass concentration measurements. The main limitations of the observer design are: (i) bounded disturbances are not considered in the dynamics of the observation error for the known state; (ii) some conditions of a Riccati differential equation must be satisfied.

In [23], a super-twisting observer is designed for a two-dimensional system, considering disturbances in the two observation error dynamics. Two disturbance types are considered in the observation error dynamics: in the first, the upper bound is the function of the observation error for the known state (known observation error); in the second, the upper bound is constant. The observation errors converge to zero in finite time for the first disturbance type. Thus, the convergence is proved, and the convergence time is determined. The observation errors converge to a compact set for the second disturbance type. Thus, the convergence region is determined, but the time-dependent bound of the transient behavior of the observation errors and the convergence times are not determined. In addition, the observer design algorithm is proposed, which involves the selection of design parameters. Finally, the observer and the algorithm are applied to a model of microalgae culture in a photobioreactor, performing an estimation of biomass growth rate, substrate uptake rate, and internal quota. However, the observer algorithm involves an iterative solution of LMIs, and the observer involves a discontinuous signal.

In this work, a new algorithm is proposed for setting the parameters of a robust observer for second-order systems, considering persistent but bounded disturbances in the two observation error dynamics. The algorithm is applied to a model of microalgae culture in a photobioreactor for the estimation of biomass growth rate and substrate uptake rate based on known concentrations of biomass and substrate. The main contributions over closely related studies of the stability of state observers (for instance [10,21,23,25]) are:

- Ci. The width of the convergence region of the observer error for the unknown state is expressed in terms of the interaction between the observer parameters and the disturbance in terms of the observer error dynamics. Thus, the desired estimation accuracy can be defined by the user by setting the observer parameters in accordance with this relationship. In contrast:
    - In [21], the dependence of the width of the convergence region on the observer parameters and disturbance terms is not determined.
    - In [10], the width of the convergence region is expressed in terms of the bounds of the disturbances and measurement noise, but bounded disturbances are not considered in the dynamics of the estimation error of the known state, so the effect of these disturbances is not considered in the convergence region.
    - In [23], the width of the convergence region is expressed in terms of the bounds of the disturbances of the dynamics of the estimation error of the known state, but the effect of observer parameters and bounded disturbance of the dynamics of the estimation error of the unknown state are not considered.
- Cii. The properties and limits of this width are determined. It was found that this width has a minimum point and a vertical asymptote with respect to one of the observer parameters, and their coordinates were determined. Then, the highest accuracy of the state estimation can be obtained by setting the observer parameters equal or similar to the coordinates of the minimum. In contrast, in [21,23,25]: (i) the properties, limits, and minimum of the width of the convergence region of the estimation error for the unknown state are not determined; (ii) the observer parameter values that lead to the lowest width of the convergence region are not determined.
- Ciii. The algorithm considers the combined effect of disturbance terms and observer parameters on the width of the convergence region.

In addition, the advantages of the proposed algorithm over closely related algorithms are:

(i) *Advantage A1*. It involves a significantly simpler definition of observer parameters: the fulfillment of Riccati equation conditions, solution of LMI constraints, and fulfillment of eigenvalue conditions are not required, thus, reducing the trial-and-error effort. In contrast, the fulfillment of these conditions is commonly required in closely related observer strategies, for instance [10,23,26].

(ii) *Advantage A2*. Different from [10,16–22], unknown bounded terms are considered in the dynamics of the observer error for the known state.

(iii) *Advantage A3*. The time derivatives of the disturbance terms of the plant model are not required to be bounded, whereas this condition is required in [25,27–30].

(iv) *Advantage A4*. Different from [23,31], discontinuous signals are not used in the observer, thus, avoiding problematic numerical solutions.

The work is organized as follows. The bioreactor model is presented in Section 2. The preliminaries in Section 3 include the observer equations and the bound of the transient and asymptotic behavior of the observer error. The main results presented in Section 4 include the formulation of the algorithm for setting the observer parameters and the determination of the width of the convergence region of the observer error in terms of the observer parameters. An application to a microalgae bioreactor is shown in Section 5, and the discussion and conclusions are drawn in Section 6.

2. Bioreactor Model

Consider the system

$$\frac{dx_1}{dt} = h_1 + bx_2 + \delta_1, \quad (1)$$

$$\frac{dx_2}{dt} = h_2 + \delta_2, \quad (2)$$

where x_1 and x_2 are the states; h_1 and h_2 are model functions; δ_1 and δ_2 are disturbance terms; and b is the x_2 gain in the dynamics of x_1. The model terms fulfill the following assumptions:

Assumption 1. *The functions h_1 and h_2 are known; the state x_1 is measured, and the coefficient b is known; the state x_2 and the terms δ_1 and δ_2 are unknown.*

Assumption 2. *The coefficient b is bounded away from zero:*

$$|b| \geq b_{min} > 0$$

where b_{min} is an unknown positive constant.

Assumption 3. *The disturbance terms δ_1 and δ_2 are bounded.*

3. Preliminaries: Observer and Bounds for the Transient and Steady Behavior of the Observer Error

In this section, the observer equations and the bounds for the transient and asymptotic behavior of the observer error for the unknown state ($\overline{x}_2$) are recalled from [24]. The detailed mathematical procedure of the Lyapunov-based formulation of the observer is provided in [24].

3.1. Observer

The observer equations are [24]:

$$\frac{d\hat{x}_1}{dt} = b\hat{x}_2 - |b|\left(\omega\overline{x}_1 + \left(k + \frac{1}{4\omega}\right)\psi_{x_1} + sat_{x_1}\hat{\theta}\right) + h_1, \quad (3)$$

$$\frac{d\hat{x}_2}{dt} = -b\omega\left(\left(k + \frac{1}{4\omega}\right)\psi_{x_1} + sat_{x_1}\hat{\theta}\right) + h_2, \quad (4)$$

$$\frac{d\hat{\theta}}{dt} = \gamma|b||\psi_{x_1}|. \quad (5)$$

where

$$\overline{x}_1 = \hat{x}_1 - x_1, \quad (6)$$

$$\psi_{x_1} = \begin{cases} \overline{x}_1 - \varepsilon & \text{for } \overline{x}_1 \geq \varepsilon \\ 0 & \text{for } \overline{x}_1 \in [-\varepsilon, \varepsilon] \\ \overline{x}_1 + \varepsilon & \text{for } \overline{x}_1 \leq -\varepsilon \end{cases} \quad (7)$$

$$sat_{x_1} = \begin{cases} 1 & \text{for } \overline{x}_1 \geq \varepsilon \\ \frac{1}{\varepsilon}\overline{x}_1 & \text{for } \overline{x}_1 \in [-\varepsilon, \varepsilon] \\ -1 & \text{for } \overline{x}_1 \leq -\varepsilon \end{cases} \quad (8)$$

$$\sigma = sign(b)$$

where $\hat{x}_1$ is the estimate of x_1, $\hat{x}_2$ is the estimate of x_2, $\hat{\theta}$ is the updated parameter, and: (i) γ, k, ω are user-defined positive constants; (ii) the width of the convergence region of $\overline{x}_1$, that is, ε, is user-defined, positive, and constant.

3.2. Mathematical Definitions

The main mathematical definitions are given as follows. b, h_1, h_2, δ_1 and δ_2 are terms of the model (1) and (2) described after Equations (1) and (2), satisfying Assumptions 1, 2, and 3. In addition, $\bar{x}_1 = \hat{x}_1 - x_1$ is the observer error for the known state, $\bar{x}_2 = \hat{x}_2 - x_2$ is the observer error for the unknown state; x_1 is the known state, x_2 is the unknown state, and $z = \bar{x}_2 - \sigma \omega \bar{x}_1$.

Mathematical definitions related to the function V_z:

$$V_z = \frac{1}{2}\psi_z^2$$

$$\psi_z = \begin{cases} z + \delta_{min} & \text{for } z \geq -\delta_{min} \geq 0 \\ 0 & \text{for } z \in (-\delta_{max}, -\delta_{min}) \\ z + \delta_{max} & \text{for } z \leq -\delta_{max} \leq 0 \end{cases}$$

where δ_{min} and δ_{max} are constants that satisfy

$$\delta \geq \delta_{min}, \quad \delta_{min} \in (-\infty, 0]; \delta \leq \delta_{max}, \quad \delta_{max} \in [0, \infty),$$

where δ is defined as

$$\delta = \frac{1}{b}\left(\frac{\delta_2}{\sigma \omega} - \delta_1\right),$$

and ψ_{z0} is the value of ψ_z at the initial time.

Mathematical definitions related to the overall Lyapunov function:

$$V_{z\theta x1} = V_z + V_{x1} + V_\theta,$$

$$V_{x1} = \frac{1}{2}\psi_{x1}^2; \quad V_\theta = \frac{1}{2}\gamma^{-1}\tilde{\theta}^2; \quad \tilde{\theta} = \hat{\theta} - \theta$$

where θ is a positive constant fulfilling:

$$|-\delta_{zt} - \delta_1/b| \leq \theta; \quad \delta_{zt} = \psi_z - z.$$

Mathematical definitions of convergence regions:

$$\Omega_{x1} = \{\bar{x}_1 : -\varepsilon \leq \bar{x}_1 \leq \varepsilon\}$$

$$\Omega_{x2} = \{\bar{x}_2 : |\bar{x}_2| \leq max\{-\delta_{min}, \delta_{max}\} + \omega\varepsilon\}$$

3.3. Convergence of the Observer Error for the Known State

The combined state z is defined as:

$$z = \bar{x}_2 - \sigma \omega \bar{x}_1, \qquad (9)$$

The Lyapunov function for z is defined as

$$V_z = \frac{1}{2}\psi_z^2, \qquad (10)$$

$$\psi_z = \begin{cases} z + \delta_{min} & \text{for } z \geq -\delta_{min} \geq 0 \\ 0 & \text{for } z \in (-\delta_{max}, -\delta_{min}) \\ z + \delta_{max} & \text{for } z \leq -\delta_{max} \leq 0 \end{cases}.$$

where δ_{min} and δ_{max} are constant limits for the disturbance term

$$\delta = \frac{1}{b}\left(\frac{\delta_2}{\sigma \omega} - \delta_1\right),$$

that satisfy

$$\delta \geq \delta_{min}, \quad \delta_{min} \in (-\infty, 0],$$
$$\delta \leq \delta_{max}, \quad \delta_{max} \in [0, \infty).$$

Differentiating V_z with respect to time, yields

$$\frac{dV_z}{dt} \leq -2\omega|b|V_z \leq 0.$$

The overall Lyapunov function is:

$$V_{z\theta x1} = V_z + V_{x1} + V_\theta,$$

$$V_{x1} = \frac{1}{2}\psi_{x1}^2; \; V_\theta = \frac{1}{2}\gamma^{-1}\tilde{\theta}^2; \; \tilde{\theta} = \hat{\theta} - \theta$$

where V_z is given by Equation (10), γ is a user-defined positive constant, $\hat{\theta}$ is provided by Equation (5) and θ is a positive constant fulfilling

$$|-\delta_{zt} - \delta_1/b| \leq \theta; \; \delta_{zt} = \psi_z - z.$$

The time derivative of $V_{z\theta x1}$ leads to

$$\frac{dV_{z\theta x1}}{dt} = \frac{d}{dt}(V_z + V_{x1} + V_\theta) \leq -kb_{min}\psi_{x1}^2 \leq 0. \tag{11}$$

This indicates the asymptotic convergence of the observer error $\bar{x}_1$ to the compact set $\Omega_{x1} = \{\bar{x}_1 : -\varepsilon \leq \bar{x}_1 \leq \varepsilon\}$.

Remark 1. *The ψ_z definition given after Equation (10) indicates that ψ_z, ψ_z^2 and $d\psi_z^2/dz$ exist and are continuous. The ψ_{x_1} definition (7) indicates that ψ_{x_1}, $\psi_{x_1}^2$, and $d\psi_{x_1}^2/d\bar{x}_1$ exist and are continuous. Consequently, V_z, V_{x1} and the overall Lyapunov function $V_{z\theta x1}$ exist and are continuous. A detailed determination of $dV_{z\theta x1}/dt$, dV_z/dt, dV_{x1}/dt, dV_θ/dt is given in [24].*

Remark 2. *The term 'overall Lyapunov function' is used for the Lyapunov function that results from the addition of several quadratic or positive forms and whose time derivative indicates the convergence result of some state. This term is also used in [32,33]. Notice that this condition is only fulfilled by $V_{z\theta x1}$, as follows from Equation (11).*

3.4. Bounds for the Transient and Steady Behavior of the Observer Error for the Unknown State

From the definition of z (9), it follows that the observer error $\bar{x}_2$ can be rewritten in terms of z and $\bar{x}_1$:

$$\bar{x}_2 = z + \sigma\omega\bar{x}_1.$$

This leads to

$$|\bar{x}_2| \leq |z| + \omega|\bar{x}_1|.$$

Combining the dynamics of z and $\bar{x}_1$, yields

$$|\bar{x}_2| \leq |\psi_{zo}|e^{-\omega b_{min}(t-t_o)} + \max\{-\delta_{min}, \delta_{max}\} + \omega|\bar{x}_1| \tag{12}$$

where ψ_{zo} is the value of ψ_z at the initial time, and δ_{min} and δ_{max} are constant limits for the disturbance term

$$\delta = \frac{1}{b}\left(\frac{\delta_2}{\sigma\omega} - \delta_1\right), \tag{13}$$

that satisfy

$$\begin{aligned}\delta &\geq \delta_{min}, \; \delta_{min} \in (-\infty, 0], \\ \delta &\leq \delta_{max}, \; \delta_{max} \in [0, \infty).\end{aligned} \tag{14}$$

b_{min} is a constant limit for b that satisfies Assumption 2.

Despite the fact that the convergence of $\bar{x}_1$ to $\Omega_{x1} = \{\bar{x}_1 : -\varepsilon \leq \bar{x}_1 \leq \varepsilon\}$ is asymptotic, one can consider that $\bar{x}_1 \in \Omega_{x1}$ for some $t \geq T_1$, that is, $|\bar{x}_1| \leq \varepsilon$. Combining with

Equation (12) yields the time-dependent bound for the transient behavior of the observer error $\bar{x}_2$:

$$|\bar{x}_2| \leq |\psi_{zo}|e^{-\omega b_{min}(t-t_o)} + max\{-\delta_{min}, \delta_{max}\} + \omega\varepsilon \text{ for } t \geq T_1 \qquad (15)$$

Hence, $\bar{x}_2$ converges asymptotically to the compact set

$$\Omega_{x2} = \{\bar{x}_2 : |\bar{x}_2| \leq max\{-\delta_{min}, \delta_{max}\} + \omega\varepsilon\} \qquad (16)$$

so that the limits of the convergence region Ω_{x2} are $max\{-\delta_{min}, \delta_{max}\} + \omega\varepsilon$ and $-max\{-\delta_{min}, \delta_{max}\} - \omega\varepsilon$.

4. Formulation of the Algorithm for Setting the Observer Parameters and Determination of the Width of the Convergence Region of the Observer Error in Terms of the Observer Parameters

In this section: (i) the width of the convergence region Ω_{x2} (16) is expressed in terms of the interaction between the parameters of the observer (3)–(5) and δ_1, δ_2, the disturbance terms of the observer error dynamics; (ii) an algorithm is formulated for setting the observer parameters $\omega, \varepsilon, \gamma, k$.

4.1. Determination of the Width of the Convergence Region of the Observer Error

From the definition of δ in Equation (13), it follows that

$$|\delta| \leq \frac{1}{\omega}d_2 + d_1 \qquad (17)$$

where d_1 and d_2 are positive constants that satisfy

$$\left|\frac{\delta_2}{b}\right| \leq d_2; \ \left|\frac{\delta_1}{b}\right| \leq d_1 \qquad (18)$$

From Equation (17) and the conditions on δ_{min} and δ_{max} (14), it follows that the δ_{min} and δ_{max} values can be chosen to be:

$$\delta_{max} = \frac{1}{\omega}d_2 + d_1; \ \delta_{min} = -\delta_{max}$$

so that the terms in Equation (14) are fulfilled. Then, the convergence set Ω_{x2} (16) becomes

$$\Omega_{x2} = \{\bar{x}_2 : |\bar{x}_2| \leq f_w\} \qquad (19)$$

$$f_w = \frac{1}{\omega}d_2 + d_1 + \omega\varepsilon \qquad (20)$$

so that the width of the convergence set Ω_{x2} is f_w and the limits of Ω_{x2} are $-f_w$ and $+f_w$. The main features of the f_w function are:

$$f_w > 0; \ f_w \text{ has a vertical asymptote, at } \omega = 0$$
$$\lim_{\omega \to \infty} f_w = \infty; \ f_w > d_1 \geq \sup_{t \geq t_o}|\delta_1/b|; \ \lim_{\omega \to 0^+} f_w = \infty \qquad (21)$$

From these properties, it follows that f_w has a minimum point with respect to ω. Its coordinates are determined by differentiating f_w expression (20) with respect to ω, which yields:

$$\omega^* = \sqrt{d_2}\frac{1}{\sqrt{\varepsilon}}; \ f_w^* = 2\sqrt{d_2}\sqrt{\varepsilon} + d_1 \qquad (22)$$

Therefore, the relationship between f_w^* and ω^* is given by

$$f_w^* = 2d_2\frac{1}{\omega^*} + d_1 \qquad (23)$$

Remark 3. The properties (21) of the f_w function and its minimum (22) indicate that $\omega = \omega^*$ and a low ε value leads to low f_w, which implies a low width of the convergence region Ω_{x2}, and consequently, a high quality of x_2 estimation, as follows from Equations (19) and (20).

Remark 4. An overlarge ω value fulfilling $\omega \gg \omega^*$ leads to: (i) fast convergence of the upper bound of $\bar{x}_2$, as follows from Equation (15); (ii) a large f_w value, which implies a low quality of $\bar{x}_2$ estimation, as follows from Equations (19) and (20). Therefore, the choice of ω must take into account both the convergence rate and the width of the convergence region of $\bar{x}_2$.

Remark 5. A low ε value leads to low f_w^*, since f_w^* increases with respect to ε, as follows from Equation (22). However, overly small ε values lead to steeper slopes in the shape of the sat_{x_1} signal (8) of the observer, which implies that the numerical solution of the differential equation must use a smaller step size.

Remark 6. The f_w^* function (23) increases with d_1, whereas ω^* is independent of d_1, as follows from Equation (22).

In the case that $\delta_1 = 0$ in Equation (1), we have

$$|\delta| \leq \frac{1}{\omega}d_2$$

and one can use

$$\delta_{max} = \frac{1}{\omega}d_2; \ \delta_{min} = -\delta_{max}$$

Then, Equation (19) becomes

$$\Omega_{x2} = \{\bar{x}_2 : |\bar{x}_2| \leq f_w\} \quad (24)$$

$$f_w = \frac{1}{\omega}d_2 + \omega\varepsilon \quad (25)$$

The resulting features of f_w for $\delta_1 = 0$ are:

$f_w > 0$; f_w has a vertical asymptote, at $\omega = 0$;

$$\lim_{\omega \to \infty} f_w = \infty; \ \lim_{\omega \to 0^+} f_w = \infty$$

From these properties, it follows that f_w has a minimum point with respect to ω. The coordinates of this minimum are determined by differentiating f_w expression (22) with respect to ω, which yields:

$$\omega^* = \sqrt{d_2}\frac{1}{\sqrt{\varepsilon}}; \ f_w^* = 2\sqrt{d_2}\sqrt{\varepsilon} \quad (26)$$

4.2. Formulation of the Algorithm for Setting the Observer Parameters

The algorithm presented in Algorithm 1 allows us to set the observer parameters ω, ε, γ, and k, so as to define: (i) the convergence rate of $\bar{x}_2$; (ii) the value of $f_w = \frac{1}{\omega}d_2 + d_1 + \omega\varepsilon$, which is the width of the $\bar{x}_2$ convergence set $\Omega_{x2} = \{\bar{x}_2 : |\bar{x}_2| \leq f_w\}$.

Algorithm 1: Algorithm for setting the parameters of the observer (3)–(5).

Step	Description
1	Cast the system model in the form (1)–(2) and identify the known state x_1, the unknown state x_2, and the terms b, h_1, h_2, δ_1, δ_2.
2	Obtain the values of b_{min} that satisfy Assumption 2 and the values of d_2, d_1, satisfying Equation (18). To this end, the values of d_2, d_1 can be obtained by the simulation of δ_2/b, δ_1/b, based on the x_1, x_2 model, with model parameter values obtained from either closely related studies or offline fitting.
3	Set the values of ω, ε to define: — The time-dependent bound for the transient evolution of $\bar{x}_2$, given by Equation (15): $\lvert \bar{x}_2 \rvert \leq \lvert \psi_{zo} \rvert e^{-\omega b_{min}(t-t_o)} + max\{-\delta_{min}, \delta_{max}\} + \omega\varepsilon$; for $t \geq T_1$ — The limit of the convergence region of $\bar{x}_2$, given by Equations (19) and (20): $\Omega_{x2} = \{\bar{x}_2 : \lvert \bar{x}_2 \rvert \leq f_w\}$; $f_w = \frac{1}{\omega}d_2 + d_1 + \omega\varepsilon$ where $f_w > d_1 \geq \sup_{t \geq t_o} \lvert \delta_1/b \rvert$ and the minimum point of f_w is given by Equation (22): $\omega^* = \sqrt{d_2}\frac{1}{\sqrt{\varepsilon}}$; $f_w^* = 2\sqrt{d_2}\sqrt{\varepsilon} + d_1$
4	Set a high value of γ to define the update rate of $\hat{\theta}$, according to Equation (5). Set a high value of k to define the convergence rate of $\bar{x}_1$, according to Equation (11).

Remark 7. *The proposed algorithm and the observer (3)–(5) lead to a more practical and simpler real-time state estimation in either laboratory or industrial applications, according to the advantages A1 to A4, which are due to the observer of [24]. They can be applied to systems whose model can be cast in the second-order form (1) and (2), which includes a wide range of mechanical and physical systems. Some examples are:*

- *Microalgae reactor represented by the Droop model: (i) estimation of specific bio-mass growth rate based on known biomass concentration; (ii) estimation of specific substrate uptake rate based on known substrate concentration—see [8,23].*
- *Anaerobic bioreactor for hydrogen production via the dark fermentation of glucose: estimation of influent glucose concentration based on known reactor glucose con-centration—see [3].*
- *Fed-batch bioreactor for ethanol production: (i) estimation of the rate of enzymatic hydrolysis based on known substrate (starch) concentration; (ii) estimation of the glucose consumption rate based on known glucose concentration—see [4].*
- *Membrane fuel cell: estimation of stack temperature based on known oxygen pres-sure—see [34].*
- *Photovoltaic system: estimation of the power gradient based on known generated electric power—see [35].*
- *DC-DC buck converter: estimation of the time derivative of the output tracking er-ror based on the known average output voltage—see [36].*
- *Second-order underactuated mechanical system: estimation of the time derivative of the pole angle—see [20].*

Remark 8. *The convergence rate and the width of the $\bar{x}_2$ convergence set (f_w) can be properly defined by setting the observer parameters ω, ε, γ, k in accordance with the proposed procedure, with ω, ε values corresponding to the minimum point of f_w, that is, ω^*, f_w^*.*

Remark 9. *The proposed observer algorithm deals with the combined effect of disturbance terms and observer parameters on the width of the convergence region for the estimation error of the unknown state, as follows:*

(a) *The convergence region is expressed as a function of the combined effect of observer parameters and disturbance terms—see Equations (19) and (20). Then, the desired estimation accuracy can be defined by the user by properly setting the observer parameters in accordance with this relationship.*

(b) *The properties of this expression are determined in terms of the observer parameters, including the limits and the coordinates of the minimum—see Equations (21)–(23). In turn, these properties allow choosing ω, ε values to avoid an undesired overlarge f_w value, and the lowest*

f_w value is obtained by using the coordinates of the minimum, that is, $\omega = \omega^*$, according to Equation (22). Thus, the highest accuracy of the state estimation is obtained by setting the observer parameters equal or similar to the coordinates of the minimum.

5. Application to Microalgae Bioreactor

The developed algorithm for setting parameters of the observer (3)–(5) is used to estimate the substrate uptake rate ρ and specific growth rate μ in a continuous microalgae bioreactor. The concentrations of substrate and biomass are considered to be known, and the system is described by the Droop model [23,37]:

$$\frac{dx}{dt} = \mu x - Dx \tag{27}$$

$$\frac{ds}{dt} = -\rho x + D(s_i - s) \tag{28}$$

$$\frac{dq}{dt} = \rho - \mu q \tag{29}$$

where x is the biomass concentration, s is the substrate concentration, and q is the cell quota of assimilated nutrient; $D = F_i/v$ is the dilution rate, F_i is the feeding flow rate, v is the broth volume, s_i is the fed substrate concentration, μ is the specific growth rate, and ρ is the specific substrate uptake rate. The expressions for μ, ρ, and the model parameters are [23]:

$$\begin{cases} \mu(q) = \max\left\{0, \mu_m\left(1 - \frac{Q_0}{q}\right)\right\}; \rho = \rho_m\left(\frac{s}{s+K_s}\right) \\ \rho_m = 0.03 \frac{mgN}{mgC \cdot d}; K_s = 0.0010 \frac{mgN}{L}; \mu_m = 0.5 \, d^{-1}; \\ Q_0 = 0.045 \, mgN/mgC; \\ x_{to} = 0.1 \, mgC/L; s_{to} = 0.01 \, mgN/L; q_{to} = 0.06 \, mgN/mgC; \\ D = \begin{cases} 0.25\left(1 + \sin\left(\frac{2\pi}{\tau_D}t\right)\right) & d^{-1} \text{ for } t < 6 \, d; \\ 0 \text{ for } t \geq 6 \, d \end{cases} \\ \tau_D = 8 \, d; s_i = 0.05 \, mgN/L; \end{cases} \tag{30}$$

The model details, including parameters and specific growth rate expression, are given in [23].

The f_w curve as a function of ω and ε is computed using Equation (20), the curves of f_w^* and ω^* as a function of ε are computed using Equation (22), and the f_w^* vs. ω^* curve is computed using Equation (23).

The simulation of the model (27)–(29) and the observer (3)–(5) was performed using Matlab software (The Math Works Inc., Natick, MA, USA): the differential equations were numerically integrated using the ode45 routine.

Although model (27)–(29) comprises three states, it leads to the following second-order subsystems:

A)

$$\frac{ds}{dt} = -\rho x + D(s_i - s)$$

$$\frac{d\rho}{dt} = \delta_2$$

for the first example, so that $x_1 = s; x_2 = \rho$.

B)

$$\frac{dx}{dt} = \mu x - Dx$$

$$\frac{d\mu}{dt} = \delta_2$$

for the second example, so that $x_1 = x; x_2 = \mu$.

This approach is also considered in [23].

5.1. First Example: Estimation of Substrate Uptake Rate

The specific substrate uptake rate ρ is estimated using the substrate mass balance model (28) and the knowledge of substrate and biomass concentrations. The fed substrate concentration s_i is inaccurately known: $s_i = \bar{s}_i + \delta_{sin}$, where $\bar{s}_i$ is the known value of s_i, and δ_{sin} is the uncertainty; $\bar{s}_i = 0.05$ mg N/L; $\delta_{sin} = 0.1\bar{s}_i \times \sin\left(\frac{2\pi t}{\tau_{si}}\right)$; $\tau_{si} = 3$. The substrate concentration (s) is the known state, and the specific substrate uptake rate (ρ) is the unknown state, so that substrate model (28) can be cast in the form (1), (2) with

$$x_1 = s;\ x_2 = \rho;\ b = -x;\ h_1 = (\bar{s}_i - s)D;\ h_2 = 0;\ \delta_1 = D\delta_{si};\ \delta_2 = \frac{d\rho}{dt} \quad (31)$$

Additionally, the observer (3)–(5) provides the estimate of ρ, that is, $\hat{x}_2 = \hat{\rho}$. The observer structure is given in Figure 1. x is the biomass concentration, s is the substrate concentration, ρ is the specific substrate uptake rate, $D = F_i/v$ is the dilution rate, F_i is the feeding flow rate, v is the broth volume, and s_i is the fed substrate concentration. In addition, x_1 is the known state, x_2 is the unknown state, and $\hat{x}_2$ is the estimate of x_2.

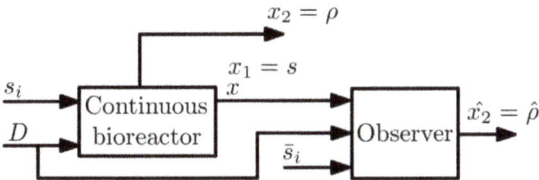

Figure 1. Structure of the observer application to microalgae bioreactor for estimating the specific substrate uptake rate ρ.

To examine the f_w function (20), the d_1, d_2 bounds of the disturbance terms δ_1/b, δ_2/b are obtained by simulation based on the x_1, x_2 model, yielding $d_1 = 0.04$, $d_2 = 0.11$. The curves of f_w, f_w^*, ω^* for different ε, ω values are shown in Figure 2.

Low f_w values are obtained for $\omega = \omega^*$ and low ε value (see Figure 2b,d), which is in accordance with remark 4.1. A minimum of the f_w function is characterized by $\omega^* = 8.564$, $f_w^* = 0.0657$ for $\varepsilon = 0.0015$, as follows from Equation (22). The observer parameters are chosen to be:

$$\varepsilon = 0.0015;\ \omega = 8.56;\ k = 40;\ \gamma = 100;\ \hat{x}_{1|t_0} = 0.1;\ \hat{x}_{2|t_0} = 0\ d^{-1};\ \hat{\theta}_{t_0} = 0 \quad (32)$$

So that $f_w \approx f_w^*$. The bioreactor is simulated using model (27)–(29) with plant model terms and parameters (30), whereas the observer (3)–(5) is simulated using the definition of the terms of the system model given by Equation (31), and the values of observer parameters given by Equation (32), and it is observed that (Figure 3):

- The observer error $\tilde{x}_1$ converges faster than $\tilde{x}_2$.
- The observer error $\tilde{x}_1 = \hat{x}_1 - x_1$ converges asymptotically to the compact set $\Omega_{x1} = \{\tilde{x}_1 : -\varepsilon \leq \tilde{x}_1 \leq \varepsilon\}$ and remains inside for $t \geq 2.6$ d approx. (Figure 3a,b).
- The observer error $\tilde{x}_2 = \hat{x}_2 - x_2$ converges to the computed compact set Ω_{x2} and remains inside for $t \geq 4.4$ d approx. (Figure 3c,d). The limits $(-f_w, +f_w)$ of the Ω_{x2} convergence set are indicated through dashed horizontal lines in Figure 3d.
- The low width of Ω_{x2} is owed to the small values of δ_1/b and ε.

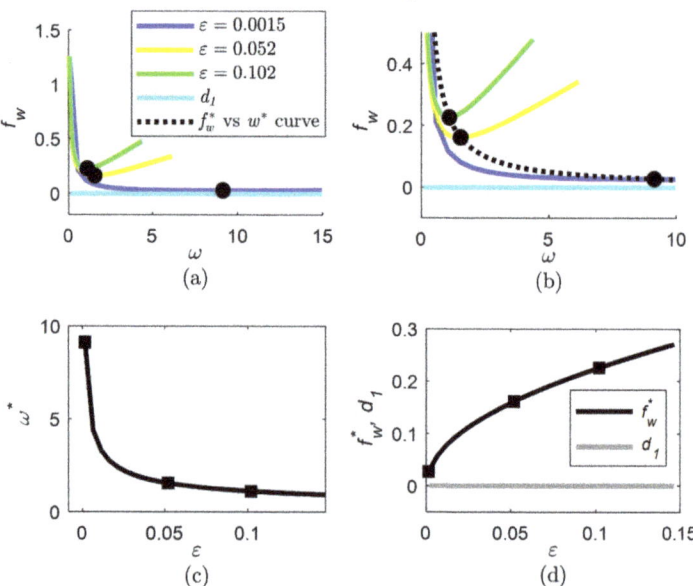

Figure 2. Effect of the observer parameters ε, ω on the f_w function (20) for estimation of the specific substrate uptake rate ρ: (**a**) f_w as a function of ω for several ε values, indicating the minimum point; (**b**) detail of f_w as a function of ω for several ε values, indicating the minimum point; (**c**) values of ω^* as a function of ε, indicating the points for the ε values considered in subfigure a; (**d**) values of f_w^* as a function of ε, indicating the points for the ε values considered in subfigure a.

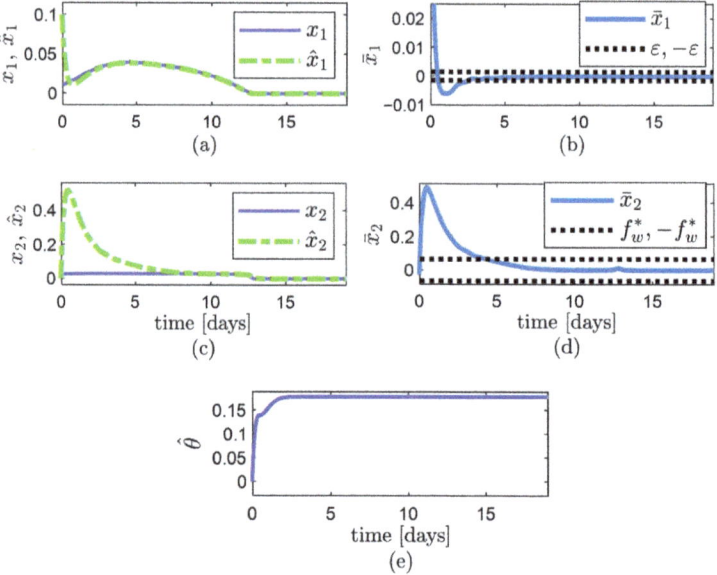

Figure 3. Performance of the observer (3)–(5) for estimation of specific substrate uptake rate ρ, using the observer parameters obtained through the proposed algorithm: (**a**) trajectory of state x_1 and estimate $\hat{x}_1$; (**b**) trajectory of the observer error for the known state, $\bar{x}_1$; (**c**) trajectory of state x_2 and estimate $\hat{x}_2$; (**d**) trajectory of the observer error for the unknown state, $\bar{x}_2$, with the limits $(-f_w, +f_w)$ of the Ω_{x2} convergence set indicated through dashed horizontal lines; (**e**) trajectory of the updated parameter $\hat{\theta}$.

The performed simulations confirm the adequacy of the parameter recommendations provided in the observer algorithm to achieve proper convergence speed and the width of the convergence region of $\bar{x}_2$.

5.2. Second Example: Estimation of Biomass Growth Rate

The specific growth rate μ is estimated using the biomass mass balance model (27) and the knowledge of biomass concentration. The biomass concentration (x) is the known state, and the specific growth rate μ is the unknown state, so the biomass model (27) can be cast in the form (1), (2) with

$$x_1 = x;\ x_2 = \mu;\ b = x;\ h_1 = -Dx;\ h_2 = 0;\ \delta_1 = 0;\ \delta_2 = \frac{d\mu}{dt} \quad (33)$$

Additionally, the observer (3)–(5) provides the estimate of μ, that is, $\hat{x}_2 = \hat{\mu}$. The observer structure is given in Figure 4. x is the biomass concentration, s is the substrate concentration, μ is the specific growth rate, ρ is the specific substrate uptake rate, $D = F_i/v$ is the dilution rate, F_i is the feeding flow rate, v is the broth volume, and s_i is the fed substrate concentration. In addition, x_1 is the known state, x_2 is the unknown state, and $\hat{x}_2$ is the estimate of x_2.

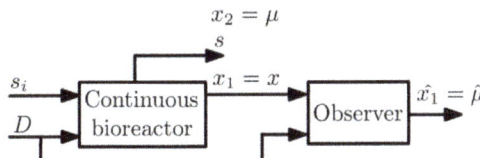

Figure 4. Structure of the observer application to microalgae bioreactor for estimation of the specific growth rate μ.

To examine the f_w function, the d_1, d_2 bounds of the disturbance terms δ_1/b, δ_2/b are obtained by simulation based on the x_1, x_2 model, yielding $d_1 = 0$, $d_2 = 0.125$. The curves of f_w, f_w^*, ω^* for different ε, ω values are shown in Figure 5.

Low f_w values are obtained for $\omega = \omega^*$ and low ε value (see Figure 5b,d), which is in accordance with remark 4.1. A minimum of the f_w function is characterized by $\omega^* = 9.129$, $f_w^* = 0.0097$ for $\varepsilon = 0.0015$. The observer parameters are chosen to be:

$$\varepsilon = 0.0015;\ \omega = 9.12;\ k = 40;\ \gamma = 100;\ \hat{x}_{1|to} = 0.1 mgC/L;\ \hat{x}_{2|to} = 0\ d^{-1};\ \hat{\theta}_{to} = 0 \quad (34)$$

So that $f_w \approx f_w^*$. The bioreactor is simulated using model (27)–(29) with plant model terms and parameters (30), whereas the observer (3)–(5) is simulated using the plant model terms and parameters given by Equation (33), and the values of observer parameters given by Equation (34), and it is observed that (Figure 6):

- The observer error $\bar{x}_1$ converges faster than $\bar{x}_2$.
- The observer error $\bar{x}_1 = \hat{x}_1 - x_1$ enters to the compact set Ω_{x1} at 4.92 days and remains inside afterward (Figure 6a,b).
- The observer error $\bar{x}_2 = \hat{x}_2 - x_2$ remains inside its compact set for $t \geq 15.3$ d approx. (Figure 6c,d). The limits $(-f_w, +f_w)$ of the Ω_{x2} convergence set are indicated through dashed horizontal lines in Figure 6d.
- A low width of Ω_{x2} is achieved by choosing ε, ω values on the basis of the proposed algorithm.

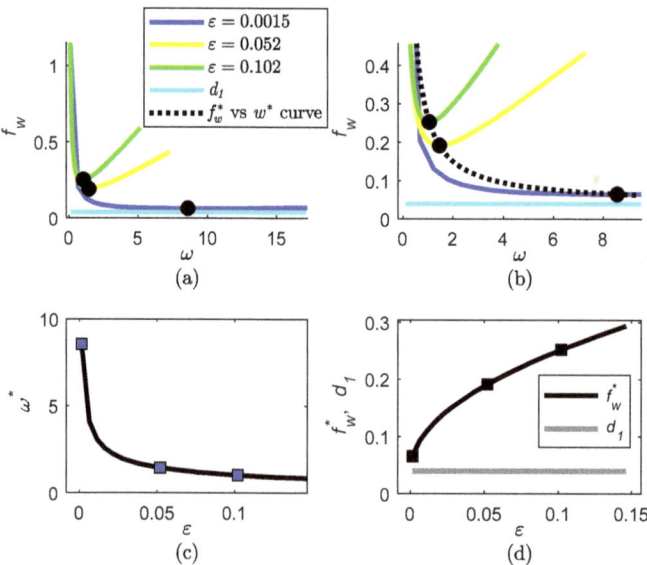

Figure 5. Effect of the observer parameters ε, ω on the f_w function (19) for estimation of the specific growth rate μ: (**a**) f_w as a function of ω for several ε values; (**b**) detail of f_w as a function of ω for several ε values, indicating the minimum point; (**c**) values of ω^* as a function of ε, indicating the points for the ε values considered in subfigure a; (**d**) values of f_w^* as a function of ε, indicating the points for the ε values considered in subfigure a.

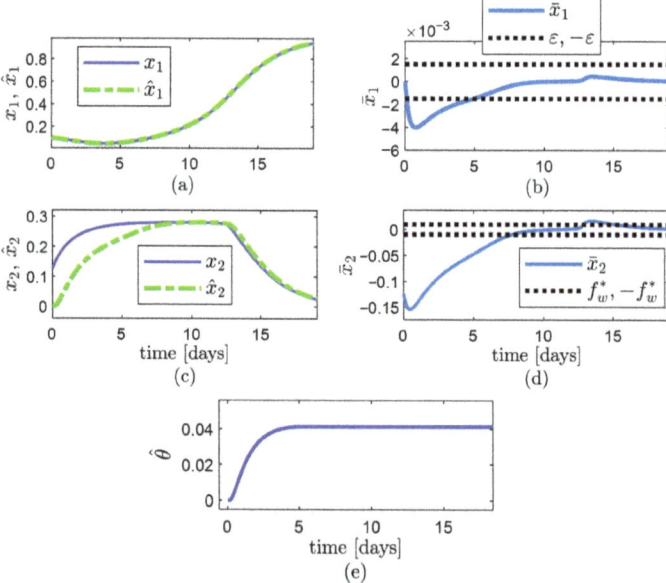

Figure 6. Performance of the observer (3)–(5) for estimation of specific growth rate μ, using the observer parameters obtained through the proposed algorithm: (**a**) trajectory of state x_1 and estimate $\hat{x}_1$; (**b**) trajectory of the observer error for the known state, $\bar{x}_1$; (**c**) trajectory of state x_2 and estimate $\hat{x}_2$; (**d**) trajectory of the observer error for the unknown state, $\bar{x}_2$, with the limits $(-f_w, +f_w)$ of the Ω_{x2} convergence set indicated through dashed horizontal lines; (**e**) trajectory of the updated parameter $\hat{\theta}$.

6. Discussion and Conclusions

6.1. Discussion

- The main contributions over closely related studies of the stability of state observers are:
- Ci. The width of the convergence region of the observer error for the unknown state is expressed in terms of the interaction between the observer parameters and the disturbance in terms of the observer error dynamics. Then, the user defines the desired estimation accuracy by properly setting the observer parameters in accordance with the aforementioned relationship.
- Cii. The properties and limits of this width are determined; it was found that this width has a minimum point and a vertical asymptote with respect to one of the observer parameters, and their coordinates were determined. Thus, the highest accuracy of the state estimation is obtained by setting the observer parameters equal or similar to the coordinates of the minimum.
- The main challenges encountered in this research work are:
- Choosing the idea of contributions Ci and Cii as the core topics of the paper required identifying contributions and limitations of high-quality works addressing observer design and stability analysis, mainly [23,25]. This implied a deep understanding of all the mathematical developments involved in the stability analysis, and also the advantages, disadvantages, and limitations of the observer and its stability properties.

The statement of the procedure for determining the constants that satisfy Equation (18). Based on several literature studies, we finally concluded that they could be obtained by the simulation of δ_2/b, δ_1/b, based on the x_1, x_2 model, with model parameter values obtained from either closely related studies or offline fitting, as stated in Algorithm 1.

6.2. Conclusions

In this work, a new algorithm is proposed for setting parameters of a robust observer for second-order systems, considering persistent but bounded disturbances in the two observation error dynamics. As the main contribution over closely related studies of the stability of state observers, the width of the convergence region of the observer error for the unknown state is expressed in terms of the interaction between the observer parameters and the disturbance terms of the observer error dynamics. Moreover, the properties and the minimum of this relationship were determined.

The proposed observer algorithm leads to a more practical and simpler state estimation in either laboratory or industrial applications. It can be used for systems whose model can be cast in second-order form, for instance, mechanical, chemical, and biochemical systems. Moreover, it can be used for multiple state estimation, in cases of several second-order systems. The choice of the observer parameters must consider both the convergence rate and width of the convergence region of the estimation error of the unknown state. Choosing the observer parameter values to be similar or equal to the values for the minimum leads to a high quality of state estimation.

The performed simulations confirm the adequacy of the parameter recommendations provided in the observer algorithm to achieve the proper convergence speed and width of the convergence region of the observer error for the unknown state.

Future work will include: (i) extending the observer and the algorithm to system models of third order; (ii) extending the observer and the algorithm to system models of general nth order; (iii) considering noise in the measurement of the known state.

Author Contributions: Conceptualization, A.R.; methodology, A.R.; writing—original draft preparation, A.R., J.E.C.-B. and F.E.H.; writing—review and editing, A.R., F.E.H. and J.E.C.-B.; visualization, A.R., F.E.H. and J.E.C.-B. All authors have read and agreed to the published version of the manuscript.

Funding: A. Rincón was supported by Universidad Católica de Manizales. The work of F.E. Hoyos and John E. Candelo-Becerra were supported by Universidad Nacional de Colombia—Sede Medellín.

Institutional Review Board Statement: Not applicable.

Informed Consent Statement: Not applicable.

Data Availability Statement: Not applicable.

Acknowledgments: This work was supported by Universidad Católica de Manizales and Universidad Nacional de Colombia, Sede Medellín. Fredy E. Hoyos and John E. Candelo-Becerra thank the Departamento de Energía Eléctrica y Automática. The work of Alejandro Rincón was supported by Universidad Católica de Manizales.

Conflicts of Interest: The authors declare no conflict of interest.

References

1. Reis de Souza, A.; Gouzé, J.L.; Efimov, D.; Polyakov, A. Robust Adaptive Estimation in the Competitive Chemostat. *Comput. Chem. Eng.* **2020**, *142*, 107030. [CrossRef]
2. Zalai, D.; Kopp, J.; Kozma, B.; Küchler, M.; Herwig, C.; Kager, J. Microbial Technologies for Biotherapeutics Production: Key Tools for Advanced Biopharmaceutical Process Development and Control. *Drug Discov. Today Technol.* **2020**, *38*, 9–24. [CrossRef] [PubMed]
3. Torres Zúñiga, I.; Villa-Leyva, A.; Vargas, A.; Buitrón, G. Experimental Validation of Online Monitoring and Optimization Strategies Applied to a Biohydrogen Production Dark Fermenter. *Chem. Eng. Sci.* **2018**, *190*, 48–59. [CrossRef]
4. Lyubenova, V.N.; Ignatova, M.N. On-Line Estimation of Physiological States for Monitoring and Control of Bioprocesses. *AIMS Bioeng.* **2017**, *4*, 93–112. [CrossRef]
5. Zeinali, S.; Shahrokhi, M. Observer-Based Singularity Free Nonlinear Controller for Uncertain Systems Subject to Input Saturation. *Eur. J. Control* **2020**, *52*, 49–58. [CrossRef]
6. Ibáñez, F.; Saa, P.A.; Bárzaga, L.; Duarte-Mermoud, M.A.; Fernández-Fernández, M.; Agosin, E.; Pérez-Correa, J.R. Robust Control of Fed-Batch High-Cell Density Cultures: A Simulation-Based Assessment. *Comput. Chem. Eng.* **2021**, *155*, 107545. [CrossRef]
7. Nuñez, S.; Garelli, F.; de Battista, H. Closed-Loop Growth-Rate Regulation in Fed-Batch Dual-Substrate Processes with Additive Kinetics Based on Biomass Concentration Measurement. *J. Process Control* **2016**, *44*, 14–22. [CrossRef]
8. Jamilis, M.; Garelli, F.; de Battista, H. Growth Rate Maximization in Fed-Batch Processes Using High Order Sliding Controllers and Observers Based on Cell Density Measurement. *J. Process Control* **2018**, *68*, 23–33. [CrossRef]
9. Lara-Cisneros, G.; Femat, R.; Dochain, D. An Extremum Seeking Approach via Variable-Structure Control for Fed-Batch Bioreactors with Uncertain Growth Rate. *J. Process Control* **2014**, *24*, 663–671. [CrossRef]
10. Robles-Magdaleno, J.L.; Rodríguez-Mata, A.E.; Farza, M.; M'Saad, M. A Filtered High Gain Observer for a Class of Non Uniformly Observable Systems—Application to a Phytoplanktonic Growth Model. *J. Process Control* **2020**, *87*, 68–78. [CrossRef]
11. Noll, P.; Henkel, M. History and Evolution of Modeling in Biotechnology: Modeling & Simulation, Application and Hardware Performance. *Comput. Struct. Biotechnol. J.* **2020**, *18*, 3309–3323. [CrossRef]
12. Jamilis, M.; Garelli, F.; Mozumder, M.S.I.; Castañeda, T.; de Battista, H. Modeling and Estimation of Production Rate for the Production Phase of Non-Growth-Associated High Cell Density Processes. *Bioprocess Biosyst. Eng.* **2015**, *38*, 1903–1914. [CrossRef] [PubMed]
13. Jin, Z.; Wang, Z.; Zhang, X. Cooperative Control Problem of Takagi-Sugeno Fuzzy Multiagent Systems via Observer Based Distributed Adaptive Sliding Mode Control. *J. Franklin Inst.* **2022**, *359*, 3405–3426. [CrossRef]
14. Guo, R.; Feng, J.; Wang, J.; Zhao, Y. Leader-Following Successive Lag Consensus of Nonlinear Multi-Agent Systems via Observer-Based Event-Triggered Control. *J. Franklin Inst.* **2022**. [CrossRef]
15. Xiao, Y.; Che, W.W. Neural-Networks-Based Event-Triggered Consensus Tracking Control for Nonlinear MASs with DoS Attacks. *Neurocomputing* **2022**, *501*, 451–462. [CrossRef]
16. Miranda-Colorado, R. Observer-Based Saturated Proportional Derivative Control of Perturbed Second-Order Systems: Prescribed Input and Velocity Constraints. *ISA Trans.* **2022**, *122*, 336–345. [CrossRef]
17. Borkar, A.; Patil, P.M. Super Twisting Observer Based Full Order Sliding Mode Control. *Int. J. Dyn. Control* **2021**, *9*, 1653–1659. [CrossRef]
18. ben Tarla, L.; Bakhti, M.; Bououlid Idrissi, B. Implementation of Second Order Sliding Mode Disturbance Observer for a One-Link Flexible Manipulator Using Dspace Ds1104. *SN Appl. Sci.* **2020**, *2*, 485. [CrossRef]
19. Byun, G.; Kikuuwe, R. An Improved Sliding Mode Differentiator Combined with Sliding Mode Filter for Estimating First and Second-Order Derivatives of Noisy Signals. *Int. J. Control Autom. Syst.* **2020**, *18*, 3001–3014. [CrossRef]
20. Liu, W.; Chen, S.; Huang, H. Double Closed-Loop Integral Terminal Sliding Mode for a Class of Underactuated Systems Based on Sliding Mode Observer. *Int. J. Control Autom. Syst.* **2020**, *18*, 339–350. [CrossRef]
21. Besançon, G.; Voda, A.; Popescu, A. Closed-Loop-Based Observer Approach for Tunneling Current Parameter Estimation in an Experimental STM. *Mechatronics* **2022**, *83*, 102743. [CrossRef]
22. Hu, Q.; Jiang, B.; Zhang, Y. Observer-Based Output Feedback Attitude Stabilization for Spacecraft With Finite-Time Convergence. *IEEE Trans. Control Syst. Technol.* **2019**, *27*, 781–789. [CrossRef]
23. Coutinho, D.; Vargas, A.; Feudjio, C.; Benavides, M.; Wouwer, A. vande A Robust Approach to the Design of Super-Twisting Observers—Application to Monitoring Microalgae Cultures in Photo-Bioreactors. *Comput. Chem. Eng.* **2019**, *121*, 46–56. [CrossRef]

24. Rincón, A.; Hoyos, F.E.; Restrepo, G.M. Design and Evaluation of a Robust Observer Using Dead-Zone Lyapunov Functions—Application to Reaction Rate Estimation in Bioprocesses. *Fermentation* **2022**, *8*, 173. [CrossRef]
25. Kicki, P.; Łakomy, K.; Lee, K.M.B. Tuning of Extended State Observer with Neural Network-Based Control Performance Assessment. *Eur. J. Control* **2022**, *64*, 100609. [CrossRef]
26. Wang, P.; Zhang, X.; Zhu, J. Online Performance-Based Adaptive Fuzzy Dynamic Surface Control for Nonlinear Uncertain Systems Under Input Saturation. *IEEE Trans. Fuzzy Syst.* **2019**, *27*, 209–220. [CrossRef]
27. Madonski, R.; Shao, S.; Zhang, H.; Gao, Z.; Yang, J.; Li, S. General Error-Based Active Disturbance Rejection Control for Swift Industrial Implementations. *Control Eng. Pract.* **2019**, *84*, 218–229. [CrossRef]
28. Shi, S.; Lu, J.; Hu, Y.; Sun, Y. Robust Output-Feedback SOSM Control Subject to Unmatched Disturbances and Its Application: A Fixed-Time Observer-Based Method. *Nonlinear Anal. Hybrid Syst.* **2022**, *45*, 101210. [CrossRef]
29. Hans, S.; Joseph, F.O.M. Control of a Flexible Bevel-Tipped Needle Using Super-Twisting Controller Based Sliding Mode Observer. *ISA Trans.* **2021**, *109*, 186–198. [CrossRef]
30. Meng, R.; Chen, S.; Hua, C.; Qian, J.; Sun, J. Disturbance Observer-Based Output Feedback Control for Uncertain QUAVs with Input Saturation. *Neurocomputing* **2020**, *413*, 96–106. [CrossRef]
31. Abadi, A.S.S.; Hosseinabadi, P.A.; Mekhilef, S. Fuzzy Adaptive Fixed-Time Sliding Mode Control with State Observer for A Class of High-Order Mismatched Uncertain Systems. *Int. J. Control Autom. Syst.* **2020**, *18*, 2492–2508. [CrossRef]
32. Tang, Z.-L.; Tee, K.P.; He, W. Tangent Barrier Lyapunov Functions for the Control of Output-Constrained Nonlinear Systems. *IFAC Proc. Vol.* **2013**, *46*, 449–455. [CrossRef]
33. Rozgonyi, S.; Hangos, K.M.; Szederkényi, G. Determining the Domain of Attraction of Hybrid Non–Linear Systems Using Maximal Lyapunov Functions. *Kybernetika* **2010**, *46*, 19–37.
34. Sankar, K.; Thakre, N.; Singh, S.M.; Jana, A.K. Sliding Mode Observer Based Nonlinear Control of a PEMFC Integrated with a Methanol Reformer. *Energy* **2017**, *139*, 1126–1143. [CrossRef]
35. Valenciaga, F.; Inthamoussou, F.A. A Novel PV-MPPT Method Based on a Second Order Sliding Mode Gradient Observer. *Energy Convers. Manag.* **2018**, *176*, 422–430. [CrossRef]
36. Zhang, L.; Wang, Z.; Li, S.; Ding, S.; Du, H. Universal Finite-Time Observer Based Second-Order Sliding Mode Control for DC-DC Buck Converters with Only Output Voltage Measurement. *J. Franklin Inst.* **2020**, *357*, 11863–11879. [CrossRef]
37. Muñoz-Tamayo, R.; Martinon, P.; Bougaran, G.; Mairet, F.; Bernard, O. Getting the Most out of It: Optimal Experiments for Parameter Estimation of Microalgae Growth Models. *J. Process Control* **2014**, *24*, 991–1001. [CrossRef]

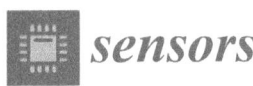

Article

Improved Individualized Patient-Oriented Depth-of-Hypnosis Measurement Based on Bispectral Index

Gorazd Karer * and Igor Škrjanc

Faculty of Electrical Engineering, University of Ljubljana, 1000 Ljubljana, Slovenia
* Correspondence: gorazd.karer@fe.uni-lj.si

Abstract: Total intravenous anesthesia is an anesthesiologic technique where all substances are injected intravenously. The main task of the anesthesiologist is to assess the depth of anesthesia, or, more specifically, the depth of hypnosis (DoH), and accordingly adjust the dose of intravenous anesthetic agents. However, it is not possible to directly measure the anesthetic agent concentrations or the DoH, so the anesthesiologist must rely on various vital signs and EEG-based measurements, such as the bispectral (BIS) index. The ability to better measure DoH is directly applicable in clinical practice—it improves the anesthesiologist's assessment of the patient state regarding anesthetic agent concentrations and, consequently, the effects, as well as provides the basis for closed-loop control algorithms. This article introduces a novel structure for modeling DoH, which employs a residual dynamic model. The improved model can take into account the patient's individual sensitivity to the anesthetic agent, which is not the case when using the available population-data-based models. The improved model was tested using real clinical data. The results show that the predictions of the BIS-index trajectory were improved considerably. The proposed model thus seems to provide a good basis for a more patient-oriented individualized assessment of DoH, which should lead to better administration methods that will relieve the anesthesiologist's workload and will benefit the patient by providing improved safety, individualized treatment, and, thus, alleviation of possible adverse effects during and after surgery.

Keywords: general anesthesia; total intravenous anesthesia; target-controlled infusion; propofol; BIS index; depth of hypnosis; improved mathematical model; population-data-based model; residual model

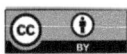

1. Introduction

Adequate general anesthesia (GA) is a prerequisite in surgeries as well as in various other medical procedures. The anesthesiologist must take care of three main aspects of the patient state during the procedure: besides considering the vital signs, they must administer substances that keep the patient deeply unconscious, prevent the patient from feeling pain, and keep the patient's muscles adequately relaxed. Furthermore, the patient must not be aware of, or even remember, what was happening during GA. Therefore, it is essential to properly administer the needed substances during the medical procedure.

GA and the dynamic response of the patient's body to anesthetic substances can be regarded as quite complex dynamic systems. Various pharmacokinetic (PK) and pharmacodynamic (PD) mechanisms take place inside the patient's body; however, it is unfortunately generally not yet possible to claim that these PK and PD systems have been completely studied or adequately modeled. Furthermore, the anesthetic depth is a controversial concept, which involves the three main aspects of hypnosis, analgesia, and muscle relaxation. In addition, amnesia must also be ensured. However, anesthetic depth cannot be directly measured.

The main job of the anesthesiologist is to monitor the patient's vital functions and properly maintain the functions of the patient's organs. Anesthetic agents are administered in various ways into the patient's body so as to achieve adequate GA: the two most commonly used methods in clinical practice are the intravenous administration induction of the anesthetic agent, i.e., injection of the anesthetic agent into a patient's vein, or the inhalatory administration of anesthetic agent, in which the substance is induced by the patient inhaling a prepared breathing mixture. If the anesthetic agents are injected intravenously, the anesthesiologic technique is known as *total intravenous anesthesia* (TIVA) [1,2]. In this article, we focus on TIVA administration exclusively.

During the medical procedure, the anesthesiologist aims to maintain the appropriate depth of hypnosis (DoH) by adjusting the dosage of the anesthetic agent. Clearly, the PK and PD of the anesthetic agent and the type of procedure must be taken into account, e.g., long-term sedation in an intensive care unit requires deeper DoH than GA during surgery. Too-deep anesthesia is manifested as a drop in blood pressure level and heart rate frequency as well as slow post-operative awakening of the patient from GA [3]. On the other hand, the opposite is also true. Moreover, inadequate depth of anesthesia results in the activation of sympathetic nerves, or, in the most unlikely event, with the patient awakening, which must be avoided at all costs [4]. In modern clinical practice, DoH is determined by assessing the relevant clinical signs (iris, sweating, movements), by interpreting hemodynamic measurements [5] and by estimating the DoH from EEG signals [6]. The latter is made possible by several established measurement systems, such as BIS index, NeuroSense, Narcotrend, Entropy (Scale and Response), WAV_{CNS}, and Patient State Index.

BIS index is a noninvasive measurement method. A BIS monitor is connected to electrodes on the patient's head and the bispectral index is calculated from the measured EEG signals. The BIS monitor provides a single dimensionless number, which ranges from 0 (equivalent to EEG silence) to 100. A BIS value between 40 and 60 indicates an appropriate level for GA, whereas a value below 40 is appropriate for long-term sedation due to head injuries. The reference can thus be set to the applicable value; the manner and speed of approaching the reference value depend on the specific characteristics of the procedure and the pharmacokinetics and pharmacodynamics of the substance in the patient's body. The BIS value can, therefore, be considered as a representation of the DoH, although some papers question the relevance of BIS measurement for representing hypnosis as a graded state during surgery [7,8]. The authors in [7] pointed out the poor correlation between BIS and serum concentrations of propofol, which calls into question the relevance of the BIS measurement in representing hypnosis as a graded state during surgery. When they included all values during anesthesia, there was a significant correlation between BIS and serum propofol, but the correlation was poor and disappeared when the outliers were removed. Their results do not seem to support the idea that BIS represents a continuous measure of DoH, assuming that elevated serum concentrations of propofol correspond to deeper hypnotic levels. However, because they have too few data points to test the correlation between serum concentration and BIS in individual patients, the reason could be that there are interindividual differences in sensitivity to propofol. They noted that a correlation could exist in a single patient but is not evident in data from many subjects.

In the literature, there are several approaches to modeling the effect of propofol, which is a hypnotic anesthetic agent. For this purpose, a number of PK and PD models have been developed, e.g., [9–12]. The models of propofol response define the general structure of the dynamic system, whereas the particular parameters depend on the individual patient's characteristics, such as gender, age, height, weight, etc., as well as the particular patient's individual sensitivity to the effects of propofol and their ability to have propofol eliminated from the body. Certain infusion pumps employ the PK models to enable *target controlled infusion* (TCI), where the pump sets the proper flow of the medication with regard to the model [13].

In the last years, an emerging paradigm in medicine seems to have grasped the idea of personalized medicine [14]. In the field of drug delivery systems, this includes modeling, control, analysis, and pharmacological studies, as well as development of novel medical devices and conducting of targeted clinical trials. In this regard, the systematic employment of dynamic-system analysis along with control theory offers a wide range of application opportunities in the medical domain [15–20]. Despite the fact that for TCI various PK models can be implemented, all having their own advantages and drawbacks, the Marsh [21] and Schnieder [22,23] models are mainly used in clinical practice. However, these models often do not reflect the actual dynamic properties that depend on individual sensitivity to the substance of the particular patient, which is generally not considered. For instance, the authors in [24] found that titration of propofol based on BIS monitoring allows a reduction in drug consumption that is associated with a similar decrease in propofol plasma concentrations compared with TCI. An inverse relationship between cardiac output and plasma propofol concentration was reported in [25]. In addition, the authors in [26] showed that remifentanil plasma concentrations during remifentanil and propofol anesthesia are influenced by cardiac output in a similar manner to propofol, although the metabolic sites are different. Because cardiac output is known not to be constant during anesthesia, this also significantly affects plasma concentrations and, thus, the effects of propofol and remifentanil. The authors concluded that actual blood concentrations of remifentanil and propofol may differ significantly from expected concentrations, especially when cardiac output is low. Cardiac output is therefore an important factor whose influence should be investigated in PK and PD models. This again supports the idea that individualized PK and PD modeling could improve anesthetic delivery methods. Therefore, approaches using population-based-data models often cannot ensure optimal performance, especially when treating a patient with a particularly considerable discrepancy from the population-data-based models. A population-data-based approach cannot yield universally usable models, even if a very large number of patients would be taken into account and despite the fact that only relatively healthy patients are considered.

The dynamic mathematical models can be directly used in clinical practice for assessing DoH-related variables by implementing them in soft sensors [27] or state observers [28], which would improve the anesthesiologist's assessment of the patient state regarding anesthetic agent concentrations and, consequently, the effects, hence benefiting the patients in the long run. In addition, the models can enable in silico testing of various potentially clinically implementable closed-loop control algorithms, e.g., PID-controller-based approaches [29–31]. Furthermore, they represent the basis for a number of advanced control approaches, such as robust control [32–34], model-predictive control [35,36], fuzzy-rule-based decision system [37], event-based control [38], etc. Despite difficulties in objective pain measurement [18,39], a number of articles also consider the inherent MIMO (or MISO) nature of the controlled system, which is due to drug interactions, especially when analgesics (such as remeifentanil) are considered [40–42].

The article introduces a novel structure for modeling DoH. The modeling framework results in an improved individualized assessment of DoH, which is reflected in better predictions of the related anesthetic agent concentrations as well as the measured BIS signal. The article is structured as follows. First, we introduce the basic three-compartmental model and the upgraded population-data-based model, namely, the PK and PD parts. Next, we introduce the improved model structure and present the residual dynamic model add-on. In Section 4, the identification procedure is presented, including the identification signals, filtering, and parameter estimation. This is further extended to online recursive parameter estimation. Next, we validate the improved model by comparing the simulated data for the particular patient to real clinically acquired data, which were logged during a surgery in a real clinical setting. We end the article with some concluding remarks.

2. Propofol Pharmacokinetic and Pharmacodynamic Modeling

The pharmacokinetics of the basic population-data-based model is described by the Schnider model [22,23]. A well-established three-compartmental model structure is used as the basis for dynamic relations. For details, see [43,44]. The internal dynamics of the model can be formulated using Equations (1)–(3).

$$\frac{dx_1}{dt} = \phi - k_{12}x_1 - k_{13}x_1 - k_{10}x_1 + k_{21}x_2 + k_{31}x_3 \qquad (1)$$

$$\frac{dx_2}{dt} = -k_{21}x_2 + k_{12}x_1 \qquad (2)$$

$$\frac{dx_3}{dt} = -k_{31}x_3 + k_{13}x_1 \qquad (3)$$

In Equations (1)–(3), the variables x_1, x_2, and x_3 represent the amount of the drug in compartments V_1, V_2, and V_3, respectively. The infusion flow rate is denoted as ϕ. As noted above, the parameters k_{12}, k_{21}, k_{13}, and k_{31} represent the partition coefficients that determine the speed at which the drug moves from one particular compartment to another. Finally, k_{10} is the rate of elimination of the drug from the patient's body. Note that the concentration in the central compartment is often referred to as plasmatic concentration.

The effect site for the drug propofol is basically the central nervous system. The effect site is thus part of the central compartment, but the effect of the drug is subject to some dynamics with regard to the (theoretical) concentration in the central compartment [44]. Therefore, a first-order model was used to describe the effect-site concentration dynamics, as given in Equation (4).

$$\frac{dx_e}{dt} = -k_{e0}x_e + k_{e0}x_1 \qquad (4)$$

The effect-site concentration of propofol is considered as the main influence on the DoH. Despite acknowledging that DoH is a multivariable and a not very easy to grasp concept, involving deep unconsciousness, analgesia, amnesia, and muscle relaxation, we want to keep the model as simple as possible, yet not too simple for our requirements. Therefore, we first assume that BIS index is an adequate measure for DoH, despite the fact that the assumption might be debatable [8,45,46]. Furthermore, we consider an SISO model, where the input represents propofol inflow, and the output represents the value of the BIS index.

Despite the fact that the PD effect mechanism has not been fully studied yet, in the literature, a sigmoid E_{max} model based on the general Hill equation [47] is usually considered, as given in Equation (5).

$$\begin{aligned} y_{BIS} &= y_{BIS}(x_e) \\ y_{BIS} &= BIS_0 - (BIS_0 - BIS_{min})\frac{x_e^\gamma}{x_{e50}^\gamma + x_e^\gamma} \end{aligned} \qquad (5)$$

In Equation (5), BIS_0 denotes the characteristic value for a fully awake patient, BIS_{min} stands for the minimum value of BIS index, and γ is the parameter that defines the nonlinear shape of the response curve.

Therefore, the combined model can be regarded structurally as a Wiener nonlinear model.

The parameters of the phamacokinetic model are taken from [22,23,48]. The values are given in Table 1.

Table 1. Parameter values.

Parameter	Value
V_c	4.271
k_{10}	$0.443 + 0.0107 \cdot (weight/\text{kg} - 77) -$ $- 0.0159 \cdot (LBM/\text{kg} - 59) +$ $+ 0.0062 \cdot (height/\text{cm} - 177)$ / min
k_{12}	$0.302 - 0.0056 \cdot (age/\text{years} - 53)$ / min
k_{13}	0.196 /min
k_{21}	$[1.29 - 0.024 \cdot (age/\text{years} - 53)] \cdot$ $\cdot [18.9 - 0.391 \cdot (age - 53)]^{-1}$ / min
k_{31}	0.0035 / min
k_{e0}	0.456 / min

Note that the values of model parameters depend on the patient's age, weight, height, and gender. Parameter LBM is calculated as given in Equation (6).

$$LBM = \begin{cases} 1.1 \cdot weight/\text{kg} - 128 \left(\frac{weight/\text{kg}}{height/\text{cm}} \right)^2 & ; \text{male} \\ 1.07 \cdot weight/\text{kg} - 148 \left(\frac{weight/\text{kg}}{height/\text{cm}} \right)^2 & ; \text{female} \end{cases} \quad (6)$$

The parameters of the BIS-index-effect output submodel (see Equation (5)) are set as suggested in [49] and are given in Table 2.

Table 2. Parameter values.

Parameter	Value
BIS_0	95.6
BIS_{min}	8.9
x_{e50}	2.23
γ	1.58

3. Residual Model Introduction—Improvement of the Population-Data-Based Model

Population-data-based mathematical models, such as the one described in the previous section, are regularly used in clinical practice, namely, for TCI propofol infusion, which has become a standard approach in administration of the anesthetic agent. In spite of this, we need to consider the fact that the available models are derived from population-based measurements, both regarding the pharmacokinetic and the pharmacodynamic part.

Prior to a medical procedure, the implemented mathematical model is always tuned to the particular patient's properties (e.g., age, weight, height, and gender). Despite this, the model is still based on a broader population sample that was involved in the measured-data gathering. Hence, it is impossible for such a model to take into account specific interpatient variabilities. Therefore, the basic population-data-based model can broadly predict DoH, but it can exhibit severe discrepancies from the actual BIS-indicated DoH of a particular patient, especially when the particular patient's sensitivity to the anesthetic agent is considerably different from the dynamics assumed in the mathematical model.

In order to improve the population-data-based model accuracy by taking into account the specific patient's individual dynamic properties, we propose an extension to the basic model structure. The whole model is then structured as follows: besides the population-data-based model, we introduce an additional residual model, which is intended to mathematically describe the dynamic discrepancy of the patient's particular sensitivity to anesthetic-agent infusion. The discrepancy signal represents the ideal residual model output. The improved model structure, with the additional residual dynamic add-on, is shown in Figure 1. The output of the improved model BIS_{sim} is, therefore, calculated as given in Equation (7).

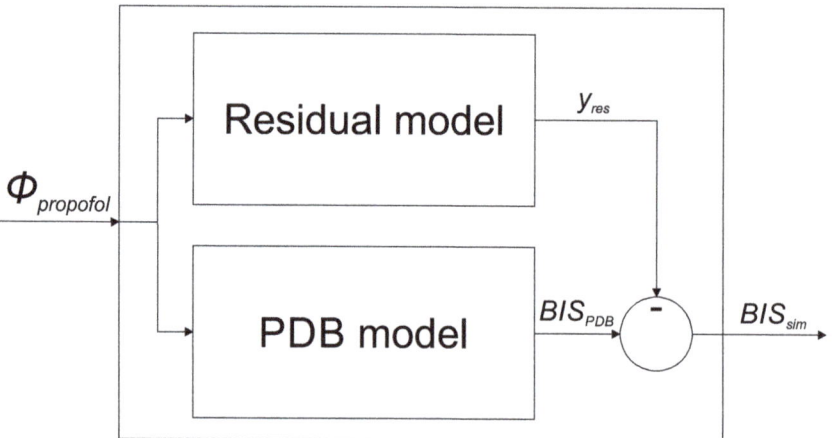

Figure 1. The improved model structure consisting of the population-data-based (PBD) model, and the residual dynamic model.

$$BIS_{sim} = BIS_{PDB} - y_{res} \qquad (7)$$

Here, BIS_{PDB} denotes the basic population-data-based model output, and y_{res} is the residual model output.

The goal of introducing the residual model is thus to improve the combined model output. This means that the combined model includes the population-data-based model as the basis for modeling the patient dynamic response to propofol. In addition, the residual model considers the particular patient's individual dynamic response to propofol, namely, the individual patient discrepancies from the population-data-based model, thus enabling a more accurate assessment of DoH expressed by BIS index. Note that the following conditions prevent a patient from being included in the study: patients with poor general condition (ASA > 3), patients with BMI > 35, drug addicts, patients taking psychotropic medicines or opioid analgesics (including tramadol), patients with a severe psychiatric disease or central nervous system disease (except the reason for surgery), patients with arrhythmia affecting or preventing the measurements (e.g., chronic atrial fibrillation), and patients that received benzodiazepines.

4. Identification of the Residual Dynamic Model

4.1. Identification Signals

The residual dynamic model is identified based on the data measured during a medical procedure treating an individual patient. The input of the residual dynamic model is the actual propofol inflow $\phi_{propofol}$, whereas its output is obtained by subtracting the actual measured BIS signal BIS_{data} from the population-data-based model output BIS_{PDB}, as shown in Equation (8). The latter is calculated according to the predefined population-data-based PK and PD model, taking into account the individual patient's properties.

Both signals are sampled using $T_s = 1$ s sampling rate. The whole experiment is therefore represented by two discrete-time signals in Equations (8) and (9).

$$y_{res,id}(z) = BIS_{PDB}(z) - BIS_{data}(z) \tag{8}$$

$$u_{res,id}(z) = \phi_{propofol}(z) \tag{9}$$

4.2. Residual Dynamic Model Structure

The structure of the residual dynamic model should be as simple as possible, but at the same time complex enough to be able to adequately model the patient's discrepancy from the population-data-based model. Despite that higher complexity of the models and possibly evolving identification could yield favorable approximations [50–52], especially if the identification data are noise-free, we established that an appropriate structure for our case is a second-order model, which is structured as an affine autoregressive model with exogenous inputs. Its discrete-time formulation is given in Equation (10).

$$y_{res}(t + T_s) = a_1 y_{res}(t) + a_2 y_{res}(t - T_s) + b_1 u_{res}(t) + c \tag{10}$$

Here, a_1, a_2, b_1, and c represent the parameters to be estimated. Note that t represents a particular time-instant of the model. A single step of the model T_s is not necessarily equal to the data-sampling rate $T_{s,data}$. In our case, it is $T_s = 5 \cdot T_{s,data} = 5$ s.

The model parameters can be gathered in the parameter vector Θ as given in Equation (11).

$$\Theta^T = [a_1, a_2, b_1, c] \tag{11}$$

The regressor is defined in Equation (12).

$$\Psi(t)^T = [y_{res}(t), y_{res}(t - T_s), u_{res}(t), 1] \tag{12}$$

In this way, Equation (10) can be rewritten in Equation (13).

$$y_{res}(t + T_s) = \Theta^T \Psi(t) \tag{13}$$

4.3. Parameter Estimation

The parameters of the residual dynamic model a_1, a_2, b_1, and c are estimated from the measured data concerning the particular patient.

As the measured BIS_{data} signal is prone to significant noise, the first step is to apply a suitable filter, which should ensure better identification results. We established that a simple first-order filter (with a filtering time-constant τ_f) is adequate. The filter can be represented by the transfer function in Equation (14). Its discrete-time equivalent is given in Equation (15).

$$\tau_f = 20 \text{ s}$$
$$H_f(s) = \frac{1}{\tau_f s + 1} = \frac{1}{20s + 1} \tag{14}$$

$$H_f(z) = \frac{0.04877}{z - 0.9512} \tag{15}$$

Finally, the filtered identification signals are given in Equations (16) and (17).

$$y_{res,id,f}(z) = H_f(z) y_{res,id}(z) \tag{16}$$

$$u_{res,id,f}(z) = H_f(z) u_{res,id}(z) \tag{17}$$

The filtered signals $y_{res,id,f}$ and $u_{res,id,f}$ are used for estimating the parameters of the residual dynamic model Θ.

The output data vector **Y** contains the output variable as given in Equation (18).

$$\mathbf{Y} = \begin{bmatrix} y_{res,id,f}(t_1) \\ \vdots \\ y_{res,id,f}(t_P) \end{bmatrix} \quad (18)$$

The regression matrix $\boldsymbol{\Psi}$ is obtained by using the whole set of measured data, as given in Equations (19) and (20).

$$\boldsymbol{\Psi} = \begin{bmatrix} \boldsymbol{\Psi}_f^T(t_1) \\ \vdots \\ \boldsymbol{\Psi}_f^T(t_P) \end{bmatrix} \quad (19)$$

$$\boldsymbol{\Psi}(t_i)_f^T = \begin{bmatrix} y_{res,id,f}(t_i), y_{res,id,f}(t_i - T_s), u_{res,id,f}(t_i), 1 \end{bmatrix} \quad (20)$$

Here, t_i represents a time instant concerning a particular identification data pair ($i = 1, \ldots, P$).

According to Equations (18)–(20) and (13), the parameters of the residual dynamic model Θ can be obtained using the least-squares identification method, as given in Equation (21).

$$\Theta = (\boldsymbol{\Psi}^T \boldsymbol{\Psi})^{-1} \boldsymbol{\Psi}^T \mathbf{Y} \quad (21)$$

5. Online Recursive Parameter Estimation

In order to implement the proposed modeling framework as an intelligent soft sensor for assessing DoH, we must be able to acquire the improved combined model for DoH during surgery. The population-data-based submodel is based on patient data and can be derived prior to surgery. On the other hand, the particular patient's individual dynamic response to propofol, namely, the individual patient discrepancies from the population-data-based model, can only be assessed after the measured data becomes available, i.e., either after finishing the medical procedure, as proposed in Section 4.3, which can rarely be used, or during the medical procedure as soon as new data become available. The latter approach enables the use of the improved model during the medical procedure.

The recursive parameter estimation is carried out as described below. The residual model in Equations (10) and (13) is linear in the parameters, therefore it is possible to analytically derive a least-squares estimate of the parameters. Furthermore, if the identified system parametersare expected to be time-varying, the online estimation algorithm can place more emphasis on newly acquired data and gradually discard older data. Therefore, the proposed approach implements a recursive least-squares identification with exponential forgetting [53]. The algorithm can consider a least-squares loss function for exponentially discarding older data as time passes. The model parameters are, therefore, estimated using Equations (22)–(24).

$$\hat{\Theta}(t) = \hat{\Theta}(t - T_s) + K(t)\left(y_{res,id,f}(t) - \boldsymbol{\Psi}_f^T(t)\hat{\Theta}(t - T_s)\right) \quad (22)$$

$$K(t) = P(t - T_s)\boldsymbol{\Psi}_f(t)\left(\lambda + \boldsymbol{\Psi}_f^T(t)P(t - T_s)\boldsymbol{\Psi}_f(t)\right)^{-1} \quad (23)$$

$$P(t) = \left(I - K(t)\boldsymbol{\Psi}_f^T(t)\right)P(t - T_s)/\lambda \quad (24)$$

In Equations (22)–(24), $P(t)$ denotes the covariance matrix ($P(t) \in \mathbb{R}^{n \times n}$), where n represents the length of the regressor. $\hat{\Theta}(t)$ denotes the vector of the identified or estimated process parameters, λ denotes the forgetting factor, and I is the unity matrix, where

$I \in \mathbb{R}^{n \times n}$. The recursive parameter estimation is carried out online—in every time step t—and returns the calculated parameters of the model $\hat{\Theta}(t)$.

The forgetting factor λ is defined in Equation (25), where t_λ stands for the time constant for the exponential forgetting and T_s is the sampling time.

$$\lambda = e^{-\frac{T_s}{t_\lambda}} \qquad (25)$$

The regressive parameter estimation method can consider time-varying dynamics of the identified process; therefore, exponential forgetting can be employed. The forgetting factor has to be set between $0 < \lambda \leq 1$. In this manner, the data used for parameter estimation are pondered, so that the last data are pondered by factor 1, whereas the data that are $k_s \cdot T_s$ time steps old are pondered only by a factor of λ^{k_s}.

The initial covariance matrix $P(0)$ has to be positive-definite and properly sized. If the regressive parameter estimation method is interpreted as a Kalman filter, it can be regarded as ensuring that the parameters are distributed with an initial covariance $P(0)$ and initial mean-values $\hat{\Theta}(0)$ [53].

In each time step t, a new estimation is calculated. The new parameter estimations $\hat{\Theta}(t)$ are recursively based on the estimations from the previous time step $t - T_s$ and the online newly measured data. Therefore, the resulting model adapts to the new measurements as soon as they are available.

6. Model Validation Based on Real Clinical Data

In order to validate the proposed modeling approach, we gathered real data during a TIVA medical procedure. In our case, the treated patient was a 46-year-old male who weighed 59 kg and was 175 cm tall.

6.1. Recorded Signals

The signal denoting the inflow of propofol $\phi_{propofol}$ was parsed from the clinically recorded data and is shown in Figure 2. One can see that, firstly, a bolus dose is introduced in order to rapidly increase the concentration of propofol in the body. This phase is called the induction of anesthesia and results in the patient losing consciousness. Later, a suitable dose of propofol is continuously administered in order to keep the proper anesthetic depth.

The recorded BIS_{data} signal for the particular treated patient is shown in Figure 3. The plasmatic concentration of propofol c_p and effect-site concentration of propofol c_e are obtained by simulating the dynamic model defined in Equations (1)–(4) based on the measured inflow signal of propofol $\phi_{propofol}$. Next, the population-data-based BIS trajectory BIS_{PDB} is obtained according to Equation (5). Finally, it is possible to obtain the identification signals for the residual dynamic model $y_{res,id,f}$ and $u_{res,id,f}$ using Equations (8), (9), and (15)–(17). The identification signals are shown in Figure 4. Note that only the relevant interval of the measured data is considered.

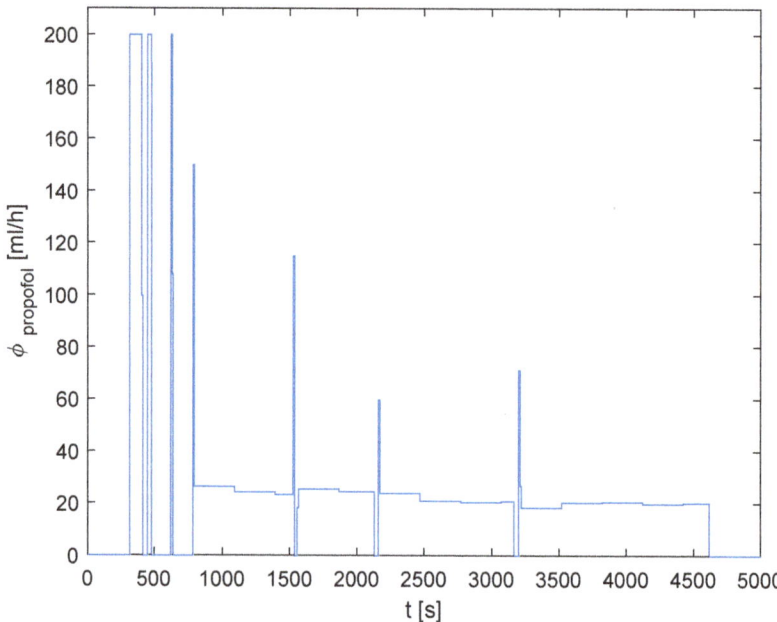

Figure 2. The inflow of propofol $\phi_{propofol}$.

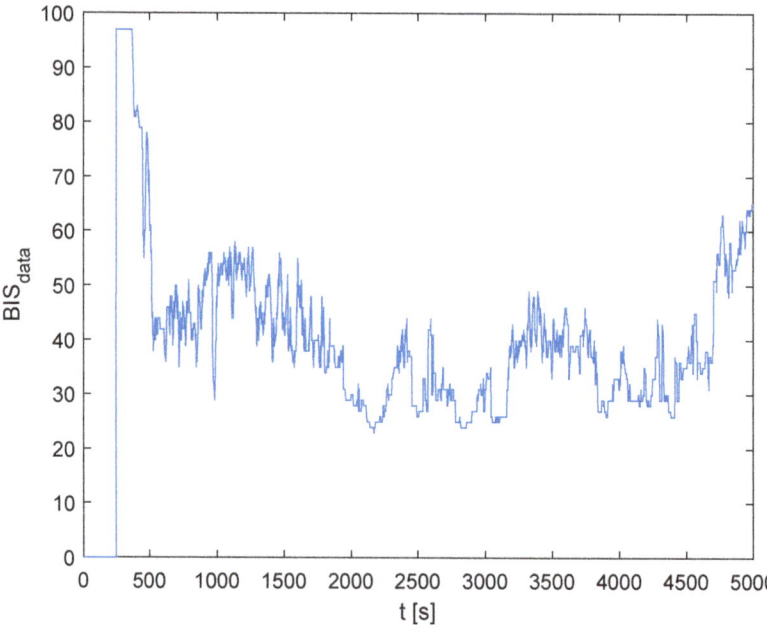

Figure 3. The measured BIS trajectory BIS_{data}.

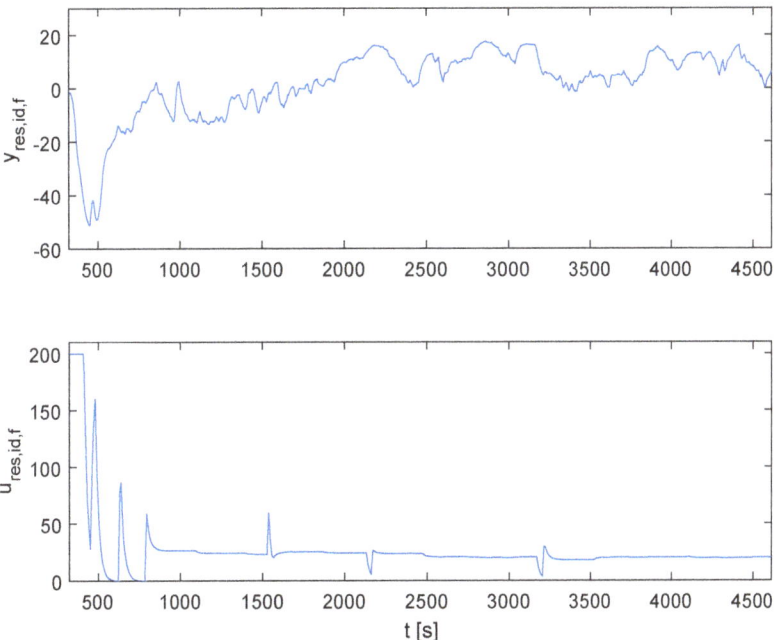

Figure 4. The identification signals for the residual dynamic model $y_{res,id,f}$ and $u_{res,id,f}$.

6.2. Identification Results

The final resulting parameters of the residual dynamic model are given in Equation (26).

$$\Theta^T = [1.7376, -0.7469, -0.0053, 0.1638] \tag{26}$$

When conducting online recursive parameter estimation, the parameters converge to the values in Equation (26). Before starting, the initial values for the algorithm are set as given in Equations (27)–(29).

$$P(0) = 100 \cdot I = \begin{bmatrix} 100 & 0 & 0 & 0 \\ 0 & 100 & 0 & 0 \\ 0 & 0 & 100 & 0 \\ 0 & 0 & 0 & 100 \end{bmatrix} \tag{27}$$

$$\hat{\Theta}^T(0) = [1.7242, -0.7356, -0.0040, 0.1729] \tag{28}$$

$$\lambda = 1 \tag{29}$$

As the recursive parameter estimation is carried out, the parameters a_1, a_2, b_1, and c change their values along the trajectories shown in Figure 5.

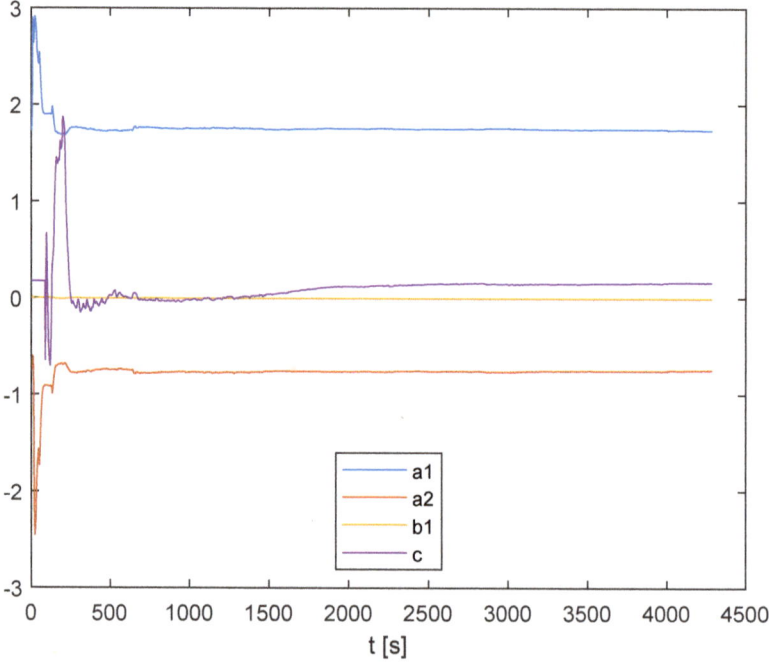

Figure 5. Online recursive parameter estimation.

6.3. Model Validation

In order to validate the obtained model, we employ a quantitative measure for predictive quality assessment, which is often used in the literature, namely, the *prediction mean square error* (PMSE). It is calculated according to Equation (30).

$$PMSE_x = \frac{1}{N}\sum_{i=1}^{N}(x_{i,sim} - x_{i,data})^2 \qquad (30)$$

Furthermore, there are two more quantitative measures that are often used in the literature to compare the simulated and the measured signal, such as the BIS-index trajectory: the *median performance error* (MDPE), which is calculated according to Equation (31), and *median absolute performance error* (MDAPE), which is calculated according to Equation (32).

$$MDPE_x = median\{\frac{x_{i,data} - x_{i,sim}}{x_{i,sim}} \cdot 100\%\}_{i=1,\ldots,N} \qquad (31)$$

$$MDAPE_x = median\{|\frac{x_{i,data} - x_{i,sim}}{x_{i,sim}}| \cdot 100\%\}_{i=1,\ldots,N} \qquad (32)$$

In Equations (30)–(32), x_{sim} and x_{data} denote the simulated and the measured data, respectively, whereas N stands for the number of data points in the dataset.

Figure 6 shows the output of the residual dynamic model y_{res} compared to the measurements-based trajectory $y_{res,id,f}$.

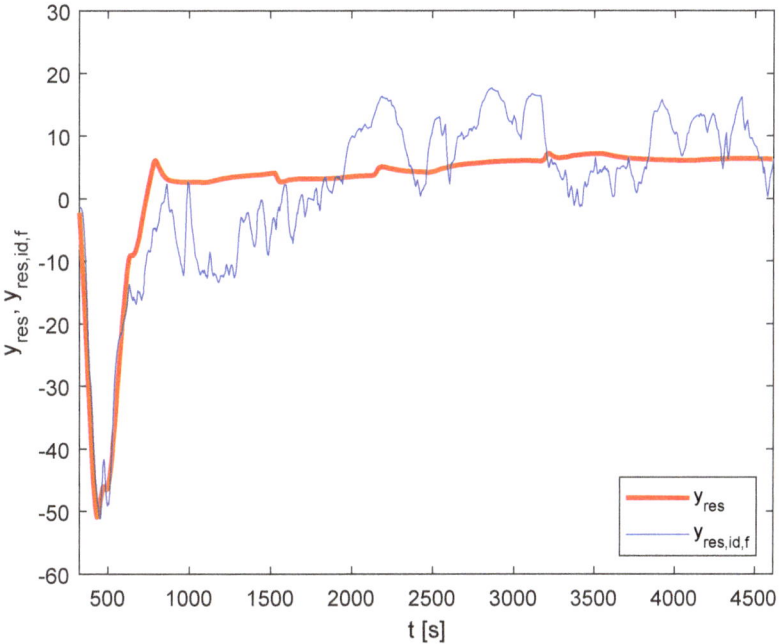

Figure 6. Residual dynamic model validation: y_{res} and $y_{res,id,f}$.

Finally, the output of the improved model is calculated according to Equation (7). The relevant *BIS* trajectories are shown in Figure 7.

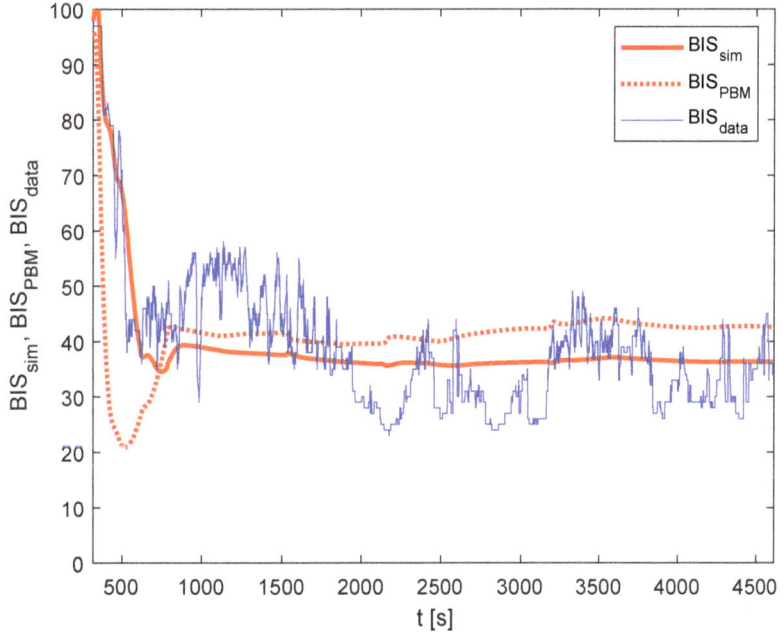

Figure 7. Improved model validation: BIS_{sim}, BIS_{PBM}, and BIS_{data}.

For the case of the particular patient and medical procedure, the calculated criteria for y_{res} and BIS are given in Table 3 and Table 4, respectively.

Table 3. Predictive quality measures for y_{res}.

y_{res}	PMSE	MDPE	MDAPE
Without residual model	166.0	N/A	N/A
With residual model	50.8	−4.88	101.4
Improvement	3.27	N/A	N/A

The presented residual dynamic model reduces the PMSE of the difference between y_{res} and $y_{res,id,f}$ from 166.0 to 50.8; therefore, the improvement factor is 3.27.

Table 4. Predictive quality measures for BIS.

BIS	PMSE	MDPE	MDAPE
Without residual model	179.8	−10.85%	22.56%
With residual model	63.3	−0.605%	16.92%
Improvement	2.84	10.24%	5.64%

The implementation of the improved model reduces the PMSE from 179.8 (BIS_{BMS} and BIS_{data}) to 63.3 (for BIS_{sim} and BIS_{data}). In this case, the improvement factor is 2.84. Furthermore, the MDPE criterion improved by 10.24%, and MDAPE by 5.64%.

The main limitation of the proposed model is that it cannot be rigorously validated for a specific patient before its implementation because of its dependence on online measurements collected during the medical procedure. Moreover, no two anesthetic applications are alike, even if the same patient undergoes the same type of surgery several times, for example. Since the dynamic characteristics of the patient may change over time, it is not possible to compare the performance in two different interventions even if the same patient is treated. Because we cannot claim that the individualized dynamic model in question is time-invariant in the long run, it cannot be validated by using a special validation dataset that is strictly separate from the dataset used for identification. Furthermore, as the goal of the additional residual model is to consider the individual patient's discrepancy from the population-data-based model, it is not sensible to cross-validate it using another patient's measurements.

On the other hand, the results suggest that a significant improvement can be achieved, compared with the approach based only on the population-data-based model. In the future, the modeling framework will be further verified with several more datasets on different individuals treated with TIVA.

7. Conclusions

The article introduces a novel structure for modeling DoH, resulting in an improved individualized assessment of DoH, which is reflected in better predictions of the measured BIS signal. The presented model structure for modeling DoH dynamics employs the residual dynamic model add-on, which is used to model a particular treated patient's individual dynamic discrepancies from the population-data-based model. In such a manner, the model can take into account the patient's individual sensitivity to the anesthetic agent, which is not the case when using the population-data-based model exclusively, e.g., when using TCI, as is often the case in clinical practice. Therefore, the proposed modeling framework provides an improved mechanism for predicting DoH measured by the BIS index.

The improved model was verified using real clinical data logged during a medical treatment of a particular patient that lasted a little more than one hour. The results show that the predictions of the BIS-index trajectory were, indeed, considerably improved. Hence, the improved model seems to provide a solid foundation for better simulations as well as for the implementation in closed-loop model-based predictive control of DoH. The modeling framework will be further verified with several more datasets concerning various individuals that have been treated with TIVA.

To sum up, the presented framework provides a basis for a more patient-oriented individualized model for assessing DoH. The model seems to provide a deeper insight into DoH dynamics, which should lead to better administration methods that will relieve the anesthesiologist's workload and will benefit the patient by providing improved safety, individualized treatment, and, thus, alleviation of possible adverse effects during and after surgery.

Author Contributions: Conceptualization, G.K. and I.Š.; methodology, G.K. and I.Š.; software, G.K. and I.Š.; validation, G.K. and I.Š.; formal analysis, G.K. and I.Š.; investigation, G.K. and I.Š.; resources, G.K. and I.Š.; data curation, G.K. and I.Š.; writing—original draft preparation, G.K. and I.Š.; writing—review and editing, G.K. and I.Š.; visualization, G.K. and I.Š.; supervision, G.K. and I.Š.; project administration, G.K. and I.Š.; funding acquisition, I.Š. All authors have read and agreed to the published version of the manuscript.

Funding: The authors acknowledge the financial support from the Slovenian Research Agency [research core funding number P2-0219].

Institutional Review Board Statement: Not applicable.

Informed Consent Statement: Informed consent was obtained from all subjects involved in the study.

Data Availability Statement: The data used are available upon request to the corresponding author.

Acknowledgments: The authors would like to thank Iztok Potočnik and Vesna Novak-Jankovič from University Medical Centre Ljubljana for providing the measured data.

Conflicts of Interest: The authors declare no conflict of interest.

References

1. Al-Rifai, Z.; Mulvey, D. Principles of total intravenous anaesthesia: Practical aspects of using total intravenous anaesthesia. *BJA Educ.* **2016**, *16*, 276–280. [CrossRef]
2. Absalom, A.R.; Glen, J.B.; Zwart, G.J.; Schnider, T.W.; Struys, M.M. Target-Controlled Infusion: A Mature Technology. *Anesth. Analg.* **2016**, *122*, 70–78. [CrossRef]
3. Wesselink, E.M.; Kappen, T.H.; Torn, H.M.; Slooter, A.J.; van Klei, W.A. Intraoperative hypotension and the risk of postoperative adverse outcomes: A systematic review. *Br. J. Anaesth.* **2018**, *121*, 706–721. [CrossRef]
4. Tasbihgou, S.R.; Vogels, M.F.; Absalom, A.R. Accidental awareness during general anaesthesia–A narrative review. *Anaesthesia* **2018**, *73*, 112–122. [CrossRef]
5. Potočnik, I.; Janković, V.N.; Štupnik, T.; Kremžar, B. Haemodynamic changes after induction of anaesthesia with sevoflurane vs. propofol. *Signa Vitae* **2011**, *6*, 52–57.
6. Musizza, B.; Ribaric, S. Monitoring the Depth of Anaesthesia. *Sensors* **2010**, *10*, 10896–10935. [CrossRef]
7. Hoymork, S.C.; Raeder, J.; Grimsmo, B.; Steen, P.A. Bispectral index, serum drug concentrations and emergence associated with individually adjusted target-controlled infusions of remifentanil and propofol for laparoscopic surgery. *Br. J. Anaesth.* **2003**, *91*, 773–780. [CrossRef]
8. Sleigh, J.W. Depth of AnesthesiaPerhaps the Patient Isn't a Submarine. *Anesthesiology* **2011**, *115*, 1149–1150. [CrossRef]
9. Kataria, B.K.; Ved, S.A.; Nicodemus, H.F.; Hoy, G.R.; Lea, D.; Dubois, M.Y.; Mandema, J.W.; Shafer, S.L. The pharmacokinetics of propofol in children using three different data analysis approaches. *Anesthesiology* **1994**, *80*, 104–122. [CrossRef]
10. Schüttler, J.; Ihmsen, H. Population pharmacokinetics of propofol: A multicenter study. *Anesthesiology* **2000**, *92*, 727–738. [CrossRef]
11. Kenny, G.N.; White, M. Intravenous propofol anaesthesia using a computerised infusion system. *Anaesthesia* **1990**, *46*, 204–209. [CrossRef]
12. Eleveld, D.J.; Colin, P.; Absalom, A.R.; Struys, M.M. Pharmacokinetic–pharmacodynamic model for propofol for broad application in anaesthesia and sedation. *Br. J. Anaesth.* **2018**, *120*, 942–959. [CrossRef]

13. Neckebroek, M.; Ionescu, C.M.; van Amsterdam, K.; Smet, T.D.; Baets, P.D.; Decruyenaere, J.; Keyser, R.D.; Struys, M.M. A comparison of propofol-to-BIS post-operative intensive care sedation by means of target controlled infusion, Bayesian-based and predictive control methods: An observational, open-label pilot study. *J. Clin. Monit. Comput.* **2019**, *33*, 675–686. [CrossRef]
14. Ionescu, C.M.; Neckebroek, M.; Ghita, M.; Copot, D. An Open Source Patient Simulator for Design and Evaluation of Computer Based Multiple Drug Dosing Control for Anesthetic and Hemodynamic Variables. *IEEE Access* **2021**. [CrossRef]
15. Brogi, E.; Cyr, S.; Kazan, R.; Giunta, F.; Hemmerling, T.M. Clinical Performance and Safety of Closed-Loop Systems. *Anesth. Analg.* **2017**, *124*, 446–455. [CrossRef]
16. Zaouter, C.; Joosten, A.; Rinehart, J.; Struys, M.M.; Hemmerling, T.M. Autonomous systems in anesthesia: Where do we stand in 2020? A narrative review. *Anesth. Analg.* **2020**, 1120–1132. [CrossRef]
17. Pasin, L.; Nardelli, P.; Pintaudi, M.; Greco, M.; Zambon, M.; Cabrini, L.; Zangrillo, A. Closed-loop delivery systems versus manually controlled administration of total IV Anesthesia: A meta-analysis of randomized clinical trials. *Anesth. Analg.* **2017**, *124*, 456–464. [CrossRef]
18. Ghita, M.; Neckebroek, M.; Juchem, J.; Copot, D.; Muresan, C.I.; Ionescu, C.M. Bioimpedance Sensor and Methodology for Acute Pain Monitoring. *Sensors* **2020**, *20*, 6765. [CrossRef]
19. Puri, G.D.; Kumar, B.; Aveek, J. Closed-loop anaesthesia delivery system (CLADS™) using bispectral index: A performance assessment study. *Anaesth. Intensive Care* **2007**, *35*, 357–362. [CrossRef]
20. Liu, N.; Chazot, T.; Trillat, B.; Pirracchio, R.; Law-Koune, J.D.; Barvais, L.; Fischler, M. Feasibility of closed-loop titration of propofol guided by the Bispectral Index for general anaesthesia induction: A prospective randomized study. *Eur. J. Anaesthesiol.* **2006**, *23*, 465–469. [CrossRef]
21. Marsh, B.; White, M.; Morton, N.; Kenny, G.N. Pharmacokinetic model driven infusion of propofol in children. *Br. J. Anaesth.* **1991**, *67*, 41–48. [CrossRef]
22. Schnider, T.W.; Minto, C.F.; Gambus, P.L.; Andresen, C.; Goodale, D.B.; Shafer, S.L.; Youngs, E.J. The influence of method of administration and covariates on the pharmacokinetics of propofol in adult volunteers. *Anesthesiology* **1998**, *88*, 1170–1182. [CrossRef]
23. Schnider, T.W.; Minto, C.F.; Shafer, S.L.; Gambus, P.L.; Andresen, C.; Goodale, D.B.; Youngs, E.J. The influence of age on propofol pharmacodynamics. *Anesthesiology* **1999**, *90*, 1502–1516. [CrossRef]
24. Bauer, M.; Wilhelm, W.; Kraemer, T.; Kreuer, S.; Brandt, A.; Adams, H.A.; Hoff, G.; Larsen, R. Impact of bispectral index monitoring on stress response and propofol consumption in patients undergoing coronary artery bypass surgery. *Anesthesiology* **2004**, *101*, 1096–1104. [CrossRef]
25. Kurita, T.; Morita, K.; Kazama, T.; Sato, S. Influence of cardiac output on plasma propofol concentrations during constant infusion in swine. *Anesthesiology* **2002**, *96*, 1498–1503. [CrossRef]
26. Kurita, T.; Uraoka, M.; Jiang, Q.; Suzuki, M.; Morishima, Y.; Morita, K.; Sato, S. Influence of cardiac output on the pseudo-steady state remifentanil and propofol concentrations in swine. *Acta Anaesthesiol. Scand.* **2013**, *57*, 754–760. [CrossRef]
27. Blažič, A.; Škrjanc, I.; Logar, V. Soft sensor of bath temperature in an electric arc furnace based on a data-driven Takagi–Sugeno fuzzy model. *Appl. Soft Comput.* **2021**, *113*, 107949. [CrossRef]
28. Nogueira, F.N.; Mendonça, T.; Rocha, P. Positive state observer for the automatic control of the depth of anesthesia—Clinical results. *Comput. Methods Programs Biomed.* **2019**, *171*, 99–108. [CrossRef]
29. Schiavo, M.; Padula, F.; Latronico, N.; Paltenghi, M.; Visioli, A. A modified PID-based control scheme for depth-of-hypnosis control: Design and experimental results. *Comput. Methods Programs Biomed.* **2022**, *219*, 106763. [CrossRef]
30. Padula, F.; Ionescu, C.; Latronico, N.; Paltenghi, M.; Visioli, A.; Vivacqua, G. Optimized PID control of depth of hypnosis in anesthesia. *Comput. Methods Programs Biomed.* **2017**, *144*, 21–35. [CrossRef]
31. Gonzalez-Cava, J.M.; Carlson, F.B.; Troeng, O.; Cervin, A.; van Heusden, K.; Dumont, G.A.; Soltesz, K. Robust PID control of propofol anaesthesia: Uncertainty limits performance, not PID structure. *Comput. Methods Programs Biomed.* **2021**, *198*, 105783. [CrossRef]
32. Hosseinzadeh, M. Robust control applications in biomedical engineering: Control of depth of hypnosis. *Control. Appl. Biomed. Eng. Syst.* **2020**, 89–125. [CrossRef]
33. Dumont, G.A.; Martinez, A.; Ansermino, J.M. Robust control of depth of anesthesia. *Int. J. Adapt. Control. Signal Process.* **2009**, *23*, 435–454. [CrossRef]
34. Heusden, K.V.; Dumont, G.A.; Soltesz, K.; Petersen, C.L.; Umedaly, A.; West, N.; Ansermino, J.M. Design and clinical evaluation of robust PID control of propofol anesthesia in children. *IEEE Trans. Control. Syst. Technol.* **2014**, *22*, 491–501. [CrossRef]
35. Sawaguchi, Y.; Furutani, E.; Shirakami, G.; Araki, M.; Fukuda, K. A model-predictive hypnosis control system under total intravenous anesthesia. *IEEE Trans. Biomed. Eng.* **2008**, *55*, 874–887. [CrossRef]
36. Pawłowski, A.; Schiavo, M.; Latronico, N.; Paltenghi, M.; Visioli, A. Model predictive control using MISO approach for drug co-administration in anesthesia. *J. Process Control* **2022**, *117*, 98–111. [CrossRef]
37. Mendez, J.A.; Leon, A.; Marrero, A.; Gonzalez-Cava, J.M.; Reboso, J.A.; Estevez, J.I.; Gomez-Gonzalez, J.F. Improving the anesthetic process by a fuzzy rule based medical decision system. *Artif. Intell. Med.* **2018**, *84*, 159–170. [CrossRef]
38. Merigo, L.; Beschi, M.; Padula, F.; Latronico, N.; Paltenghi, M.; Visioli, A. Event-Based control of depth of hypnosis in anesthesia. *Comput. Methods Programs Biomed.* **2017**, *147*, 63–83. [CrossRef]

39. Neckebroek, M.; Ghita, M.; Ghita, M.; Copot, D.; Ionescu, C.M. Pain Detection with Bioimpedance Methodology from 3-Dimensional Exploration of Nociception in a Postoperative Observational Trial. *J. Clin. Med.* **2020**, *9*, 684. [CrossRef]
40. Janda, M.; Schubert, A.; Bajorat, J.; Hofmockel, R.; Nöldge-Schomburg, G.F.; Lampe, B.P.; Simanski, O. Design and implementation of a control system reflecting the level of analgesia during general anesthesia. *Biomed. Tech.* **2013**, *58*, 1–11. . [CrossRef]
41. Hemmerling, T.M.; Arbeid, E.; Wehbe, M.; Cyr, S.; Taddei, R.; Zaouter, C.; Reilly, C.S. Evaluation of a novel closed-loop total intravenous anaesthesia drug delivery system: A randomized controlled trial. *Br. J. Anaesth.* **2013**, *110*, 1031–1039. [CrossRef] [PubMed]
42. Peñaranda, C.C.; Arroyave, F.D.C.; Gómez, F.J.; Corredor, P.A.P.; Fernández, J.M.; Botero, M.V.; Bedoya, J.D.B.; Toro, C.M. Technical and clinical evaluation of a closed loop TIVA system with SEDLineTM spectral density monitoring: Multicentric prospective cohort study. *Perioper. Med.* **2020**, *9*, 1–11. [CrossRef] [PubMed]
43. Karer, G. Modelling of Target-Controlled Infusion of Propofol for Depth-of-Anaesthesia Simulation in Matlab-Simulink. In *Proceedings of The 9th EUROSIM Congress on Modelling and Simulation, EUROSIM 2016, The 57th SIMS Conference on Simulation and Modelling SIMS 2016*; Linköping University Electronic Press: Linköping, Sweden, 2018; Volume 142, pp. 49–54. [CrossRef]
44. Karer, G.; Novak-Jankovič, V.; Stecher, A.; Potočnik, I. Modelling of BIS-Index Dynamics for Total Intravenous Anesthesia Simulation in Matlab-Simulink. *IFAC PapersOnLine* **2018**, *51*, 355–360. [CrossRef]
45. Ni, K.; Cooter, M.; Gupta, D.K.; Thomas, J.; Hopkins, T.J.; Miller, T.E.; James, M.L.; Kertai, M.D.; Berger, M. Paradox of age: older patients receive higher age-adjusted minimum alveolar concentration fractions of volatile anaesthetics yet display higher bispectral index values. *Br. J. Anaesth.* **2019**, *123*, 288–297. [CrossRef]
46. Kreuzer, M.; Stern, M.A.; Hight, D.; Berger, S.; Schneider, G.; Sleigh, J.W.; Garciá, P.S. Spectral and Entropic Features Are Altered by Age in the Electroencephalogram in Patients under Sevoflurane Anesthesia. *Anesthesiology* **2020**, *132*, 1003–1016. [CrossRef]
47. Goutelle, S.; Maurin, M.; Rougier, F.; Barbaut, X.; Bourguignon, L.; Ducher, M.; Maire, P. The Hill equation: A review of its capabilities in pharmacological modelling. *Fundam. Clin. Pharmacol.* **2008**, *22*, 633–648. [CrossRef]
48. *Operator's Guide*: Infusion Workstation: Orchestra Base Primea. Available online: https://www.google.com.hk/url?sa=t&rct=j&q=&esrc=s&source=web&cd=&ved=2ahUKEwiUuIrb1Jb8AhWmr1YBHV7oAjAQFnoECAkQAQ&url=http%3A%2F%2Fwww.frankshospitalworkshop.com%2Fequipment%2Fdocuments%2Finfusion_pumps%2Fuser_manuals%2FFresenius%2520Orchestra%2520Base%2520Unit%2520-%2520User%2520manual.pdf&usg=AOvVaw0-StEgOXitUKevQvWEwzsx (accessed on 26 October 2022).
49. Martín-Mateos, I.; Méndez, J.A.; Reboso, J.A.; León, A. Modelling propofol pharmacodynamics using BIS-guided anaesthesia. *Anaesthesia* **2013**, *68*, 1132–1140. [CrossRef]
50. Andonovski, G.; Lughofer, E.; Skrjanc, I. Evolving Fuzzy Model Identification of Nonlinear Wiener-Hammerstein Processes. *IEEE Access* **2021**, *9*, 158470–158480. [CrossRef]
51. Škrjanc, I.; Andonovski, G.; Iglesias, J.A.; Sesmero, M.P.; Sanchis, A. Evolving Gaussian on-line clustering in social network analysis. *Expert Syst. Appl.* **2022**, *207*, 117881. [CrossRef]
52. Ožbot, M.; Lughofer, E.; Škrjanc, I. Evolving Neuro-Fuzzy Systems based Design of Experiments in Process Identification. *IEEE J. Mag. | IEEE Xplore* **2022**. [CrossRef]
53. Åström, K.J.; Wittenmark, B. *Adaptive Control*, 2nd ed.; Addison-Wesley Publishing Company: Boston, MA, USA, 1995.

Disclaimer/Publisher's Note: The statements, opinions and data contained in all publications are solely those of the individual author(s) and contributor(s) and not of MDPI and/or the editor(s). MDPI and/or the editor(s) disclaim responsibility for any injury to people or property resulting from any ideas, methods, instructions or products referred to in the content.

Hybrid Feature Fusion-Based High-Sensitivity Fire Detection and Early Warning for Intelligent Building Systems

Shengyuan Xiao [1], Shuo Wang [2], Liang Ge [3,*], Hengxiang Weng [3], Xin Fang [3], Zhenming Peng [1] and Wen Zeng [4]

[1] School of Information and Communication Engineering, University of Electronic Science and Technology of China, Chengdu 611731, China
[2] School of Chemistry and Chemical Engineering, Southwest Petroleum University, Chengdu 610500, China
[3] School of Mechanical and Electronic Engineering, Southwest Petroleum University, Chengdu 610500, China
[4] School of Materials Science and Engineering, Chongqing University, Chongqing 400044, China
* Correspondence: cgroad@swpu.edu.cn

Abstract: High-sensitivity early fire detection is an essential prerequisite to intelligent building safety. However, due to the small changes and erratic fluctuations in environmental parameters in the initial combustion phase, it is always a challenging task. To address this challenge, this paper proposes a hybrid feature fusion-based high-sensitivity early fire detection and warning method for in-building environments. More specifically, the temperature, smoke concentration, and carbon monoxide concentration were first selected as the main distinguishing attributes to indicate an in-building fire. Secondly, the propagation neural network (BPNN) and the least squares support vector machine (LSSVM) were employed to achieve the hybrid feature fusion. In addition, the genetic algorithm (GA) and particle swarm optimization (PSO) were also introduced to optimize the BPNN and the LSSVM, respectively. After that, the outputs of the GA-BPNN and the PSO-LSSVM were fused to make a final decision by means of the D-S evidence theory, achieving a highly sensitive and reliable early fire detection and warning system. Finally, an early fire warning system was developed, and the experimental results show that the proposed method can effectively detect an early fire with an accuracy of more than 96% for different types and regions of fire, including polyurethane foam fire, alcohol fire, beech wood smolder, and cotton woven fabric smolder.

Keywords: early fire warning; hybrid feature fusion; intelligent building system; D-S evidence theory

1. Introduction

Over the past few years, building fires have been one of the most common and frequent types of fire, causing severe property losses and fatalities [1–3]. Thus, it has become extremely important and imperative to effectively decrease and control the risk of fire in buildings. One of the most critical technologies is early fire warning, and both academia and industry are exploring approaches that enable the prompt detection and accurate determination of scene conditions in the early stages of building fires [4]. Furthermore, with the development of intelligent buildings, an effective early fire detection and warning system is also an essential prerequisite to provide safe, healthy, and comfortable residential or working conditions.

For achieving early fire detection and warning inside building environments, many algorithms have been presented, which can be mainly divided into three categories, namely optical, smoke, and carbon-monoxide sensors. Li et al. [5,6] conducted a fire detection algorithm performance evaluation based on image complexity, which could accurately determine the detection level of the detection algorithm under different image complexity conditions. Li et al. [7] proposed a new hybrid model for fire prediction based on the visual information of RGB images. The model achieves promising performance, which also shows the potential to monitor the constant changes in a building fire through the continuous processing of images of flames. Xie et al. [8] employed an early fire detection method for shielded indoor environments based on fire light reflection characteristics and established a multi-expert system by extracting the change characteristics of the fire area with light reflection. They then verified the method based on a large data evaluation system. However, in the above methods, they ignored the early stages of the fire that may not involve the open flame but cannot determine the correct scene conditions in time. The temperature, another major feature of fire, has also attracted significant attention. Ji et al. [9] proposed a machine-learning-based real-time prediction method for monitoring physical parameters for early fire warnings based on temperatures. The results show that the trained intelligences improve the accuracy and reliability of building fire warnings. Sun et al. [10] verified a bio-inspired artificial intelligence algorithm driven by temperature data to detect fire in 3D spaces. Yusuf et al. [3] presented a linearly regressive artificial-neural-network-based technique to predict temperature increases caused by building fire environments. This method predicts temperature ranges in a burning compartment based on the historic fire behavior data modelled via a neural network algorithm. Garrity et al. [11] exploited a compact embedded artificial neural network (ANN) with a second-stage classifier, reading temperature data from the in-built thermocouple, to produce the output of predicted temperatures. However, this technical approach, namely its ability to judge temperature fluctuations in special environments, still requires further improvement. To compensate for the deficiencies of the feature parameter, Zhang et al. [12] proposed DBN-R-LSTM-NN to classify and predict fire smoke and other features based on data collected from IoT sensors. Pincoot et al. [13] designed a vision-based indoor fire and smoke detection system with small training and test datasets, whereby different pixel density images, high-density smoke environments, and flame density scenes were recognized. Qiu et al. [14] developed a distributed feedback carbon monoxide (CO) sensor based on lasers used for the early warning detection of fire and verified the reliability of this sensor via different experiments. Li et al. [15] studied and proposed an early fire detection method based on a gas turbulent diffusion (GTD) model and particle swarm optimization (PSO). The experimental results verify that the sensor system has good fire detection and location performance. Chen et al. [16] proposed a fast and cost-effective indoor fire alarm system, which is used to find the fire, carbon monoxide, smoke, temperature, and humidity data in real time and conduct effective data analysis and classification. For smoke detection, the influence of smoke and dust in the environment represents a challenge.

Although vision-based sensing systems have shown good performance, massive and complex datasets often delay the time in the decision-making process [17]. Thus, visual-based sensing systems are not appropriate for early fire detection where decision making needs to be conducted in limited time. Additionally, vision-based sensing systems are inappropriate inside buildings because of the size and cost of devices, as well as privacy concerns that make them unsuitable for installation in multiple rooms and private homes. Meanwhile, single chemical sensor fire detectors are susceptible to interference from environmental conditions such as electromagnetic waves, water vapor, dust, cigarette smoke, and cooking smoke [18], which means that most smoke detectors will have false alarms when they detect these interfering conditions. Similarly, single temperature sensor devices still suffer from the misjudgment of environmental temperature fluctuations. They cannot effectively distinguish between early fire signals and environmental interference signals and cannot properly send early fire warning signals.

Due to the rapid development of machine learning, many intelligent algorithms have been presented to fuse several fire feature parameters [19–22]. This method overcomes the singularity and instability of the traditional threshold judgment method, which can significantly improve the accuracy of fire detection. Therefore, this paper proposes a hybrid feature fusion-based early fire detection method. First, by means of the distributed wireless sensing network, a hybrid feature collection system is developed to collect the smoke concentration, temperature, and CO concentration. On this account, a hybrid feature fusion algorithm, combining an error back propagation (BP) neural network with a least square support vector machine (LSSVM), is proposed. Then, the genetic algorithm (GA) and particle swarm optimization (PSO) are applied to obtain the optimal parameters in the data fusion process of the two algorithms, in order to achieve the optimized feature-level fusion results. Furthermore, the two algorithms are treated as subevidence bodies and the output results are adopted as the basic probability assignment of the D-S evidence theory for decision-level fusion to realize highly sensitive and reliable early fire warnings.

2. Suggestions and Methodology

The process of the hybrid feature data fusion algorithm is shown in Figure 1. The smoke concentration, temperature, and carbon monoxide concentration are obtained after collecting nodes and they are then transmitted to the data processing center via LoRa as inputs of the genetic algorithm–back propagation neural network (GA-BPNN) and the particle swarm optimization–least squares support vector machine (PSO-LSSVM). The two models both obtain three outputs: fire, smolder, and no fire. Then, the results of the feature layer fusion are integrated by the D-S evidence theory to output the final decision.

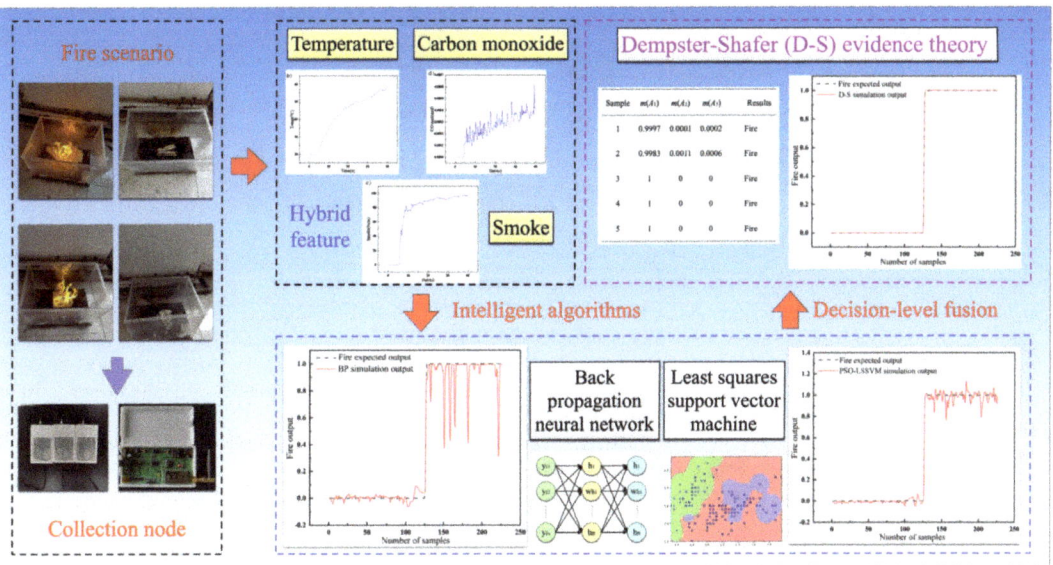

Figure 1. Overall design of the early fire detection and warning system.

2.1. Genetic Algorithm–Back Propagation Neural Network Fire Warning Model

The BPNN algorithm optimized by GA is a continuous and iterative process used for searching the best weight and threshold [19]. The process of the BPNN algorithm optimized by GA is shown in Figure 2.

The BPNN is a multi-layer forward feedback network for error correction, which includes the forward propagation of the signal and backward propagation of the error. The error excitation function is a sigmoid function, as shown in Equation (1).

$$Y_i = \frac{1}{1 + \exp\left[-\left(\sum_{i=1}^{n} w_{ij}x_i + w_{j0}\right)\right]}$$

$$Y_k = \sum_{k=1}^{N} w_{kj}Y_j + w_{k0}$$

(1)

where Y_k is the kth variable of the output layer, Y_j is the jth variable of the hidden layer, x_i is the ith input variable, N is the number of output neurons, n is the number of hidden neurons, w_{kj} is the weight between the output layer and the hidden layer, and w_{ji} is the weight between the input layer and the hidden layer.

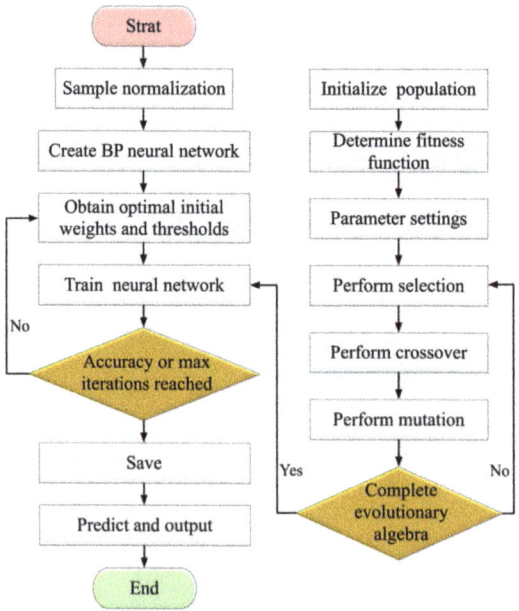

Figure 2. The BPNN process with GA optimization.

The gradient descent method is often used to optimize the parameters of neural networks. However, BPNN is difficult to converge and may fall into local extremes. Since the GA [23] can reduce the solution space of the neural network, the global optimal solution can be obtained more quickly and stably by the GA-BPNN [24]. The GA uses selection, crossover, and mutation to generate several initial populations of defined encoding lengths in a random number [25].

In the GA optimization strategy, the best realized individuals of the new generation will be considered as a result of the execution and GA setups shown in Table 1. The optimal parameters obtained by GA are then brought into the BPNN for training.

Table 1. The GA setups.

Types	Symbols	Interval
The coding length	N	20~200
The crossover probability	P_c	0.4~0.99
The mutation probability	\	0.005~0.1
The number of terminated evolutionary generations	\	100~1000

2.2. Particle Swarm Optimization–Least Squares Support Vector Machine Fire Warning Model

The inputs to the LSSVM are the smoke concentration, temperature, and carbon monoxide concentration. The penalty factor C and the kernel parameter σ of the LSSVM are optimized by PSO. The simulation outputs are compared with the expected outputs to verify the feasibility of the algorithm, and the design is shown in Figure 3.

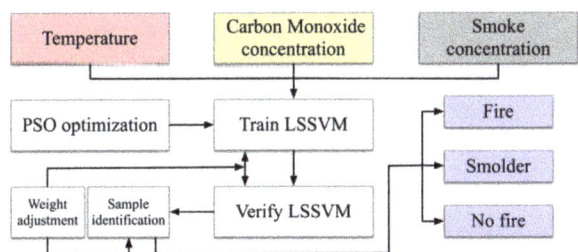

Figure 3. The PSO-LSSVM fire warning algorithm model.

In support vector machines (SVMs), the dot product algorithm in the high-level feature is replaced by the kernel function [26].

SuykensJ and Vandewalle [27] further proposed the least squares support vector machine (LSSVM) for solving pattern classification and regression prediction problems [28]. A nonlinear function $\varphi(x_i)$ is used to map the input to the feature space, and the nonlinear function estimation modeling is shown in Equation (2).

$$f(x) = b + (\varnothing(x), w) \qquad (2)$$

where w is the weight vector and b is the bias term.

The evaluation problem is described as the optimization problem based on the principle of structured risk minimization and the Lagrange function is constructed, as shown in Equation (3), to solve the optimization problem.

$$L_{LSSVM} = \frac{1}{2}w^2 + \frac{1}{2}\gamma \sum_{i=1}^{N} e_i^2 - \sum_{i=1}^{N} \alpha_i[(w, \varnothing(x_i)) + b + e_i - y_i] \qquad (3)$$

where a_i is the Lagrange multiplier.

The linear problems can be simplified by eliminating w and e_i, as described in Equation (4).

$$\begin{bmatrix} 0 & E^T \\ E & \Omega + \frac{1}{\gamma}E \end{bmatrix} \begin{bmatrix} b \\ a \end{bmatrix} = \begin{bmatrix} 0 \\ y \end{bmatrix} x \qquad (4)$$

where $y = [y_1, \ldots, y_N]^T$, $a = [a_1, \ldots, a_N]^T$, $E = [1, \ldots, 1]^T$, and Ω is a symmetric matrix equation for the $N \times N$ as shown in Equation (5).

$$\Omega_{ij} = K(x_i, x_j) = \varnothing(x_i)^T \varnothing(x_j) i, j = 1, 2, \ldots, N \qquad (5)$$

where $K(x_i, y_j)$ is the kernel function that satisfies the Meser condition [29].

Finally, the LSSVM can be described, as shown in Equation (6).

$$y(x) = (w, \varnothing(x)) + b = \sum_{i=1}^{n} \alpha_i \varnothing(x_i) \cdot \varnothing(x) + b = \sum_{i=1}^{n} \alpha_i K(x_i, x) + b \qquad (6)$$

The four main forms of the LSSVM kernel function are shown in Table 2.

Table 2. The forms of the kernel function.

Kernel Function	Forms
The polynomial kernel function	$K(x, x_i) = (x \cdot x_i + c)^N$
The radial basis kernel function	$K(x, x_i) = \exp\left(\frac{\|x - x_i\|^2}{2\sigma^2}\right)$
The sigmoid kernel function	$K(x, x_i) = \tanh(\tau \cdot (x, x_i) + t), (\tau > 0, t > 0)$
The linear kernel function	$k(x, x_i) = x * x_i$

The PSO algorithm simulates a bird in a flock by designing a massless particle with position and velocity attributes [30]. The individual extremes are matched with the current global optimal solution shared by other particles in the global to adjust the speed and position [31].

The PSO will initialize to a group of random particles and find the optimal solution by iteration [21]. The particle update is tracked (p_{best}, g_{best}) in iteration by Equations (7) and (8).

$$v_i = v_i + c_1 \times rand() \times (pbest_i - x_i) + c_2 \times rand() \times (gbest_i - x_i) \tag{7}$$

$$x_i = x_i + v_i \tag{8}$$

where $i = 1, 2, \ldots, N$, and N is the total number of particles. V_i is the speed of the particle. Rand ( ) is a random number between 0 and 1. X_i is the current position of the particle. C_1 and c_2 are the learning factors of $c_1 = c_2 = 2$. The maximum value of v_i is $Vmax$ (>0); if $v_i > Vmax$, then $v_i = Vmax$.

According to the update of the velocity v, c_1 is aimed towards the local optimal solution and c_2 is aimed towards the global optimal solution. The representation is shown in Figure 4.

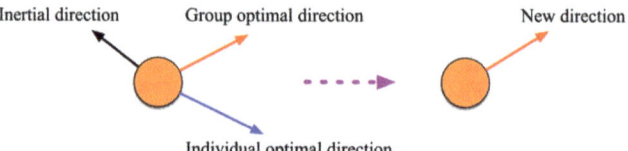

Figure 4. Schematic diagram of particle search for optimization.

The design steps of the PSO are shown in Figure 5.

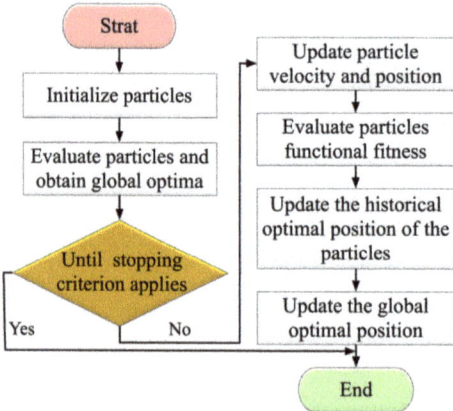

Figure 5. Particle swarm optimization process.

The initialization of the PSO algorithm is shown in Table 3. The fire detection uses the smoke concentration, temperature, and carbon monoxide concentration as inputs for training and testing samples. Then, the samples are trained by the LSSVM. The optimal penalty factor c and the optimal kernel function width factor σ of the LSSVM are obtained by the PSO optimization search. The partial fusion results of another group of samples can be obtained as the original fusion results for adjustment.

Table 3. The PSO algorithm initialization parameters.

Types	Symbols	Interval
The acceleration factor	c_1	1.5
	c_2	1.7
The maximum number of population evolution	\	300
The population size	\	30
The penalty factor range	\	0.1~1000
The kernel function width factor range	σ	0.01~1000

To assess the performance of the BPNN, the GA-BPNN, and the PSO-LSVM model, three evaluation indicators, i.e., the mean square error (MSE), the root mean square error (RMSE), and the mean absolute error (MAE), are adopted [20]. The MSE, RMSE, and MAE are calculated, as shown in Equations (9)–(11). The smaller the MSE, RMSE, and MAE, the smaller the error.

$$RSE = \frac{1}{N} \sum_{m=1}^{N_d} (\hat{y}_m - y_m)^2 \quad (9)$$

$$RMSE = \sqrt{\frac{1}{N_d} \sum_{m=1}^{N_d} (\hat{y}_m - y_m)^2} \quad (10)$$

$$MAE = \frac{1}{N_d} \sum_{m=1}^{N_d} |(\hat{y}_m - y_m)| \quad (11)$$

where N_d is the amount of data, y_m is the actual value of data, and $\hat{y}_m$ is the simulation output of the model.

2.3. Decision-Level Feature Data Fusion

The D-S evidence theory [32,33] is specialized in solving uncertainty problems [34,35]. It fuses confidence functions obtained by different algorithms to make decisions using the combination rules of the evidence theory. The system will make a final decision based on new evidence according to the decision rules.

Suppose U is an identification frame, the function $m: 2^\Theta \to [0, 1]$ satisfies Equation (12).

$$m(\phi) = 0, \sum_{A \subseteq \Theta} m(A) = 1 \quad (12)$$

m is the basic probability assignment function based on 2^Θ and $m(A)$ is the basic probability assignment of proposition A, indicating the degree of confidence in the probability assignment

The confidence function indicates the total degree to which the obtained evidence supports the information grading. The function Bal is defined by $\forall A \subseteq \Theta$ and $Bal(A) = \sum_{B \subseteq A} m(B)$. $2^\Theta \to [0, 1]$ is the reliability function on Θ. For $\forall A \subseteq \Theta$ if $m(A) > 0$, A is the focal element of the reliability function Bel and the union of all the focal elements in the frame Θ is the kernel.

The likelihood function describes the degree to which the obtained evidence cannot reject the score. A $pl: 2^\Theta \to [0, 1]$ is defined in Equation (13):

$$pl(A) = 1 - Bel(A) = \sum_{B \cap A \neq \phi} M(B) \quad (13)$$

The confidence functions of $Bel1$ and $Bel2$ are demonstrated. M_1 and m_2 are the corresponding basic probability assignment functions. The focal elements are $A_1, A_2, \ldots,$

A_n and $B_1, B_2, \ldots, B_n$. The new probability M can be obtained according to the D-S evidence theory shown in Equation (14):

$$M = \begin{cases} 0, C = \phi \\ \frac{1}{1-K} \sum_{A_i \cap B_j = C} m_1(A_i)m_2(B_j), C \neq \Phi \end{cases} \quad (14)$$

The calculation of K is shown in Equation (15).

$$K = \sum_{A \cap B = \phi} m_1(A)m_2(B) \quad (15)$$

On the one hand, if $K \neq 1$, the two are compatible, and basic probability assignment can be conducted. On the other hand, if $K = 1$, then m_1 and m_2 are contradictory or cannot combine.

The decision of the D-S evidence theory followed the rules shown below, assuming that $A_1 \subset \Theta, A_2 \subset \Theta$ satisfies Equations (16) and (17).

$$m(A_1) = \max[m(A_i), A \subset \Theta] \quad (16)$$

$$m(A_2) = \max[m(A_i), A_i \subset \Theta], A_i \neq A_1 \quad (17)$$

If Equations (18) and (20) are satisfied as below:

$$m(A_1) - m(A_2) > \varepsilon_1 \quad (18)$$

$$m(\Theta) < \varepsilon_2 \quad (19)$$

$$m(A_1) > m(\Theta) \quad (20)$$

where ε_1 and ε_2 are the preset thresholds, then A_1 is the determined result by the D-S evidence theory.

The training error e of the GA-BPNN and the PSO-LSSVM is calculated as part of the basic probability assignment shown in Equation (21).

$$e = \frac{1}{2}\sum (t_i - y_i)^2 \quad (21)$$

where t_i and y_i are the expected and simulated outputs in the GA-BP and the PSO-LSSVM.

The identification framework of the evidence theory $\Theta = \{A_1, A_2, A_3\}$, A_1, A_2, A_3 represents the fire, smolder, and no fire. In the portfolio of evidence $E = \{E_1, E_2\}$, E_1 and E_2 denote the outputs of the GA-BP and the PSO-LSSVM, respectively. $m_1(A_1)$, $m_1(A_2)$, and $m_1(A_3)$ represent the basic probability assignments of the GA-BP for the three outputs of fire, smolder, and no fire, respectively. $m_2(A_1)$, $m_2(A_2)$, and $m_2(A_3)$ represent the basic probability assignments of the PSO-LSSVM for the three outputs of fire, smolder, and no fire, respectively.

The final basic probability assignment of each element obtained from Equation (21) is shown in Equation (22) below:

$$m_j(A_i) = \frac{y(A_i)}{\sum_{i=1}^{3} y(A_i) + e} (j = 1, 2) \quad (22)$$

Then, the D-S evidence theory fusion rule is described in Equation (23).

$$m(A_z) = m_1(A_i) \oplus m_2(A_j) = \begin{cases} \frac{1}{1-K} \sum_{A_i \cap A_j = A_z} m_1(A_i)m_2(A_j), \forall A_Z \subseteq \Theta, A_z \neq \phi \\ 0, A_Z = \phi \end{cases} \quad (23)$$

Equation (24) is then used to calculate K:

$$K = \sum_{A_i \cap A_j = \phi} m_1(A_i) m_2(A_j) \tag{24}$$

3. Results and Discussions

3.1. Experimental Setup

Firstly, the fire dynamics simulator (FDS) [36,37] was employed to simulate in-building fires, as shown in Figure 6a. The large eddy simulation (LES) in the FDS was used by the Smagorinsky subgrid model to solve the Navier–Stokes equations for the turbulence with a low Mach number caused by the fire phenomenon. The simulated setting was a no-wind scenario. In this figure, the burning duration was set to 40 s, and the combustion products in the space are presented in Figure 6b–d. We can see that the temperature, smoke concentration, and CO concentration changed slowly in the first five seconds, and then they began to rise significantly. At the end of the 40 s burn time, the temperature achieved the maximum, while the smoke variation stabilized, and the CO concentration continued to increase. Therefore, according to the results of the building fire simulation, these three feature parameters were selected as the monitoring parameters of the fire warning system.

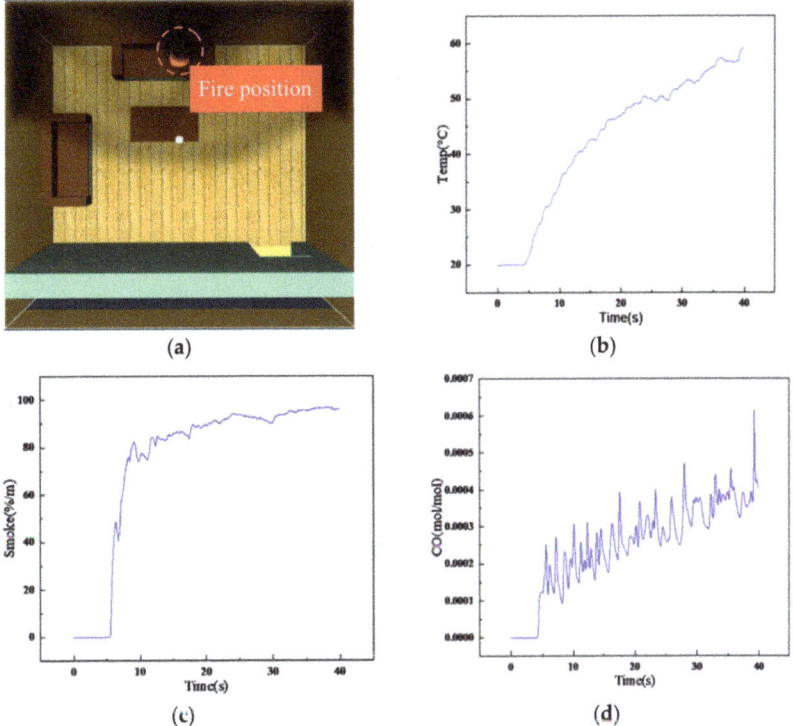

Figure 6. The simulation analysis of in-building fire features: (**a**) fire model; (**b**) temperature change; (**c**) smoke concentration change; and (**d**) carbon monoxide concentration.

Three key parameters, i.e., temperature, smoke concentration, and carbon monoxide concentration, were extracted from the experimental data to form the basic datasets. Then, we divided the outputs of the hybrid feature fusion model into three classes (open fire, smolder, and no fire). On this basis, (1,0,0), (0,1,0), and (0,0,1) were modeled as the ideal representations of open fire, smolder, and no fire, respectively. Subsequently, we developed a combustion product collection system, including the combustion product collection node and gateway node, as shown in Figure 7, to obtain the real experimental data generated by small simulated in-building fires, where 800 sets of data were collected. The feature data in the datasets were derived from combustion products of different materials, while each dataset included the temperature (Temp), smoke concentration (Smoke), and carbon monoxide concentration (CO). After that, these data were further divided into 600 sets of training data and 200 groups of test data. The training data were utilized to train the model and the optimal network training model could be obtained after consecutive iterations with learning rates of 0.001. The test data were employed to demonstrate the effectiveness.

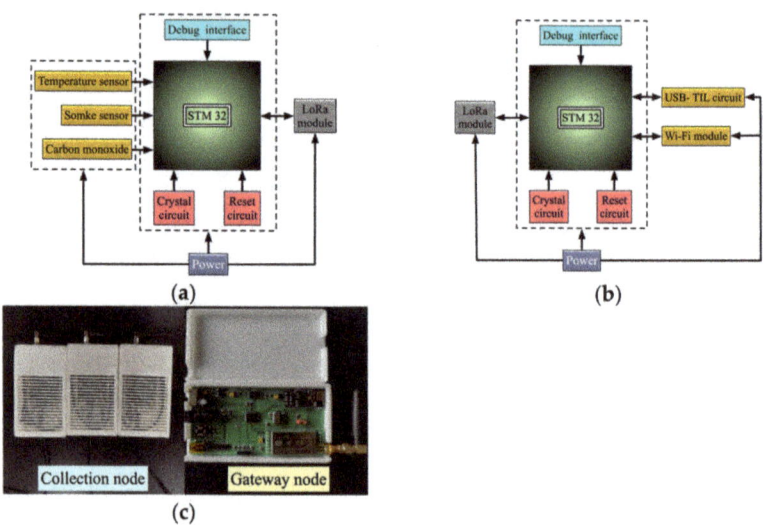

Figure 7. The fire detection and warning system: (**a**) collection node design; (**b**) gateway node design; (**c**) hardware.

3.2. Results of Open Fire

The fire test data were substituted into the already trained BPNN, and the results are shown in Figure 8a. The comparison reveals that the simulation output of the BPNN differed significantly from the expected output of fire. However, the network model optimized by the GA could obtain the optimal weights and thresholds, which we inputted into the BPNN for training. The outputs are shown in Figure 8b. It can be seen that the difference between the simulated and expected outputs was reduced.

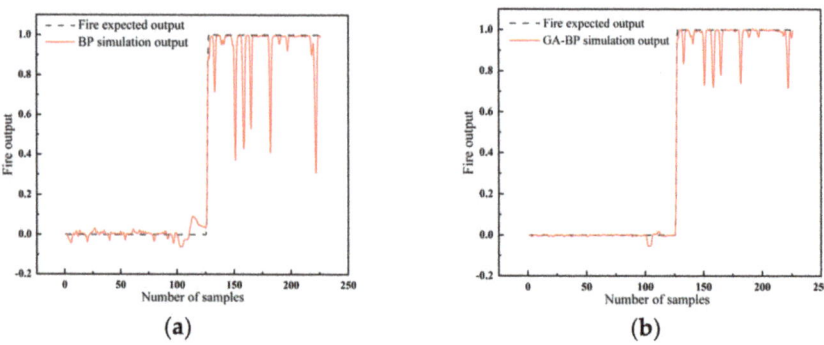

Figure 8. The output results of fire with (**a**) the BPNN and (**b**) the GA-BPNN.

The PSO-LSSVM fire warning model adopted four kernel functions: (1) the radial basis kernel function; (2) the sigmoid kernel function; (3) the polypolynomial kernel function;

(4) and the linear kernel function. The simulation results of fire based on the four types of kernel functions were compared and analyzed with the expected outputs, as shown in Figure 9a–d. It is clear that the radial basis kernel function could perform better than the other three kernel functions. Thereby, it delivered the best data fusion effects.

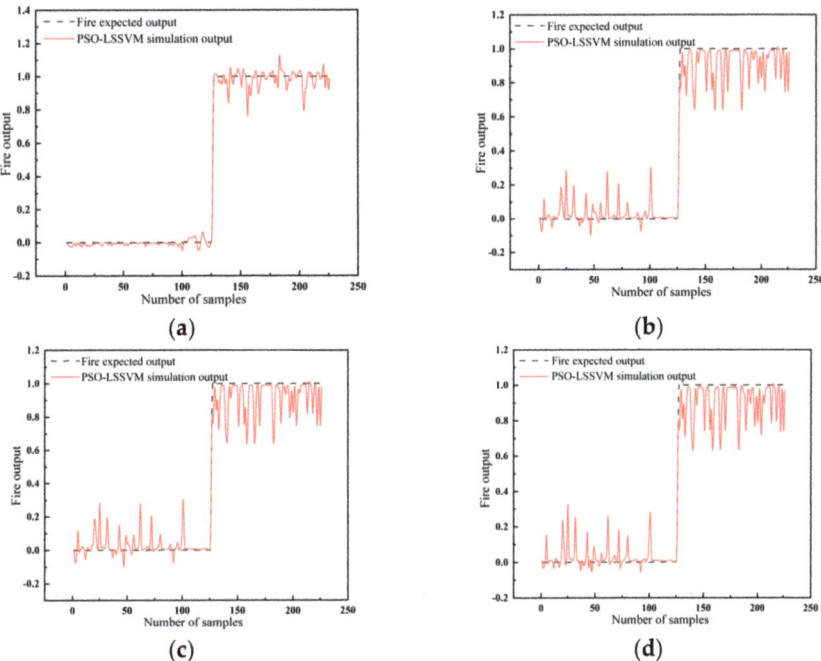

Figure 9. The output results of fire with the LSSVM for different kernel functions: (**a**) the radial basis kernel function; (**b**) the sigmoid kernel function; (**c**) the polypolynomial kernel function; (**d**) the linear kernel function.

3.3. Results of the Smolder

Figure 10 shows that the simulation results of the BPNN optimized by GA had better stability. Compared with the original model, the difference between the simulation results and the expected results was significantly reduced.

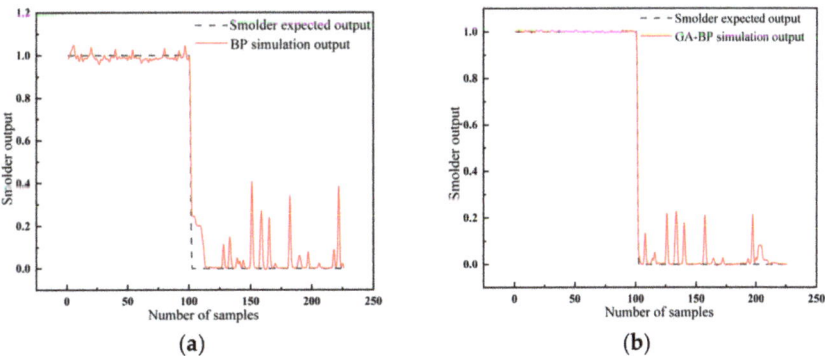

Figure 10. The output results of smolder with (**a**) the BPNN and (**b**) the GA-BPNN.

Figure 11 illustrates the different output results of smolder with the LSSVM. It can be seen that the radial basis kernel function also obtained the most stable output results, representing the highest reliability and the best data fusion effects.

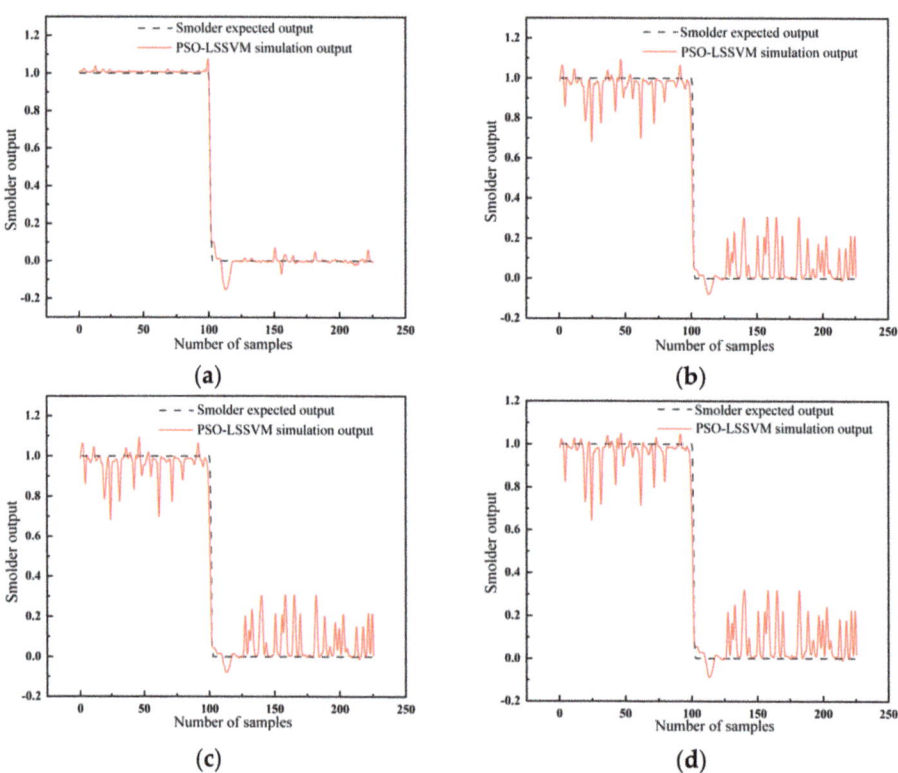

Figure 11. The output results of smolder with the LSSVM for different kernel functions: (**a**) radial basis kernel function; (**b**) sigmoid kernel function; (**c**) polypolynomial kernel function; (**d**) linear kernel function.

3.4. Model Performance Analysis

Table 4 shows the error MSE, RMSE, and MAE of the BPNN and the GA-BPNN to quantify the model performance. Table 4 also shows that the GA-BPNN had the smallest MSE, RMSE, and MAE, which indicates that the simulation output of the GA-BPNN was more suited to the expected output. The GA-BPNN also performed better than the original BPNN. Therefore, the GA-BPNN could also fuse the fire feature data in the feature layer.

Table 4. The output error analysis.

Algorithm Model	Fire			Smolder		
	MSE	RMSE	MAE	MSE	RMSE	MAE
BP	0.0185	0.1361	0.0412	0.0083	0.0910	0.0362
GA-BP	0.0037	0.0612	0.0164	0.0025	0.0498	0.0140

Table 5 illustrates the calculation analysis of the MSE, RMSE, and MAE for different kernel functions. As shown in Tables 4 and 5, the algorithm based on the RBF had the smallest MSE, RMSE, and MAE, indicating that the simulation output was closer to the expected output and the model performance was better than the others. Therefore, the

PSO-LSSVM model based on the RBF was selected to fuse the feature layer data for the fire feature.

Table 5. The output error analysis.

Kernel Function	Fire			Smolder		
	MSE	RMSE	MAE	MSE	RMSE	MAE
RBF	0.0028	0.0529	0.0293	0.000984	0.0314	0.0152
Sigmoid	0.0188	0.1370	0.0639	0.0155	0.1247	0.0603
Poly	0.0172	0.1310	0.0640	0.0146	0.1209	0.0619
Linear	0.0192	0.1386	0.0694	0.0169	0.1300	0.0681

3.5. Results of the Proposed Method

According to the empirical definition $\varepsilon_1 = 0.5$, the simulation outputs of five groups of test sample data were selected for comparison and analysis with the expected outputs using Equation (24). Table 6 shows three uncertainty data outputs from the GA-BPNN and one uncertainty output from the PSO-LSSVM. These results are ambiguous. So, these five groups of results were then assigned and calculated by the probability of the D-S evidence theory, and the results are shown in Table 7. The evidence indicates that the results of the fusion based on the D-S evidence theory were consistent with the expected outputs. Thus, the results of the D-S evidence theory fusing the two model treatments effectively addressed the ambiguity of the evidence and improved the reliability of the fused data.

Table 6. Neural network simulation output results and expected output results.

Algorithm Model	Simulation Output			Expected Output			Results
The GA-BP neural network	0.62745	0.00138	0.37117	1	0	0	Uncertainty
	0.68278	0.01471	0.30251	1	0	0	Uncertainty
	0.9969	0.0025	0.0006	1	0	0	Fire
	0.5986	0.3927	0.0087	1	0	0	Uncertainty
	0.99792	0.002	0.00008	1	0	0	Fire
The PSO-LSSVM network	0.86354	0.07689	0.07941	1	0	0	Fire
	0.87026	0.04597	0.0794	1	0	0	Fire
	0.64114	0.29953	0.05933	1	0	0	Uncertainty
	0.87451	0.11074	0.07941	1	0	0	Fire
	0.97166	0.00114	0.02283	1	0	0	Fire

Table 7. The results of the D-S evidence theory fusion approach.

Sample	$m(A_1)$	$m(A_2)$	$m(A_3)$	Results
1	0.9997	0.0001	0.0002	Fire
2	0.9983	0.0011	0.0006	Fire
3	1	0	0	Fire
4	1	0	0	Fire
5	1	0	0	Fire

A comparison of the simulated and expected outputs of the D-S evidence theory incorporating the GA-BP fire warning algorithm and the PSO-LSSVM fire warning algorithm is shown in Figure 12. The expected output and the fused output were basically the same. Additionally, the inferred results of the D-S evidence theory enabled the accurate determination of fire hazards. The combined prediction method, used to fuse the information from the above two networks after identification, provided results with higher accuracy than each single model.

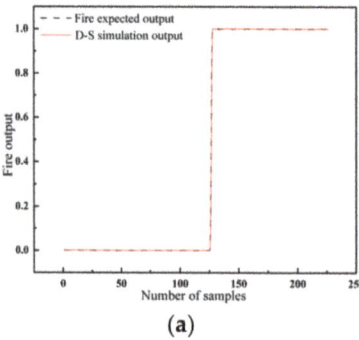
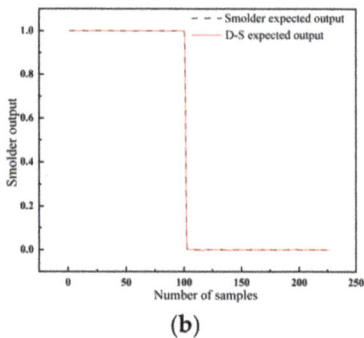

Figure 12. Comparative results of the D-S evidence theory fusion approach: (**a**) expected fire output and simulation outputs; (**b**) desired smolder output and simulation outputs.

4. Early Fire Warning Experiments

To verify the real-time performance of the presented early fire detection and warning system, we conducted four early fire warning experiments with different fire classes, i.e., polyurethane foam fire, alcohol fire, beech wood smolder, and cotton woven fabric smolder. A combustion experiment box was then placed inside the building and the fire detector was installed at 2.0 m above the combustion box.

4.1. Results of the Warning Time

Figure 13a shows the combustion process of polyurethane foam, and Figure 13b shows the fire scene. The polyurethane burned slowly at the beginning. However, a period later, the flame became larger, with a gradually increasing temperature and producing much smoke. The PC alarmed after 16 s.

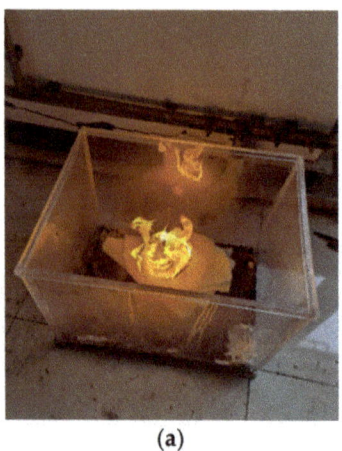
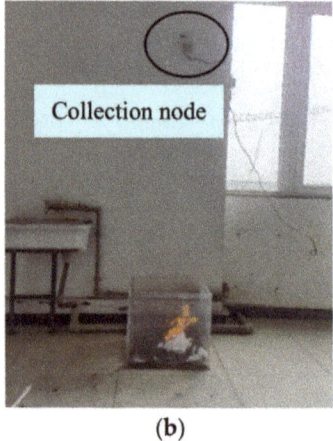

Figure 13. The polyurethane fire test: (**a**) the process of polyurethane combustion; (**b**) the fire scene.

Figure 14a shows the process of alcohol burns, and Figure 14b shows the scene of alcohol fire. The alcohol immediately burned when ignited. The flame became large and released a lot of heat, resulting in the temperature rising rapidly. However, there was no visible smoke. The PC alarmed after 18 s.

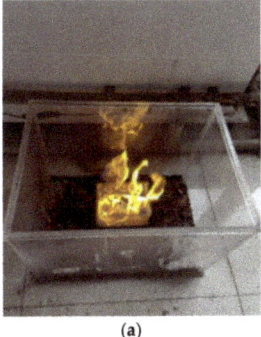 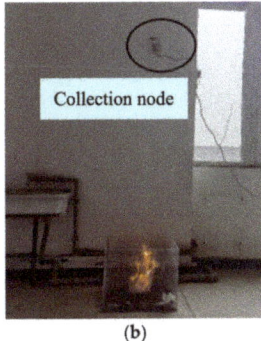

Figure 14. The alcohol fire test: (**a**) the process of alcohol combustion; (**b**) the fire scene.

Figure 15a shows the burn process of beech wood and Figure 15b shows the beech wood experiment with smolder. The smolder had no obvious fire but produced smoke particles with a slow rise in temperature. The PC alarmed after 22 s.

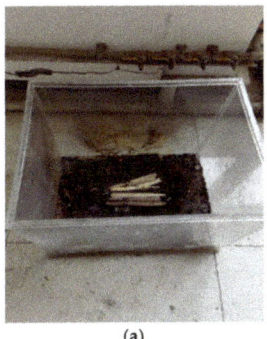 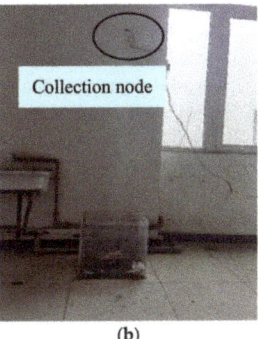

Figure 15. The beech wood smolder test: (**a**) the process of beech wood combustion; (**b**) the smolder scene.

Figure 16a shows the process when the cotton rope is ignited and smoldered, and Figure 16b shows the overall state of the cotton rope smolder. The smolder process produced a large amount of smoke, but the temperature did not rise significantly with a few sparks. The PC alarmed after 20 s.

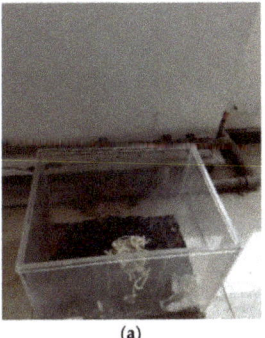 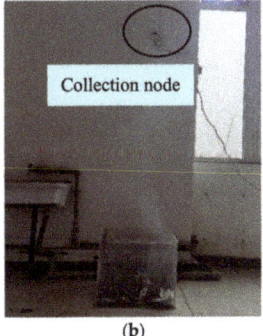

Figure 16. The cotton rope smolder test: (**a**) the process of cotton rope combustion; (**b**) the smolder scene.

4.2. Accuracy Verification of Alarm System

Fifty experiments were conducted on the above scenarios to verify the accuracy of the fire warning system. The data were collected using a single acquisition node for the features information generated from each burn experiment to verify whether the results in the PC match the real situation. A comparison between the realistic case and the fire warning system is shown in Table 8. The alarm accuracy of each type of experiment was shown to exceed 96%. The results show that the early fire warning model can ensure the detection and warning of different types of fire hazards.

Table 8. A comparison of the real situation and system recognition.

Fire Types	Experiments/n	Alarms/n	Missed Alarms/n	Accuracy/%
Polyurethane fire	50	49	1	98%
Alcohol fire	50	48	2	96%
Beech wood smolder	50	48	2	96%
Cotton rope smolder	50	49	1	98%

4.3. Distributed Network Fire Response

The main purpose of the distributed network fire warning experiment is to verify whether the early fire warning system consisting of three data collection nodes can achieve the simultaneous detection of fires in multiple regions. Three fire feature data collection nodes were used to detect fires in three different regions (see Figure 17). Each collection node was connected to a gateway node via LoRa wireless spread spectrum technology, and the gateway node collected the environmental feature data acquired by each collection node. The fusion results of the GA-BP algorithm are shown in Table 9, the fusion results of the PSO-LSSVM algorithm are shown in Table 10, and the fusion results of the D-S evidence theory are shown in Table 11.

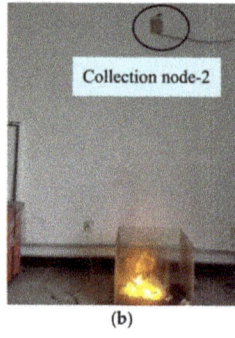
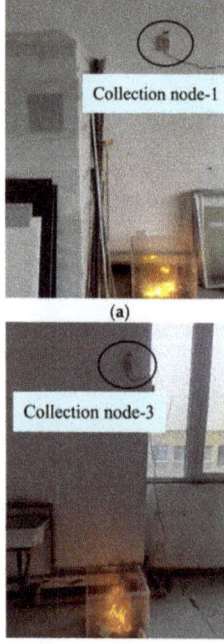

Figure 17. Distributed networking experiments: (**a**) Node 1; (**b**) Node 2; (**c**) Node 3.

Table 9. The GA-BP algorithm fusion results.

	Temperature/°C	Smoke/10^3 ppm	CO/ppm	Fire Output	Smolder Output	No Fire Output
Node 1	25.6	2.36	6	0.6949	0.0532	0.2519
	31.6	3.68	26	0.7247	0.0513	0.2239
	35.9	2.56	17	0.9296	0.0011	0.0692
Node 2	26.3	1.84	2	0.6762	0.1522	0.1716
	33.7	2.28	14	0.8124	0.0524	0.1350
	36.9	2.44	7	0.9456	0.0325	0.0219
Node 3	25.3	2.6	6	0.7025	0.2305	0.0670
	32.4	1.95	23	0.7952	0.1248	0.0800
	37	1.6	9	0.9033	0.0362	0.0605

Table 10. The PSO-LSSVM algorithm fusion results.

	Temperature/°C	Smoke/10^3 ppm	CO/ppm	Fire Output	Smolder Output	No Fire Output
Node 1	25.6	2.36	6	0.6314	0.1250	0.2436
	31.6	3.68	26	0.7615	0.0215	0.2171
	35.9	2.56	17	0.8703	0.0460	0.0838
Node 2	26.3	1.84	2	0.7043	0.1453	0.1504
	33.7	2.28	14	0.8021	0.1320	0.0659
	36.9	2.44	7	0.9382	0.0044	0.0573
Node 3	25.3	2.6	6	0.6125	0.2310	0.1566
	32.4	1.95	23	0.7493	0.0816	0.1691
	37	1.6	9	0.8853	0.0333	0.0814

Table 11. The D-S evidence theory fusion results.

	Temperature/°C	Smoke/10^3 ppm	CO/ppm	Fire Output	Smolder Output	No Fire Output
Node 1	25.6	2.36	6	0.8658	0.0131	0.1211
	31.6	3.68	26	0.9174	0.0018	0.0808
	35.9	2.56	17	0.9928	0.0001	0.0071
Node 2	26.3	1.84	2	0.9086	0.0422	0.0492
	33.7	2.28	14	0.9763	0.0104	0.0133
	36.9	2.44	7	0.9984	0.0002	0.0014
Node 3	25.3	2.6	6	0.8710	0.1078	0.0212
	32.4	1.95	23	0.9617	0.0164	0.0218
	37	1.6	9	0.9924	0.0015	0.0061

It is evident that the data obtained from different sensor nodes collected by the GA-BP and PSO-LSSVM algorithms were also ambiguous after calculation. However, the fusion of different results using the D-S evidence theory was shown to improve the reliability of the evidence.

5. Conclusions

This paper proposes a data fusion method with multiple features to achieve an in-building fire detection and early warning system. Firstly, the GA-BPNN and the PSO-LSSVM were employed to translate the smoke concentration, temperature, and CO concentration into probabilities of fire, smolder, and no fire. Subsequently, the feature data of the GA-BPNN and the PSO-LSSVM were fused by the D-S evidence theory to further improve the accuracy and the reliability of the fire warning algorithm. Finally, an early fire detection and warning system was developed. Small-scale in-building fire experiments have confirmed the effectiveness of the method, and the combined algorithm of the D-S evidence theory could significantly improve early fire detection. Additionally, the early fire warning system could accurately identify the fire signals from different types and regions. The early fire detection accuracy also exceeded 96%. However, the proposed method can only achieve fire recognition. It cannot be utilized to indicate the severity of fire. In addition, in this paper, limited kinds of experimental materials were employed for fire combustion. As a result, in future work, we plan to develop an end-to-end approach that can not only achieve fire detection but also predict the fire levels based on the featured data, and more kinds of experimental materials will be presented to demonstrate the effectiveness. Moreover, another valuable research interest is to identify the smoking behavior for avoiding false fire alarm by utilizing the hybrid feature fusion-based method.

Author Contributions: Conceptualization, S.X. and Z.P.; data curation, S.W.; formal analysis, S.W.; funding acquisition, L.G., X.F. and Z.P.; investigation, S.X.; methodology, S.X. and H.W.; project administration, L.G.; resources, L.G.; software, S.X.; supervision, L.G., Z.P. and W.Z.; validation, S.X., L.G. and H.W.; visualization, S.X. and S.W.; writing—original draft, S.X.; writing—review and editing, S.X., X.F. and W.Z. All authors have read and agreed to the published version of the manuscript.

Funding: This research was funded part by the National Natural Science Foundation of China, grant number 52174209 and the Scientific Research Starting Project of SWPU under Grant 2021QHZ022.

Institutional Review Board Statement: Not applicable.

Informed Consent Statement: Not applicable.

Data Availability Statement: Not applicable.

Conflicts of Interest: The authors declare no conflict of interest. The funders had no role in the design of the study; in the collection, analyses, or interpretation of data; in the writing of the manuscript; or in the decision to publish the results.

References

1. Zheng, X.; Chen, F.; Lou, L.; Cheng, P.; Huang, Y. Real-Time Detection of Full-Scale Forest Fire Smoke Based on Deep Convolution Neural Network. *Remote Sens.* **2022**, *14*, 536. [CrossRef]
2. Abdusalomov, A.; Baratov, N.; Kutlimuratov, A.; Whangbo, T.K. An improvement of the fire detection and classification method using YOLOv3 for surveillance systems. *Sensors* **2021**, *21*, 6519. [CrossRef]
3. Yusuf, S.A.; Alshdadi, A.A.; Alghamdi, R.; Alassafi, M.O.; Garrity, D.J. An autoregressive exogenous neural network to model fire behavior via a naïve bayes filter. *IEEE Access* **2020**, *8*, 98281–98294. [CrossRef]
4. Lou, L.; Chen, F.; Cheng, P.; Huang, Y. Smoke root detection from video sequences based on multi-feature fusion. *J. For. Res.* **2022**, *33*, 1841–1856. [CrossRef]
5. Li, P.; Yang, Y.; Zhao, W.; Zhang, M. Evaluation of image fire detection algorithms based on image complexity. *Fire Saf. J.* **2021**, *121*, 103306. [CrossRef]
6. Li, P.; Zhao, W. Image fire detection algorithms based on convolutional neural networks. *Case Stud. Therm. Eng.* **2020**, *19*, 100625. [CrossRef]
7. Li, Y.; Ko, Y.; Lee, W. RGB image-based hybrid model for automatic prediction of flashover in compartment fires. *Fire Saf. J.* **2022**, *132*, 103629. [CrossRef]
8. Xie, Y.; Zhu, J.; Guo, Y.; You, J.; Feng, D.; Cao, Y. Early indoor occluded fire detection based on firelight reflection characteristics. *Fire Saf. J.* **2022**, *128*, 103542. [CrossRef]
9. Ji, W.; Li, G.Q.; Zhu, S. Real-time prediction of key monitoring physical parameters for early warning of fire-induced building collapse. *Comput. Struct.* **2022**, *272*, 106875. [CrossRef]
10. Sun, B.; Liu, X.; Xu, Z.-D.; Xu, D. Temperature data-driven fire source estimation algorithm of the underground pipe gallery. *Int. J. Therm. Sci.* **2022**, *171*, 107247. [CrossRef]
11. Garrity, D.J.; Yusuf, S.A. A predictive decision-aid device to warn firefighters of catastrophic temperature increases using an AI-based time-series algorithm. *Saf. Sci.* **2021**, *138*, 105237. [CrossRef]
12. Zhang, Y.; Geng, P.; Sivaparthipan, C.B.; Muthu, B.A. Big data and artificial intelligence based early risk warning system of fire hazard for smart cities. *Sustain. Energy Technol. Assess.* **2021**, *45*, 100986. [CrossRef]
13. Pincott, J.; Tien, P.W.; Wei, S.; Calautit, J.K. Indoor fire detection utilizing computer vision-based strategies. *J. Build. Eng.* **2022**, *61*, 105154. [CrossRef]
14. Qiu, X.; Wei, Y.; Li, N.; Guo, A.; Zhang, E.; Li, C.; Peng, Y.; Wei, J.; Zang, Z. Development of an early warning fire detection system based on a laser spectroscopic carbon monoxide sensor using a 32-bit system-on-chip. *Infrared Phys. Technol.* **2019**, *96*, 44–51. [CrossRef]

15. Li, Y.; Yu, L.; Zheng, C.; Ma, Z.; Yang, S.; Song, F.; Zheng, K.; Ye, W.; Zhang, Y.; Wang, Y.; et al. Development and field deployment of a mid-infrared CO and CO_2 dual-gas sensor system for early fire detection and location. *Spectrochim. Acta Part A Mol. Biomol. Spectrosc.* **2022**, *270*, 120834. [CrossRef] [PubMed]
16. Chen, S.; Ren, J.; Yan, Y.; Sun, M.; Hu, F.; Zhao, H. Multi-sourced sensing and support vector machine classification for effective detection of fire hazard in early stage. *Comput. Electr. Eng.* **2022**, *101*, 108046. [CrossRef]
17. Hsu, T.W.; Pare, S.; Meena, M.S.; Jain, D.K.; Li, D.L.; Saxena, A.; Prasad, M.; Lin, C.T. An Early Flame Detection System Based on Image Block Threshold Selection Using Knowledge of Local and Global Feature Analysis. *Sustainability* **2020**, *12*, 8899. [CrossRef]
18. Cao, C.-F.; Yu, B.; Guo, B.-F.; Hu, W.-J.; Sun, F.-N.; Zhang, Z.-H.; Li, S.-N.; Wu, W.; Tang, L.-C.; Song, P.; et al. Bio-inspired, sustainable and mechanically robust graphene oxide-based hybrid networks for efficient fire protection and warning. *Chem. Eng. J.* **2022**, *439*, 134516. [CrossRef]
19. Tian, Z.; Gan, W.; Zou, X.; Zhang, Y.; Gao, W. Performance prediction of a cryogenic organic Rankine cycle based on back propagation neural network optimized by genetic algorithm. *Energy* **2022**, *254*, 124027. [CrossRef]
20. Al-Jarrah, R.; AL-Oqla, F.M. A novel integrated BPNN/SNN artificial neural network for predicting the mechanical performance of green fibers for better composite manufacturing. *Compos. Struct.* **2022**, *289*, 115475. [CrossRef]
21. Álvarez Antón, J.C.; García Nieto, P.J.; García Gonzalo, E.; Viera Pérez, J.C.; González Vega, M.; Blanco Viejo, C. A New Predictive Model for the State-of-Charge of a High-Power Lithium-Ion Cell Based on a PSO-Optimized Multivariate Adaptive Regression Spline Approach. *IEEE Trans. Veh. Technol.* **2016**, *65*, 4197–4208. [CrossRef]
22. Wu, L.; Chen, L.; Hao, X. Multi-Sensor Data Fusion Algorithm for Indoor Fire Early Warning Based on BP Neural Network. *Information* **2021**, *12*, 59. [CrossRef]
23. Zhu, J.; Wang, G.; Li, Y.; Duo, Z.; Sun, C. Optimization of hydrogen liquefaction process based on parallel genetic algorithm. *Int. J. Hydrog. Energy* **2022**, *47*, 27038–27048. [CrossRef]
24. Cao, H.; Liu, L.; Wu, B.; Gao, Y.; Qu, D. Process optimization of high-speed dry milling UD-CF/PEEK laminates using GA-BP neural network. *Compos. Part B Eng.* **2021**, *221*, 109034. [CrossRef]
25. Mota, B.; Faria, P.; Vale, Z. Residential load shifting in demand response events for bill reduction using a genetic algorithm. *Energy* **2022**, *260*, 124978. [CrossRef]
26. Jain, P.; Coogan, S.C.P.; Subramanian, S.G.; Crowley, M.; Taylor, S.; Flannigan, M.D. A review of machine learning applications in wildfire science and management. *Environ. Rev.* **2020**, *28*, 478–505. [CrossRef]
27. Suykens, J.A.K.; Vandewalle, J. Least squares support vector machine classifiers. *Neural Process. Lett.* **1999**, *9*, 293–300. [CrossRef]
28. Chamkalani, A.; Zendehboudi, S.; Bahadori, A.; Kharrat, R.; Chamkalani, R.; James, L.; Chatzis, I. Integration of LSSVM technique with PSO to determine asphaltene deposition. *J. Pet. Sci. Eng.* **2014**, *124*, 243–253. [CrossRef]
29. Song, Y.; Niu, W.; Wang, Y.; Xie, X.; Yang, S. A Novel Method for Energy Consumption Prediction of Underwater Gliders Using Optimal LSSVM with PSO Algorithm. In Proceedings of the Global Oceans 2020: Singapore–U.S. Gulf Coast, Biloxi, MS, USA, 5–30 October 2020; pp. 1–5. [CrossRef]
30. Kennedy, J.; Eberhart, R. Particle swarm optimization. In Proceedings of the ICNN'95—International Conference on Neural Networks, Perth, WA, Australia, 27 November–1 December 1995; Volume 4, pp. 1942–1948. [CrossRef]
31. Amirteimoori, A.; Mahdavi, I.; Solimanpur, M.; Ali, S.S.; Tirkolaee, E.B. A parallel hybrid PSO-GA algorithm for the flexible flow-shop scheduling with transportation. *Comput. Ind. Eng.* **2022**, *173*, 108672. [CrossRef]
32. Dempster, A.P. Upper and Lower Probabilities Induced by a Multivalued Mapping. *Ann. Math. Stat.* **1967**, *38*, 325–339. [CrossRef]
33. Shafer, G. *A Mathematical Theory of Evidence*; Princeton University Press: Princeton, NJ, USA, 1976. [CrossRef]
34. Sung, W.T.; Chang, K.Y. Evidence-based multi-sensor information fusion for remote health care systems. *Sens. Actuators A Phys.* **2013**, *204*, 1–19. [CrossRef]
35. Feng, Z.; Che, S.; Wang, X.; Yu, N. Trust Management Scheme Based on D-S Evidence Theory for Wireless Sensor Networks. *Int. J. Distrib. Sens. Netw.* **2013**, *9*, 948641. [CrossRef]
36. Wang, W.; He, T.; Huang, W.; Shen, R.; Wang, Q. Optimization of switch modes of fully enclosed platform screen doors during emergency platform fires in underground metro station. *Tunn. Undergr. Sp. Technol.* **2018**, *81*, 277–288. [CrossRef]
37. Mi, H.; Liu, Y.; Jiao, Z.; Wang, W.; Wang, Q. A numerical study on the optimization of ventilation mode during emergency of cable fire in utility tunnel. *Tunn. Undergr. Sp. Technol.* **2020**, *100*, 103403. [CrossRef]

Disclaimer/Publisher's Note: The statements, opinions and data contained in all publications are solely those of the individual author(s) and contributor(s) and not of MDPI and/or the editor(s). MDPI and/or the editor(s) disclaim responsibility for any injury to people or property resulting from any ideas, methods, instructions or products referred to in the content.

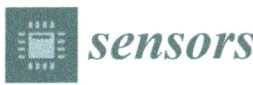

Article

Stress Detection Using Frequency Spectrum Analysis of Wrist-Measured Electrodermal Activity

Žiga Stržinar [1,2,*], Araceli Sanchis [3], Agapito Ledezma [3], Oscar Sipele [3], Boštjan Pregelj [1] and Igor Škrjanc [2]

1 "Jožef Stefan" Institute, Jamova cesta 39, 1000 Ljubljana, Slovenia
2 Faculty of Electrical Engineering, University of Ljubljana, Tržaška cesta 25, 1000 Ljubljana, Slovenia
3 Computer Science Department, University Carlos III of Madrid, 28911 Leganés, Madrid, Spain
* Correspondence: ziga.strzinar@ijs.si

Abstract: The article deals with the detection of stress using the electrodermal activity (EDA) signal measured at the wrist. We present an approach for feature extraction from EDA. The approach uses frequency spectrum analysis in multiple frequency bands. We evaluate the proposed approach using the 4 Hz EDA signal measured at the wrist in the publicly available Wearable Stress and Affect Detection (WESAD) dataset. Seven existing approaches to stress detection using EDA signals measured by wrist-worn sensors are analysed and the reported results are compared with ours. The proposed approach represents an improvement in accuracy over the other techniques studied. Moreover, we focus on time to detection (TTD) and show that our approach is able to outperform competing techniques, with fewer data points. The proposed feature extraction is computationally inexpensive, thus the presented approach is suitable for use in real-world wearable applications where both short response times and high detection performance are important. We report both binary (stress vs. no stress) as well as three-class (baseline/stress/amusement) results.

Keywords: affective computing; EDA; stress detection; physiological signals; frequency analysis

1. Introduction

Affect recognition is an interdisciplinary field that touches on signal processing, machine learning, psychology and physiology. Affective state recognition is useful in a number of scenarios. One affective state that has received a lot of attention recently is stress [1–6], especially since it has been demonstrated that frequent and prolonged stress has negative effects on mental and physical well-being, immune system, lower employee efficiency, lower employee engagement, more sick days, etc. [1,7,8].

The field of affect recognition aims to identify and label different affective states. Since the affective state of a subject is a psychological state inherent to the observed subject, it is not directly observable. Therefore, affect recognition uses several other observable variables to achieve its goal. These include (1) physiological signals such as electrocardiogram (ECG), EDA, electromyography (EMG), respiratory rate and subject temperature [5,9–11]; (2) subject context data such as accelerometer data, behaviour patterns, GPS data and smartphone usage [12]; (3) alternative subject data such as video or audio recordings [11]; (4) environmental contexts such as ambient temperature and humidity [13]

Recent advances in wearable technology [6,14] have led to increased research interest in wearables-focused affect recognition, e.g., [4–6,12,15,16]. With the increasing popularity of wearable electronics, algorithms that aim to detect affect using wearable sensors have a greater chance of being used in practice.

In real-world applications, two aspects of any proposed solution are important: (1) detection performance and (2) algorithm responsiveness—the time from onset of the affective state to detection (time to detection—TTD). Our goal is to present an approach to stress detection that provides competitive performance while improving responsiveness.

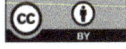

In Sections 1.1–1.4, we provide background information on affective state detection with wearable sensors. In Section 2, we first show some recent results on stress detection using wearable EDA sensors and then present and explain our proposed method. Results and discussion can be found in Section 3.

1.1. WESAD

Several datasets on affect recognition are publicly available, for example, DEAP [9], NonEEG [10], WESAD [5] and MAHNOB-HCI [11]. While some datasets work in valence-arousal space (Russel's circumplex model [17]), WESAD works with the categorical model. It is more focused on stress than some of the other datasets; the main purpose of the dataset is stress detection. WESAD also focuses on wearable sensors, making it perfect for our needs. The multimodal dataset includes both chest and wrist-based measurements of acceleration, ECG, BVP, EDA, EMG, respiration and temperature. The dataset includes fifteen subjects and three major affective states: baseline, stress and amusement.

Some advantages of the WESAD dataset are:

1. Chest and wrist measurement: the same type of physiological signals are measured at two sites, allowing comparison and validation
2. Real-world tasks: The tasks that the subjects performed are likely to occur in real life, such as public speaking or job interviews. Although WESAD was recorded in a laboratory environment, the dataset is comparable in this respect to data generated in the field.
3. High sampling frequency: data collected with a chest-worn device were sampled at 700 Hz; data from the wrist-worn Empatica E4 (http://www.empatica.com/research/e4/, accessed on: 20 November 2022) were sampled at lower frequencies, up to 64 Hz.
4. The authors present a reference classification approach and give a baseline accuracy and F1 scores.

A number of stress detection methods have been evaluated using WESAD. Their results are given in Section 2.1.

1.2. EDA

EDA broadly refers to any change in the electrical properties of the skin' Greco et al. [18], skin conductance (SC) is a commonly used measure of EDA. Activation of the sweat glands by the autonomic nervous system (ANS) is reflected in SC.

Skin conductance is usually interpreted as an aggregation of two components: the slower 'tonic' (SCL—skin conductance level, EDL—electrodermal level) and the faster 'phasic' (SCR—skin conductance response, EDR—electrodermal response). The latter is interpreted as a short-term reaction to stimuli and is, therefore, of particular interest in affect recognition. In [18], the disaggregation problem is formulated as a convex optimization problem and a solution is provided.

In [15], the drawbacks of using EDA in wearable stress detection research are pointed out. The basis of the critique is that EDA was not supported in the most widely used wearable operating systems at the time. For example, in [5] the EDA signal is measured at the wrist with the Empatica E4, which is not actually a consumer-oriented product. However, since the article was published, new smartwatches have hit the market, some of which include an EDA sensor (Fitbit Charge 5, Fitbit Sense). Furthermore, a patent filed by Apple [14] indicates the possible future inclusion of EDA sensors in the smartwatch product range in the future. Therefore, we believe that the use of EDA for stress detection in wearables should be explored and appropriate methods developed.

1.3. EDA Feature Extraction

In [19], three EDA-based features for stress detection are presented. The features are also used in [5,15]. The three features are:

$$\mu_{SCL} = \frac{1}{N}\sum_{i=1}^{N} \hat{X}_{SCL}(t-i) \tag{1}$$

$$\rho_{SCL} = \rho(t, \hat{X}_{SCL}) \tag{2}$$

$$\sigma_{SCR} = \left(\frac{1}{N}\sum_{i=1}^{N} \hat{X}_{SCR}^2(t-i)\right)^{1/2} \tag{3}$$

μ_{SCL} is the average SCL trend over the last N samples, ρ_{SCL} captures the degree of linearity of SCL and σ_{SCR} captures the standard deviation in SCR.

Four skin conductance features are defined in [20]. The four features are calculated from the absolute value of skin conductance by determining and analysing the local minima and maxima of the measurements. The four features are calculated for a sliding window and give the number of peaks, the sum of the peak values, the sum of the minima values and the estimated area under the response of the skin conductance. The features are also used in [5,15].

The FLIRT toolkit [21] is an open-source Python package for data processing and feature extraction for wearable sensor data. According to the authors, the contribution of the package lies in its holistic approach—the package includes methods for loading datasets, preprocessing, segmentation and feature extraction. The package focuses on four signals: ECG, IBI (inter-beat interval), EDA and ACC (accelerometer).

The EDA features included in FLIRT are statistical, entropy-based, time domain, frequency domain, time-frequency domain and SCR peak-based features:

- time domain: 29 SCR and 21 SCL features are calculated, including statistical (mean, standard deviation, minimum, maximum, percentile values, interquartile range), energy, entropy, number of peaks, SCR peak properties, etc.
- frequency domain: 10 SCR and 10 SCL features including energy, interquartile range, variance and spectral powers at specific frequencies.
- time-frequency domain: 6 statistical features for each EDA component, 12 in total.

Another Python toolkit for EDA feature extraction is available—pyEDA [22]. The authors propose statistical features based on peak detection and raw RDA signal. The authors also propose the use of an autoencoder for feature extraction. The autoencoder is an unsupervised artificial neural network. A total of 64 features are obtained by the authors in this way.

The EDA signal, like any other measured physical signal, is continuous. Most data processing pipelines and algorithms work with data vectors of limited length, often of a fixed length. Therefore, the continuous EDA signal must be segmented and converted into fixed-length segments. The commonly used approach is the sliding window. In sliding window segmentation, the window length and the segmentation step are the two parameters. Many researchers do not give much thought to these, in EDA analysis, 60 s windows are the most commonly used. In [15], different window lengths are analysed for feature extraction. It is reported that longer windows lead to better stress detection, with the longest window studied, 120 s, performing better than the others.

1.4. Evaluation of Stress Detection

The goal of affect recognition and stress detection is to develop algorithms for use in the real world. The generalization property of an algorithm refers to its ability to perform *well* on unseen data. In the case of affect recognition, *unseen* can mean a new user who was not present during training. To evaluate an algorithm for this scenario, the leave one subject out (LOSO) cross-validation approach is used.

LOSO requires that the training dataset comes from a set of subjects. The dataset must also be appropriately labelled. For J subjects, J models M are trained: $M_j, 1 \leq j \leq J$. The j-th model is trained on training data without the data of subject j. Subject j's data are only used for model validation. In this way, J models are trained and scored to produce J scores. The scores are then averaged to determine the total score of the algorithm.

The most common score for classifiers is the accuracy score (4). It is calculated based on the number of true positives (TP), false positives (FP), true negatives (TN) and false negatives (FN).

However, for unbalanced datasets, the F1 score (5) is usually used in such scenarios. WESAD is unbalanced.

$$Accuracy = \frac{TP + TN}{TP + TN + FP + FN} \quad (4)$$

$$F1 = \frac{2TP}{2TP + FP + FN} \quad (5)$$

2. Materials and Methods

In the following sections, we give an overview of the state of the art in EDA-based stress detection with wearable sensors (Section 2.1), describe segmentation and frequency analysis (Section 2.2), and then present our approach in Sections 2.3–2.6.

2.1. Stress Detection Using EDA from Wearable Sensors

Several authors have used WESAD to evaluate their stress detection algorithms. This section lists the results obtained by these authors.

2.1.1. Reference WESAD Classification Results

In WESAD [5], the authors provide reference classification results. Binary (stress vs. no stress) and three-class classification results (stress vs. baseline vs. amusement) are provided. As this is a multimodal dataset (10 sensors), each sensor is used both independently and in groups (all wrist-based, all chest-based, etc.). Five classifiers are evaluated (decision tree, random forest, AdaBoost with decision tree, linear discriminant analysis and K-nearest neighbours). For each, both the F1 score and the accuracy are reported.

The best results for three-class classification were obtained with chest-based ECG, EDA, EMG, respiratory rate and temperature data. The best classifiers for three-class classification were AdaBoost and linear discriminant analysis for accuracy (80.34%) and F1 score (74.43%), respectively.

The best binary classification was obtained using chest-based ECG, EDA, EMG, respiratory and temperature data from the chest. The best classifier for both accuracy and F1 score was linear discriminant analysis, achieving 93.12% and 91.47%, respectively.

The best results of the WESAD authors focusing only on the wrist EDA signal are shown in Table 1. All other approaches aim to outperform this reference.

Table 1. Reference WESAD classification scores [5] for stress detection from wrist-based EDA measurements. AB: AdaBoost with decision trees; LDA: linear discriminant analysis.

	Best F1-Score (%) (Classifier)	Best Accuracy (%) (Classifier)
binary	75.34 ± 0.57 (AB)	79.71 ± 0.43 (AB)
three-class	49.06 ± 0.59 (AB)	62.32 (LDA)

2.1.2. Analysis by Siirtola

In [15], the same features are used as in [5]. The aim of the study is to investigate the effect of window size in the calculation of the features. The conclusion is that longer window sizes lead to better stress detection. The longest window size studied, 120 s, performs better than the other options (15 s and above). Three classifiers are used—LDA, QDA (linear and quadratic discriminant analysis, respectively) and RF (random forest). The best (binary) classification results (for WESAD) are obtained by LDA using skin temperature, BVP and HR signals—87.4%. F1 scores are not reported. The author uses the LOSO approach. Using EDA only, the author reports the best accuracy of 78.3% with the random forest classifier. No other hyperparameters are reported. All results were obtained using a 120 s window, which the authors consider optimal for their feature calculation and choice of classifier.

The reported accuracies are consistent with those of the WESAD authors.

2.1.3. Deep Fusion Network

In [16], an explainable deep neural network approach to affect recognition is presented. The authors demonstrate their approach using the WESAD dataset. The model used is the 'Multimodal-Multisensory Sequential Fusion' (MMSF) model. The results show that the approach performs better than the benchmark dataset [5] in terms of both accuracy and F1 scores. The authors use a very short window—only one second. The authors use both chest and wrist modalities. Since they are dealing with a multimodal problem, signal fusion is required. After experimenting with early and late fusion, they decide to use late fusion, i.e., each modality trains its own model (neural network) and the results of all modalities are fused with an additional model (random forest). The reported results are an accuracy of 83% and an F1 score of 81% (in the three-class problem, using all chest modalities of WESAD). On further analysis, the authors found that EDA measured at the chest was the most important modality. In contrast, EDA measured at the wrist was found to be insignificant. This stark difference can be attributed to the different sampling rates. The EDA measured at the chest in WESAD is sampled at 700 Hz, whereas the Empatica E4, which is used to measure EDA at the wrist, samples at a much lower frequency. This results in too few measurements in the one-second window and thus poorer performance.

2.1.4. StressNAS

In [3], deep neural networks (DNNs) are applied to the WESAD dataset. The proposed StressNAS is a data-driven approach for deep neural network design. The authors report a significant improvement in performance over the reference implementation in [5] and manual DNN design approaches. The results are presented in Table 2. The experiments were performed with a sliding window of 60 s width and 0.25 s step size.

Table 2. StressNAS: Accuracy of stress detection (WESAD). All wrist signals: BVP, EDA and temperature. (Δ [5]): an improvement over reference implementation.

	All Wrist Signals (Accuracy %)	EDA (Δ [5]) (Accuracy %)
Stress vs. No stress	93.14	79.24 (−0.47)
Three-class	83.43	66.89 (+4.57)

The three-class classification accuracy obtained using StressNAS-designed DNNs (using the EDA signal) is 4.57% higher than the reference results.

2.1.5. FLIRT Toolkit

FLIRT is a feature generation toolkit for wearable sensor data. The authors provide WESAD results [21]. They use 60 s windows with a step of 0.25 s, just as in [5]. The authors use LOSO cross-validation and the same classifiers as in [5] (LDA, RF, AB, DT). F1 scores for three class classifications are reported.

The three-class classification F1 score by the authors of FLIRT using EDA is reported as 51.96% (compared to 49.06% in [5]). Other values (binary, accuracy) are not given.

2.1.6. XGBoost

The contributions of [23] to EDA stress detection are the use of the XGBoost classifier, an alternative segmentation approach, the use of a high number of features (almost 200) and the use of feature selection algorithms. The results related to improved segmentation are of interest as the authors found an improvement of about 15% over the reference (binary classification, F1 score, chest and wrist EDA, independently) just by using an alternative segmentation strategy. In [3,5,21], the authors used a 60 s sliding window with 0.25 s steps. In [23], the authors also used a 60 s sliding window but a 30 s step. (The authors report that they obtained only 1041 segments using this approach. Our calculations show that about 8000–9000 segments should be extracted).

In addition, the authors obtain relatively small improvements (a few percentage points) by using the XGBoost classifier and using (almost 200) additional features. The authors also propose a feature selection approach to reduce the number of features and thus improve the efficiency of the classification task without significantly degrading the performance.

The final result is 89.92% F1 score of the binary classification task when using the wrist-based EDA signal and 92.38% with the chest-based EDA.

2.1.7. pyEDA

The authors of pyEDA [22], a Python library for EDA manipulation, also provide stress detection results for WESAD. However, the results reported by the authors cannot be compared with those of [3,5,15,16,21,23] because the authors do not use LOSO cross-validation and, more importantly, they define the binary classification problem as follows: 'Baseline section labels as "not stressed" (0), and EDA data in the Stress section labeled as "stressed" (1)', in this approach all data labelled as 'Amusement' are seemingly ignored.

The authors report an accuracy of 88–90% when only statistical characteristics are used. The accuracy increases to 95–97% when the autoencoder-generated features are used.

2.1.8. Summary

The results of seven papers were listed. Of the seven, only the authors of the WESAD dataset gave F1 scores *and* accuracy for the binary *and* three-class problems (see Table 3). Most of the results were obtained without giving much importance to the choice of window size in the segmentation. The exception is [15], where an increase in accuracy is reported when the window size is increased. In our work, we focus on using the EDA signal measured at the wrist. Therefore, we only compare our results with EDA-based results from other authors. Deep fusion network results obtained using only EDA are not reported and, therefore, cannot be directly compared with our results.

Among the reported results, the deep fusion network, XGBoost and pyEDA stand out for their reported values. (1) For the deep fusion network, this improvement can be attributed to the use of more signals (all chest measurements). (2) pyEDA's performance results are not directly comparable to the other results because they define the binary case differently than other authors. They do not report three-class classification. (3) The authors of XGBoost report the largest performance gain when using a thirty-second step in the segmentation. This result is surprising, but unfortunately, we could not replicate their results by combining their segmentation and our feature extraction.

Table 3. WESAD results as reported by other authors. ACC: accuracy. * The authors use a 30 s step with the sliding window, this results in prolonged time from stress onset to detection (60 s window + up to 30 s waiting period, in total up to 90 s). ** The results are with chest-measured signals (results using only wrist-measured EDA were not reported).

Approach	2 Class ACC (%)	2 Class F1 (%)	3 Class ACC (%)	3 Class F1 (%)	Window [s]
Siirtola [15]	78.3	-	-	-	120
DFN [16] **	-	-	83	81	1
StressNAS [3]	79.24	-	66.89	-	60
FLIRT [21]	-	-	-	51.96	60
XGBoost [23]	-	89.92	-	-	60 *

2.2. Segmentation and Frequency Analysis

The original dataset contains continuous, non-segmented measurements. The dataset is segmented using the sliding window approach, just as in [5]. It is ensured that each segment contains only measurements related to a single affective state. The window width and step are configurable parameters whose choice we discuss later. Figure 1 shows examples of segments for each of the affective states in WESAD.

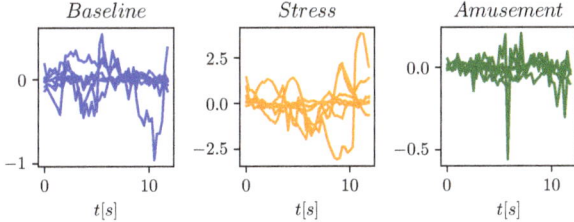

Figure 1. Examples of the three WESAD classes.

Much of the research focuses on temporal features, but we are exploring the use of frequency-based features. To obtain a frequency spectrum of a signal, the Fourier transform is performed. The transformation of the signal $x(t)$ in the time domain to $X(f)$ in the frequency domain is given in (6). For the discrete signal $x(k), k \in \mathbb{N}$, the discrete Fourier transform (DFT) is used as given in (7).

$$X(f) = \int_{-\infty}^{\infty} x(t) e^{-2\pi i f} dt \qquad (6)$$

$$X(f) = \sum_{k=0}^{N-1} x(k) e^{-i 2\pi f k / N} \qquad (7)$$

For a non-periodic discrete signal $x(k)$ of finite length $0 \leq k \leq N-1$, the DFT is discrete and periodic. For the analysis, we can restrict ourselves to the first period only and ignore the rest. Since the resulting DFT is an even function, the values at negative f may be ignored. We are left with $X = \{X_1, ..., X_{\frac{N}{2}}\}$. The frequency resolution of X is $\frac{1}{t_s N}$ (t_s is the sampling interval of x, N is the number of samples).

The Fourier transform generally results in a complex signal. The signal consists of the absolute value (absolute spectra $|X(f)|$) and the phase (phase spectra $\angle X(f)$).

We are interested in the DFT of the three affective states contained in WESAD. Each segment of the normalized dataset is labelled (stress, amusement, baseline). For each segment, DFT can be run and the absolute spectra computed. Figure 2 shows the power-normalized absolute spectra of the three classes. The mean and standard deviation envelopes are shown. It can be seen that the three classes differ in their amplitude spectra.

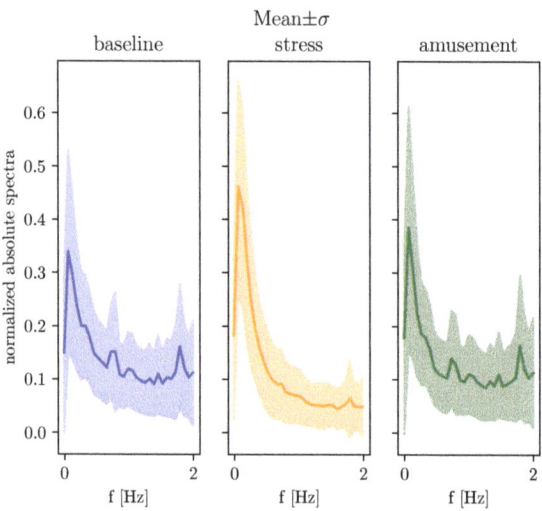

Figure 2. Normalized amplitude spectra of three classes from WESAD: mean and standard deviation.

2.3. Feature Extraction

Following the time series analysis pipeline of (1) segmentation, (2) feature extraction and (3) classification, appropriate features should be extracted. Figure 2 suggests that the absolute spectra could be used to obtain features relevant to affect recognition. In the following sections, the features are introduced and explained.

2.3.1. Frequency Band Selection

In Figure 2 the distinction between stress and the other two classes can be seen. A subset of the spectra (a frequency band) could be used to extract useful features. $|X^b|$ denotes the spectra X with amplitudes above and below the cut-off frequencies (f_{low} and f_{high}) set to 0. We propose to divide the amplitude spectra into several frequency bands and calculate features for each band. Since the EDA signal measured at the wrist is sampled at 4 Hz, we propose two frequency bands: (1) $f_{low} = 0.0$ Hz, $f_{high} = 1.0$ Hz, (2) $f_{low} = 1.0$ Hz, $f_{high} = 2.0$ Hz. In this way, one set of features describes the low frequencies and a second set of features describes the higher frequencies.

$$|X^b|(f) = \begin{cases} 0, & \text{if } f < f_{low} \\ 0, & \text{if } f > f_{high} \\ |X|(f), & \text{otherwise} \end{cases} \tag{8}$$

2.3.2. Mean and Standard Deviation

For each amplitude spectrum $|X^b_{i,j,k}|(f)$ (class i, person j, exemplar k) the mean $\overline{|X^b|}_{i,j,k}$ and the standard deviation $\sigma_{i,j,k}(|X^b|)$ of the selected frequency band are calculated:

$$N_b = (f_{high} - f_{low})f_s \tag{9}$$

$$\overline{|X^b|}_{i,j,k} = \frac{1}{N_b} \sum_f |X^b_{i,j,k}|(f) \tag{10}$$

$$\sigma_{i,j,k}(|X^b|) = \sqrt{\frac{1}{N_b - 1} \sum_f \left| |X^b_{i,j,k}|(f) - \overline{|X^b_{i,j,k}|} \right|^2} \tag{11}$$

2.3.3. Max Amplitude Spectra

In addition to the mean and the standard deviation, other features can also be obtained. Figure 2 shows that the maximum value in highlighted frequency band can be used. (12) defines $\alpha_{i,j,k}^b$ as the maximum value of $|X_{i,j,k}^b(f)|$ in the selected frequency band.

$$\alpha_{i,j,k}^b = \max_f |X_{i,j,k}^b(f)| \qquad (12)$$

2.3.4. Half-Energy Frequency

The amplitude spectra in Figure 2 show that higher frequencies are less present in the class 'stress' than in the other classes. This observation is exploited to obtain an additional feature.

According to the laws of signal processing, the square of the amplitude spectrum of a signal corresponds to the energy density spectrum of the signal—a description of the energy distribution of the signal over different frequencies [24]. The law is presented in (13). In (14) the normalized cumulative energy sum $Psi_f(f)$ is introduced.

$$\Psi(f) = |X(f)|^2 \quad \to \quad \Psi_{i,j,k}(f) = |X_{i,j,k}(f)|^2 \qquad (13)$$

$$\Psi_f(f) = \frac{1}{\int_0^\infty \Psi(\omega) d\omega} \int_0^f \Psi(\omega) d\omega \qquad (14)$$

The frequency $f_{P/2}$ that satisfies the Equation (15) is calculated and used as a new feature.

$$\int_0^{f_{P/2}} \Psi(f) df = \int_{f_{P/2}}^\infty \Psi(f) df \quad \to \quad \Psi_f(f_{P/2}) = 0.5 \qquad (15)$$

This feature is calculated using the full amplitude spectrum and does not depend on the frequency band in (8).

2.4. Feature Space

The exemplars from Figure 1 can be represented in the feature space. Figure 3 shows the features calculated for $f_{low} = 1.0$ Hz, $f_{high} = 2.0$ Hz. As expected, the stress samples (yellow) are partially separable from the other two classes.

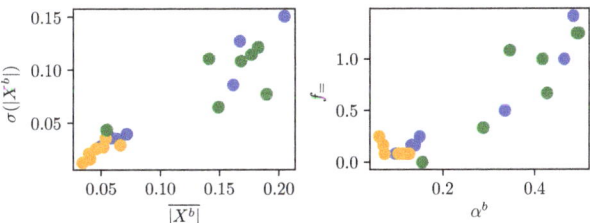

Figure 3. Seven exemplars from Figure 1 in feature space. Colours are analogous to Figure 2. The frequency band is set to $f_{low} = 1.0$ Hz, $f_{high} = 2.0$ Hz.

2.5. Sequence Analysis

Figure 4 shows 30 randomly selected examples from each of the WESAD classes in the feature space. It shows that although the samples of baseline, stress and amusement may overlap in the feature space, the samples of stress have lower variance. In this section, we exploit this observation to obtain additional features.

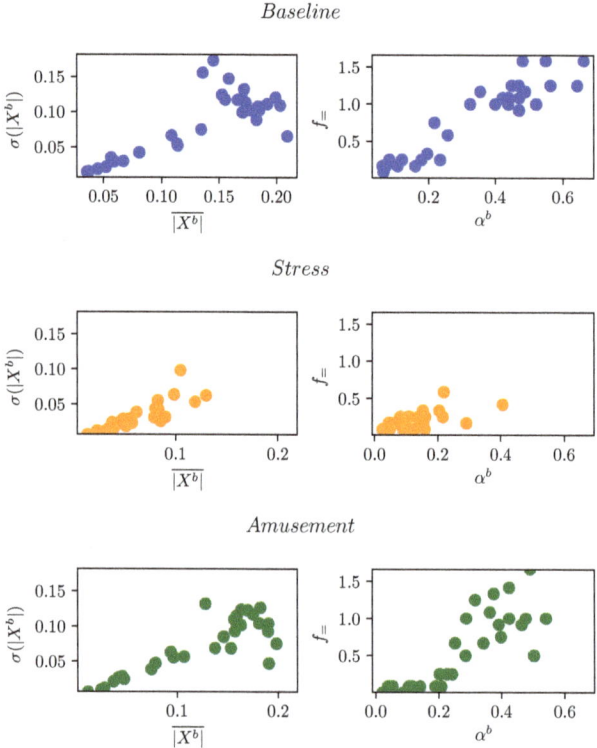

Figure 4. Thirty samples of each class from WESAD in feature space. Stress samples exhibit lower variance.

To calculate the variance, an observation window w is defined. Then w successive samples are evaluated and mean and variance are calculated for each feature. This increases the number of features from 4 to 12 for each frequency band. Equations (16) and (17) show the calculations for feature $a_{i,j,m}$, where $a_{i,j,m}$ is one of $\overline{|X^b|}_{i,j,k}$, $\sigma_{i,j,k}(|X^b|)$, $\alpha^b_{i,j,k}$, $f_{P/2}$.

$$M_w(a_{i,j,k}) = \frac{1}{w}\sum_{m=k-w}^{k} a_{i,j,m} \qquad (16)$$

$$V_w(a_{i,j,k}) = \frac{1}{w}\sum_{m=k-w}^{k} \left(a_{i,j,m} - M_w(a_{i,j,k})\right)^2 \qquad (17)$$

2.6. Multiple Bands

The features derived in (10)–(12) are calculated for a single frequency band. However, multiple frequency bands can also be defined. For m frequency bands, a total of $3*m+1$ features are derived, since (8) is independent of frequency bands.

Applying (16) and (17) results in $3*(3*m+1)$ total features.

3. Results and Discussion

3.1. Evaluation

In Sections 2.1–2.5, we presented our approach to segmentation, analysis and feature extraction for stress detection using the EDA signal measured at the wrist. In this section, the results are presented, followed by a discussion of their relevance.

3.1.1. Classifiers

The contribution of this work is the processing pipeline suitable for WESAD and the features derived in Sections 2.3 and 2.5. To evaluate our contribution, a classification task is used. Different classifiers are used for classification, similar to [5,15,21–23].

Usually, classifiers are subjected to intensive hyperparameter tuning, but this is beyond the scope of this paper. Our goal is to show how the proposed pipeline and features can be used to achieve good performance in stress detection, rather than our ability to fine-tune a classifier. Therefore, our classifiers were not fine-tuned with respect to their hyperparameters. Moreover, we compare the results of the different classifiers used with the *best performing* classifier of the reference implementation in [5]. Therefore, an improvement in accuracy and F1 score would indicate that one of the classifiers using the presented pipeline and features presented, outperformed *all* classifiers used by Schmidt et al.

The following classifiers were selected for evaluation in our work:
- Decision tree, with a maximum depth of 10;
- 1-NN;
- kNN, where k (the number of neighbours) is set to 10;
- Random forest, where the number of trees is set to either 10 or 100, the maximum depth is 10 in both cases, and the class weights are balanced;
- Support vector machine (SVM) with radial kernel and balanced class weights;
- Bagged SVM;
- AdaBoost with random forest, with 10 estimators and each random forest consisting of 100 trees of depth 10 and balanced class weights.

For all the above classifiers, their implementations in Scikit-learn [25] (version 1.1.2) are used.

3.1.2. Time to Detection

For practical stress detection, time to detection (TTD) is crucial. We define TTD as the difference between the timestamps of the first and the last sample used for classification. The time series used for training and evaluation were obtained using a sliding window approach with step t_{step} and window width t_{length}. TTD is calculated as shown in Equation (18).

$$TTD = t_{length} + (w-1) * t_{step} \tag{18}$$

3.2. Classification Results

Table 1 shows the results of the reference classification of Schmidt et al. [5]. The results were obtained using a LOSO approach and are presented for both the three-class and binary cases.

Table 4 shows the classification results obtained using the approach described in this paper. Segment length and overlap were set to $t_{length} = 48 * t_s$, $t_{overlap} = 20 * t_s$ (t_s is the sampling time $t_s = \frac{1}{4\,\text{Hz}} = 0.25$ s). To achieve a TTD of less than one minute, a window with $w = 7$ segments was chosen. This results in a TTD of 54 s. A summary of the results:

1. For the binary case, *every* tested classifier, using the approach proposed by us, *outperforms, in terms of both accuracy and F1 score, the best performing* wrist-measured EDA classifier as reported by Schmidt et al.
2. For the three-class case, only the decision tree and the nearest neighbour classifiers lead to lower accuracy than the best-performing wrist-measured EDA classifier using the established EDA features. In all other cases tested, the proposed approach performs better than the established features.

Table 4. Classification results of our proposed approach, and comparison to best results achieved by Schmidt et al. [5]. Δ is the absolute difference in accuracy or F1 score. Positive values of Δ indicate better performance by our approach. NNL nearest neighbour; RF: random forest; SVM: support vector machine.

	Binary Case			
	Accuracy (%)		F1 (%)	
	Score	Δ [5]	Score	Δ [5]
Decision Tree	84.15	4.44	81.58	6.24
1NN	81.95	2.24	78.58	3.24
10NN	83.82	4.11	80.54	5.20
RF 10	84.87	5.16	82.13	6.79
RF 100	84.84	5.13	81.82	6.48
SVM	82.69	2.98	80.08	4.74
Bagged SVM	82.12	2.41	79.93	4.59
AdaBoost RF 100	83.86	4.15	80.29	4.95
	Three-Class Case			
	Accuracy (%)		F1 (%)	
	Score	Δ [5]	Score	Δ [5]
Decision Tree	58.53	−3.79	52.68	4.62
1NN	62.21	−0.11	53.74	4.68
10NN	69.89	7.57	54.34	5.28
RF 10	65.75	3.43	56.08	7.02
RF 100	66.86	4.54	56.36	7.30
SVM	67.08	4.76	56.78	7.14
Bagged SVM	67.56	5.24	56.20	7.14
AdaBoost RF100	67.00	4.68	54.67	5.61

3.3. Constant TTD

In Section 3.2, a single t_{length}, t_{step}, w combination was evaluated. We are interested in a more comprehensive evaluation of the method as well as a comparison of a range of possible values.

$t_{length}, t_{overlap}, w$ and TTD are linked in Equation (18). For a fixed TTD, w can be determined for each t_{length} and $t_{overlap}$. In this section, the TTD was set to either 30 s (Figure 5a) or 60 s (Figure 5b). t_{length} and $t_{overlap}$ were iterated in a grid search (requiring $t_{overlap} < t_{length}$). At each combination, w was calculated (which requires $w \in \mathbb{N}$). Once w, t_{length} and $t_{overlap}$ are known, a dataset can be created and a classifier trained and evaluated. Figure 5a,b show the comparison of the classifiers with the best results of Schmidt et al.

A comparison of Figure 5a,b shows a significant drop in performance when the TTD is lowered. This is understandable as the classifier works with data that spans a shorter period of time (30 s versus 60 s).

3.4. Effect of Window Size

Figures 5a,b show the importance of choosing the correct window size. The effect of window size in stress detection has been studied before, for example in [15]. In this section, we investigate the effect of window size on classification results using our proposed features.

In Figure 6, $t_{length} = 48, t_{overlap} = 20$ are used and different window sizes are evaluated. For each calculated TTD, the accuracy and F1 scores are calculated for both the binary and three-class cases. The aim of this experiment is to show how changes in TTD affect detection performance. In this experiment, only one classifier was used, the simple kNN ($k = 10$) classifier. The classifier was chosen because of its high three-class accuracy in Table 4.

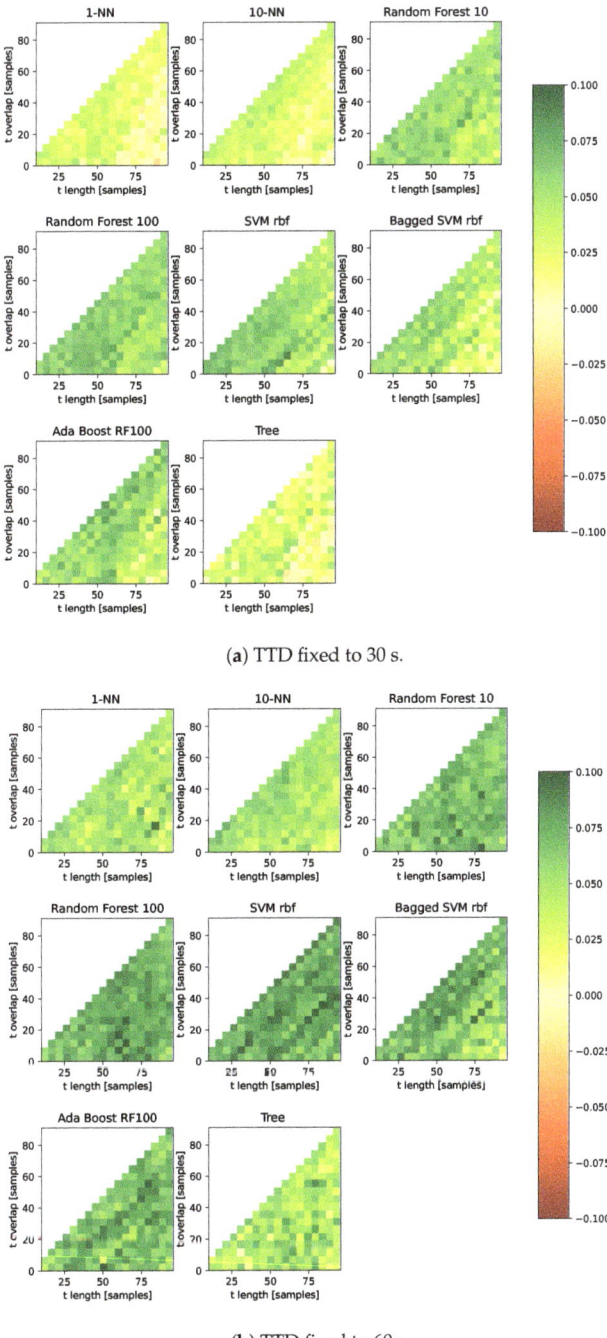

Figure 5. Improvement over Schmidt et al. (green = better), F1 score, three classes (baseline, stress, amusement).

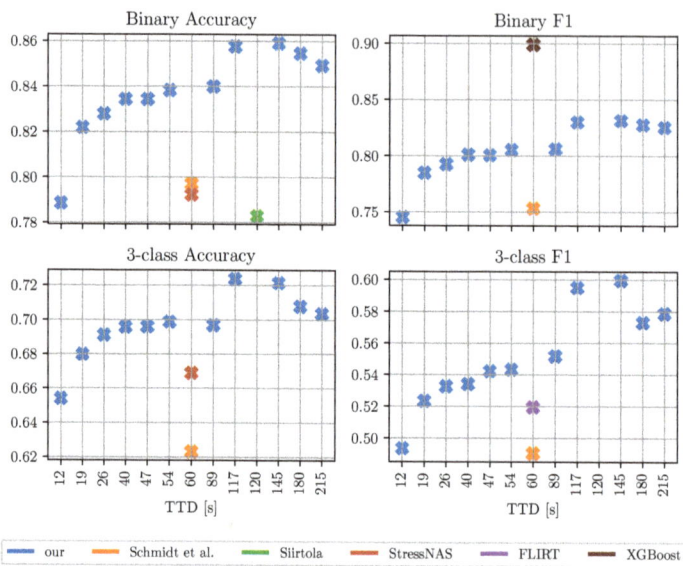

Figure 6. Effect of window size. $t_{length} = 48$, $t_{overlap} = 20$. Blue crosses: our results at various times to detection (x-axis (s)), using kNN classifier (k = 10). Orange, green, red, purple and brown crosses: results by other authors. Siirtola uses 120 s segments, while others authors use 60 s. See Table 3 for further details on results from other authors.

Figure 6 shows a positive trend with increasing TTD. Therefore, a balance between performance and short TTD must be found when choosing the window size. The figures also show the results of Schmidt et al., Siirtola, StressNAS, FLIRT and XGBoost. The figure shows that the results of the other authors were obtained with window sizes of 60 s or more. The approach we present outperforms the other approaches, even when it provides faster stress detection (shown as lower TTD in Figure 6)! Moreover, we use the simple kNN classifier, while some of the other authors use much more complex classifiers.

3.5. Discussion of Results

In Sections 3.2–3.4, we have demonstrated considerable improvements over the results of other authors. We focused only on the EDA signal measured at the wrist. The results show that the features defined in Section 2.3 provide improved classification performance.

Most other authors have used a 60 s window to obtain their features, Siirtola uses a 120 s window. We have investigated other window widths and have shown that our method performs well with shorter windows reducing the time from the onset of stress to first detection (TTD). As the window increases, the performance improves.

It is worth noting that for all other authors, we used their *best* results with the wrist-measured EDA in WESAD, even so, the proposed method clearly outperformed them on many occasions.

4. Conclusions

Affective state recognition is an active area of research, and with advances in wearable technology, recognition using wearable sensors is becoming increasingly important. Among affective states, stress has been extensively researched, in part because of its impact on productivity and well-being.

This paper explores the use of frequency analysis of EDA signals obtained from wearable sensors for stress detection.

The main contribution of this paper is the proposed method for extracting features in the frequency domain. Throughout the article, the idea is explored and validated several times. The approach is validated using data from the publicly available WESAD dataset for stress detection by wearable sensors. Our results are compared with existing techniques and those published by several other authors. The proposed approach improves the accuracy and F1 scores of some existing techniques for stress detection from (wearable measured) EDA signals.

For any detection algorithm (fault, stress, etc.), the time from onset to detection is an important performance metric in addition to the accuracy of detection. The proposed approach allows for a customizable window length and thus a large number of possible values for time to detection (TTD). A trade-off between a short detection time and accuracy has been demonstrated. The proposed method has been shown to provide higher detection accuracy with a lower TTD than other comparable methods.

The work presented in our paper is an improvement over some of the commonly used methods and can be used in practical applications for stress detection.

Author Contributions: Conceptualization, A.S., A.L., O.S. and I.Š.; methodology, B.P. and I.Š.; software, Ž.S.; validation, Ž.S.; formal analysis, A.S., A.L., O.S. and I.Š.; investigation, Ž.S., A.S., A.L., B.P. and I.Š.; resources, B.P.; data curation, Ž.S.; writing—original draft preparation, Ž.S.; writing—review and editing, Ž.S., A.S., A.L., O.S., B.P. and I.Š.; visualization, Ž.S.; supervision, B.P. and I.Š.; project administration, B.P. and I.Š.; funding acquisition, B.P. All authors have read and agreed to the published version of the manuscript.

Funding: This research was funded by the Program Chair of Excellence of Universidad Carlos III de Madrid and Bank of Santander and the Spanish Ministry of Economy, Industry and Competitiveness, projects TRA2015-63708-R, TRA2016-78886-C3-1-R, PID2019-104793RB-C31 and PDC2021-121517-C31. This research was funded by the Slovenian Research Agency, core research funding No. P2-0001 and L2-4454.

Institutional Review Board Statement: Not applicable.

Informed Consent Statement: Not applicable.

Data Availability Statement: The data presented in this study are openly available in the WESAD dataset at https://doi.org/10.1145/3242969.3242985.

Conflicts of Interest: The authors declare no conflict of interest.

References

1. O'Connor, D.B.; Thayer, J.F.; Vedhara, K. Stress and health: A review of psychobiological processes. *Annu. Rev. Psychol.* **2021**, *72*, 663–688. [CrossRef] [PubMed]
2. Makowski, D.; Pham, T.; Lau, Z.J.; Brammer, J.C.; Lespinasse, F.; Pham, H.; Schölzel, C.; Chen, S.H.A. NeuroKit2: A Python toolbox for neurophysiological signal processing. *Behav. Res. Methods* **2021**, *53*, 1689–1696. [CrossRef] [PubMed]
3. Huynh, L.; Nguyen, T.; Nguyen, T.; Pirttikangas, S.; Siirtola, P. StressNAS: Affect State and Stress Detection Using Neural Architecture Search. In Proceedings of the Adjunct 2021 ACM International Joint Conference on Pervasive and Ubiquitous Computing and 2021 ACM International Symposium on Wearable Computers, Virtual, 21–26 September 2021; pp. 121–125.
4. Gjoreski, M.; Kolenik, T.; Knez, T.; Luštrek, M.; Gams, M.; Gjoreski, H.; Pejović, V. Datasets for Cognitive Load Inference Using Wearable Sensors and Psychological Traits. *Appl. Sci.* **2020**, *10*, 3843. [CrossRef]
5. Schmidt, P.; Reiss, A.; Duerichen, R.; Marberger, C.; Van Laerhoven, K. Introducing WESAD, a Multimodal Dataset for Wearable Stress and Affect Detection. In Proceedings of the 20th ACM International Conference on Multimodal Interaction, Boulder, CO, USA, 16–20 October 2018; pp. 400–408.
6. Schmidt, P.; Reiss, A.; Dürichen, R.; Laerhoven, K.V. Wearable-based affect recognition—A review. *Sensors* **2019**, *19*, 4079. [CrossRef] [PubMed]
7. Segerstrom, S.C.; Miller, G.E. Psychological stress and the human immune system: A meta-analytic study of 30 years of inquiry. *Psychol. Bull.* **2004**, *130*, 601. [CrossRef]
8. Baptiste, N.R. Tightening the link between employee wellbeing at work and performance: A new dimension for HRM. *Manag. Decis.* **2008**, *46*, 284–309. [CrossRef]
9. Koelstra, S.; Muhl, C.; Soleymani, M.; Lee, J.S.; Yazdani, A.; Ebrahimi, T.; Pun, T.; Nijholt, A.; Patras, I. DEAP: A Database for Emotion Analysis Using Physiological Signals. *IEEE Trans. Affect. Comput.* **2011**, *3*, 18–31. [CrossRef]

10. Birjandtalab, J.; Cogan, D.; Pouyan, M.B.; Nourani, M. A non-EEG Biosignals Dataset for Assessment and Visualization of Neurological Status. In Proceedings of the 2016 IEEE International Workshop on Signal Processing Systems (SiPS), Dallas, TX, USA, 26–28 October 2016; pp. 110–114.
11. Soleymani, M.; Lichtenauer, J.; Pun, T.; Pantic, M. A Multimodal Database for Affect Recognition and Implicit Tagging. *IEEE Trans. Affect. Comput.* **2011**, *3*, 42–55. [CrossRef]
12. Wang, R.; Chen, F.; Chen, Z.; Li, T.; Harari, G.; Tignor, S.; Zhou, X.; Ben-Zeev, D.; Campbell, A.T. StudentLife: Assessing mental health, academic performance and behavioral trends of college students using smartphones. In Proceedings of the 2014 ACM International Joint Conference on Pervasive and Ubiquitous Computing, Seattle, WA, USA, 13–17 September 2014; pp. 3–14.
13. Kanjo, E.; Younis, E.M.; Ang, C.S. Deep learning analysis of mobile physiological, environmental and location sensor data for emotion detection. *Inf. Fusion* **2019**, *49*, 46–56. [CrossRef]
14. Rothkopf, F.R.; Ive, J.; Hoenig, J.; Zorkendorfer, R. Wearable Electronic Device. U.S. Patent 10,942,491, 9 March 2021.
15. Siirtola, P. Continuous Stress Detection Using the Sensors of Commercial Smartwatch. In Proceedings of the Adjunct 2019 ACM International Joint Conference on Pervasive and Ubiquitous Computing and 2019 ACM International Symposium on Wearable Computers, London, UK, 9–13 September 2019; pp. 1198–1201.
16. Lin, J.; Pan, S.; Lee, C.S.; Oviatt, S. An Explainable Deep Dusion Network for Affect Recognition Using Physiological Signals. In Proceedings of the 28th ACM International Conference on Information and Knowledge Management, Beijing, China, 3–7 November 2019; pp. 2069–2072.
17. Russell, J.A. Affective space is bipolar. *J. Personal. Soc. Psychol.* **1979**, *37*, 345. [CrossRef]
18. Greco, A.; Valenza, G.; Lanata, A.; Scilingo, E.P.; Citi, L. cvxEDA: A Convex Optimization Approach to Electrodermal Activity Processing. *IEEE Trans. Biomed. Eng.* **2015**, *63*, 797–804. [CrossRef] [PubMed]
19. Choi, J.; Ahmed, B.; Gutierrez-Osuna, R. Development and Evaluation of an Ambulatory Atress Monitor Based on Wearable Sensors. *IEEE Trans. Inf. Technol. Biomed.* **2011**, *16*, 279–286. [CrossRef]
20. Healey, J.A.; Picard, R.W. Detecting stress during real-world driving tasks using physiological sensors. *IEEE Trans. Intell. Transp. Syst.* **2005**, *6*, 156–166. [CrossRef]
21. Föll, S.; Maritsch, M.; Spinola, F.; Mishra, V.; Barata, F.; Kowatsch, T.; Fleisch, E.; Wortmann, F. FLIRT: A feature generation toolkit for wearable data. *Comput. Methods Programs Biomed.* **2021**, *212*, 106461. [CrossRef] [PubMed]
22. Aqajari, S.A.H.; Naeini, E.K.; Mehrabadi, M.A.; Labbaf, S.; Dutt, N.; Rahmani, A.M. pyEDA: An Open-Source Python Toolkit for Pre-processing and Feature Extraction of Electrodermal Activity. *Procedia Comput. Sci.* **2021**, *184*, 99–106. [CrossRef]
23. Hsieh, C.P.; Chen, Y.T.; Beh, W.K.; Wu, A.Y.A. Feature Selection Framework for XGBoost Based on Electrodermal Activity in Stress Detection. In Proceedings of the 2019 IEEE International Workshop on Signal Processing Systems (SiPS), Nanjing, China, 20–23 October 2019; pp. 330–335. [CrossRef]
24. Semmlow, J. Chapter 4—The Fourier Transform and Power Spectrum: Implications and Applications. In *Signals and Systems for Bioengineers*, 2nd ed.; Semmlow, J., Ed.; Biomedical Engineering; Academic Press: Boston, MA, USA, 2012; pp. 131–165. . [CrossRef]
25. Pedregosa, F.; Varoquaux, G.; Gramfort, A.; Michel, V.; Thirion, B.; Grisel, O.; Blondel, M.; Prettenhofer, P.; Weiss, R.; Dubourg, V.; et al. Scikit-learn: Machine Learning in Python. *J. Mach. Learn. Res.* **2011**, *12*, 2825–2830.

Disclaimer/Publisher's Note: The statements, opinions and data contained in all publications are solely those of the individual author(s) and contributor(s) and not of MDPI and/or the editor(s). MDPI and/or the editor(s) disclaim responsibility for any injury to people or property resulting from any ideas, methods, instructions or products referred to in the content.

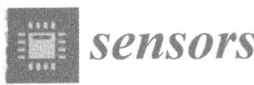

Article

Self-Sensing Variable Stiffness Actuation of Shape Memory Coil by an Inferential Soft Sensor

Bhagoji Bapurao Sul [1], Dhanalakshmi Kaliaperumal [1,*] and Seung-Bok Choi [2,3,*]

[1] Department of Instrumentation and Control Engineering, National Institute of Technology, Tiruchirappalli 620015, Tamil Nadu, India
[2] Department of Mechanical Engineering, The State University of New York, Korea (SUNY Korea), Incheon 21985, Republic of Korea
[3] Department of Mechanical Engineering, Industrial University of Ho Chi Minh City (IUH), Ho Chi Minh City 70000, Vietnam
* Correspondence: dhanlak@nitt.edu (D.K.); seungbok.choi@sunykorea.ac.kr (S.-B.C.)

Abstract: Self-sensing actuation of shape memory alloy (SMA) means to sense both mechanical and thermal properties/variables through the measurement of any internally changing electrical property such as resistance/inductance/capacitance/phase/frequency of an actuating material under actuation. The main contribution of this paper is to obtain the stiffness from the measurement of electrical resistance of a shape memory coil during variable stiffness actuation thereby, simulating its self-sensing characteristics by developing a Support Vector Machine (SVM) regression and nonlinear regression model. Experimental evaluation of the stiffness of a passive biased shape memory coil (SMC) in antagonistic connection, for different electrical (like activation current, excitation frequency, and duty cycle) and mechanical input conditions (for example, the operating condition pre-stress) is done in terms of change in electrical resistance through the measurement of the instantaneous value. The stiffness is then calculated from force and displacement, while by this scheme it is sensed from the electrical resistance. To fulfill the deficiency of a dedicated physical stiffness sensor, self-sensing stiffness by a Soft Sensor (equivalently SVM) is a boon for variable stiffness actuation. A simple and well-proven voltage division method is used for indirect stiffness sensing; wherein, voltages across the shape memory coil and series resistance provide the electrical resistance. The predicted stiffness of SVM matches well with the experimental stiffness and this is validated by evaluating the performances such as root mean squared error (RMSE), the goodness of fit and correlation coefficient. This self-sensing variable stiffness actuation (SSVSA) provides several advantages in applications of SMA: sensor-less systems, miniaturized systems, simplified control systems and possible stiffness feedback control.

Keywords: shape memory coil; joule heating effect; self-sensing actuation; variable stiffness actuation; electrical resistance; support vector machine regression model; nonlinear regression model

1. Introduction

The shape memory coil (SMC) has a larger change in force and controllable stiffness to introduce the structural elastic deformation and to be in tune with a structural load. It provides the actuation to a mechanical structure; actuation with variable load can be sensed by self-sensing the stiffness in the structure via the Shape Memory Alloy (SMA) coil's resistance. This is because of the shape memory effect phenomenon, which is an inherent property present in the nickel-titanium alloy. This inherent property is due to phase transformation from martensite to austenite and vice-versa when subjected to temperature or current. Though the SMA has same chemical composition, atomic weight and mass number, but it is different structure in the austenite and martensite phase.

Until now, none is dedicated to physical sensor or analytical models to sense the stiffness of shape memory alloy or SMA with mechanical structure. Nowadays, the sensing

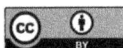

function of SMA becomes more important because the high technology for the humanoid robot, industrial automation and medical field is being progressed a lot. It has been found 30 years ago that the electrical resistance of SMA changes during phase transformation of its material [1]. The modelling of SMA resistance to stiffness as compared to the models of temperature to stiffness is very rare in literature. A linear equation only is suggested between stiffness and normalized resistance. Thus, as a need of sensing/measurement and control of stiffness accurately, it must go into details of the topic. In this case, to attenuate the surrounding environmental effect, a robust and simple adaptive control is adopted. The experimental result proved that the stiffness as well as position could be controlled to achieve the desired displacement. The stiffness of the alloy varies depending on its phase. The phase of the alloy can be estimated by measuring its electrical resistance. Electrical resistance is relatively higher in martensite and lower in the austenite phase. Furthermore, a new scheme of stiffness is implemented by considering two feedback inputs- electrical resistance and position [1].

This electrical property is useful for sensing of thermal and mechanical properties like temperature, force and strain of SMA. Since then, many research papers have proved that resistance change is sufficiently linear to measure and control displacement and strain [2]. These works intuitively explained about the relationship between displacements in the SMA wire and its resistance. Another important point is that the SMA actuator exhibits highly nonlinear behavior. Therefore, a neural network is employed to estimate the value of displacement in the SMA from its resistance change. The estimated value of displacement from resistance is used as feedback to control it [2]. The estimation of the state (contraction/displacement) of the SMA wire actuator is done with the help of its resistance. The state of the SMA wire model has been developed by using the concept of unscented Kalman filter (UKF) which uses the measured resistance. The results are compared with the work of the extended Kalman filter and show good accuracy [3]. Accurate self-sensing concept to control the flexures by controlling the SMA wire has been also developed. Then the polynomial model is used to estimate the strain value from measurement of resistance. In addition, the inaccuracies due to the presence of the hysteresis has been overcome by pretension force. By considering standard test signals such as step and sinusoidal signals, performance of the control system has been also tested [4].

The polynomial model accurately enables estimation of the SMA actuator strain by applying an electrical potential across it. The experimental results have shown that the self-sensing model can achieves a small transient error and works effectively. The self-sensing helps to develop to miniaturized devices to perform effectively and efficiently [5] in which a self-sensing concept for control has been well described by adopting an antagonistic SMA wire drive. This drive is tested under different conditions such as pre-strain and duty cycles. Then, the modeling of strain and resistance is derived with the help of a curve-fitted polynomial. It has been also realized that the accurate control of an actuator wire by self-sensing feedback with a hysteresis compensator can be done [6].

From the results of this work, it has been realized that the use of neural networks to characterize the relation between the resistance of SMA wire and its strain is very effective. The great advantage of this concept is that the single SMA wire performs dual tasks as both an actuator and a sensor. This has got great importance when the prime objectives are to reduce the overall weight, size and the cost of the actuator system [7]. Artificial neural network (ANN) is applicable to accurately establish model to develop the relationship between the electrical resistance and manipulator positions. Thus, ANN can estimate the rotary manipulator position accurately. It can be controlled by the variable structure control technique under different conditions. The effect of surrounding temperature on the ability of ANN to predict the manipulator position is thoroughly investigated [8].

It exhibits robust performance with a small tolerance and can operate without being affected by ambient temperature. In the investigation, the authors have suggested an innovative way to calculate the resistance to determine the change in length of a SMA wire. By doing this, it is possible to measure both the voltage across the entire NiTi wire and that of the fixed-length segment. These two voltages provide direct change in length of the SMA wire. This kind of sensing is used in the feedback control in unknown ambient and loading conditions. This technique is called dual measurement for self-sensing of displacement by resistance change [9]. A self-sensing technique to measure the induced force in SMA wire is developed to control the length. Therefore, it can replace the traditional load cell by the SMA wire which can work for dual purposes as actuator and sensor. A modeling technic of the SMA wire actuator is also investigated for the control of mechanical structures. While designing a controller for the motion of a mechanical structure, a dynamic model of SMA actuator may be needed. So, the relationship between resistance and displacement of SMA that is derived to determine the feasibility of self-sensing in actuator control is investigated in [10]. The stiffness is related to force and displacement linearly as well as nonlinearly according to Hooke's law. This web portal provides information about the basics of stiffness [11]. The physical, mechanical, electrical, and chemical properties are available on the web portal of Dynalloy Inc., and the portal is very helpful for calculations [12].

The sensing of displacement and stiffness without an external sensor is well described in [13]. The works [13] showed little resistance, martensite fraction, and stiffness, but not in depth like the effect of current, frequency, and pre-stress on self-sensing of the stiffness of SMA spring actuator. This enables the sensing of force without a force sensor. The direct stiffness control of the SMA actuator and sensor-less force sensing experiment is conducted successfully. Besides, several benefits of this method include simplicity of mechanism, cleanliness, silent operation, and distributed actuation system i.e., remotability, sensing ability and low driving voltage. The polynomial model of sensing the stiffness of SMA is implemented to see the influence of different activation currents and excitation/switching frequencies. It has been also shown that different activation current and excitation/switching frequencies of power transistors affected to the stiffness resistance characteristics. These experimental modeling and analyses have proved that stiffness and resistance have a sufficiently linear relation which can be easily utilized to control stiffness in a SMA spring actuator and in mechanical structures [14]. The work [14] studied the stiffness and resistance relationship with only two effects: different activation currents and switching frequencies but not the duty cycle and pre-stress. The work presented by [15,16] did not explain about the self-sensing phenomenon/concept of SMA but described modeling of stiffness-temperature and displacement with other parameters like current, temperature, resistance, and force.

A new mathematical function/model of stiffness that shows the hysteresis characteristics between the stiffness and temperature has been developed and its hysteresis characteristics between the stiffness and temperature is verified by experimental data [15]. It has been found that the hysteresis characteristics are affected by different electrical and mechanical parameters such as current, frequency, and pre-stress, respectively. The relation between stiffness and temperature in SMA spring hysteresis is experimentally verified. The hysteresis characteristics' width and height can be controlled by current, frequency and pre-stress.

As the SMA is a highly nonlinear element, its displacement/contraction changes nonlinearly with temperature. It is affected by many electrical and mechanical parameters. Hence, the modeling of the displacement in SMA spring actuator is important. The neural network is the best tool that can easily map one property with others. Therefore, the displacement of the SMA spring can be modeled by ANN and successfully verified by experimental data [16]. In this work, a systematic approach for the implementation of curve fitting models and methods is suggested to achieve an equation that precisely describes the sensor function [17].

It is known that the Support Vector Regression (SVR) technique is normally applied to forecast the tangential displacement of cement concrete dam. Thus, in general, it is tested and verified using Pearson correlation coefficient, mean absolute error (MAE) and mean squared error (MSE) with experimental data [18]. The implementation of SVR is a practical and user-friendly method for creating soft sensors for nonlinear systems. The development of a dynamic non-linear-Auto Regressive (ARX) model-based soft sensor employing SVR is suggested as a heuristic method, in which the ideal delay and order are determined automatically using the input-output data. It is noted here that an Online Support Vector Regressor (OSVR) model is effective to estimate chemical process variable. As mentioned earlier, many works investigated the self-sensing technique to relate position/length/displacement with resistance and its control. The soft sensor developed using SVR in [18–20] achieved excellent performance checked by statistical performance parameters such as MAE, MSE and correlation coefficient. The research work [21] gives the idea about the stiffness of shape memory coil in terms of resistivity and modulus of elasticity. It suggests the resistivity and shear modulus is the best alternative to existing self-sensing methods.

In research article [22], the overall stiffness is adjusted by modifying the shape of the leaf springs. Hence, the geometrical nonlinearity can be used to change global stiffness. The paper [23] method suggested in adapting stiffness in variable stiffness actuator by configuring the fluid circuits, while the humanoid robot is investigated in [24]. It has various interesting features and is a difficult mechatronics structure. Due to the close interdependence of the technological factors, it is challenging to conduct research in a specific direction. A parallel type SMA wire variable stiffness actuator with a synergistically constructed configuration that offers a small size and a wide range of stiffness adjustments in compliant structures is also studied [25]. Additionally, it provides sufficient displacement and force, making it appropriate for applications requiring peculiar soft robotic requirements. The research work [26] proposes a new type of pneumatic variable stiffness actuator (PVSA). It provides expected actuation performance with effective remote stiffness adjustment capability. A novel variable stiffness mechanism is also designed by using specially designed SMA S-spring with different thickness [27]. The actuator stiffness is discretely adjusted by changing the state combination of SMA S-spring with different thickness. The [28] work is self- sensing unique design of sandwich structure comprising active graphene coated glass fabric piezoresistive face sheets bonded to a Nomex™ honeycomb core. The research article [29] explains the design of SMA spring and how to improve the frequency of actuation. The research [30] demonstrates the ability to significantly improve the way a gripper interacts with things that are being handled and offers a path toward developing anthropomorphic grippers. The soft finger's built-in sensor may convey passive proprioceptive feelings of stiffness and curvature. While not altering the mechanics of the robotic movement, it also served as an active jamming element to adjust finger stiffness.

As evident from the literature survey, the self-sensing during actuation of SMA spring is very useful to understand the relationship between the stiffness change and force, displacement, and strain corresponding change in the electrical resistance during the phase transformation. However, so far, a comprehensive study considering several effects such as actuation current, excitation frequencies and duty cycles has not been reported yet. Consequently, the technical novelties of this study are summarized as follows: (a) achievement of the self-sensing behaviour of SMA spring during variable stiffness actuation by experimentation, (b) development of a data driven model of self-sensing variable stiffness actuation based on Support Vector Machine (SVM) regression and nonlinear regression methods, by availing the experimental data, (c) investigation the effect of different excitation/activation currents, switching/excitation frequencies and duty cycle, (d) evaluation of the cycles and pre-stresses on the stiffness-resistance characteristics during the heating cycle of SMA spring by employing SVM algorithm as a soft sensor. From the aspects of the technical novelties, several new characteristics which are significant for the development of self-sensing are found. Some of new findings are given as follows: (i) it is identified that the characteristics of the self-sensing actuation (SSA) are influenced by activation currents, switching/excitation frequencies, duty cycles and pre-stresses, (ii) both SVM regression and nonlinear regression models are acceptable to measure the self-sensing stiffness in SMC actuator during variable stiffness actuation which is experimentally validated with its significance, (iii) it is found that the electrical resistance for all factors is almost in linear relation with the stiffness of SMC during the heating cycle with a meagre hysteresis, (iv) the resistance of SMC is low under the austenite and high under the martensite phases. It is noted here that compact design of a self-sensing SMA spring/wire actuator device is feasible with the aid of the results achieved in this work.

This paper is organized as follows. After clearly describing the research motivation, literature survey and the technical contributions of this study, an experimental facility and measurement method are presented in Section 2. Section 3 provides the information about SVM regression and nonlinear regression models focusing on the usability, and the basic mathematical relations used to find the resistance and stiffness which are undertaken at various different conditions of activation/excitation current, switching/excitation frequency, duty cycle and pre-stress are given in Section 4. The detailed characteristics on the results regarding to the stiffness response, resistance response and stiffness-resistance characteristic is fully discussed in Section 5 with the brief information about application of nonlinear regression modeling, followed by conclusion in Section 6 where some of benefits achieved form this work such as robust model, cost effectiveness and reliability for compact design of self-sensing actuator.

2. Experimental Set Up

2.1. Facility

The study to self-sense the stiffness of the SMA spring during variable stiffness actuation from resistance measurement is highly significant with respect to the quality of device (in terms of accuracy, precision, sensitivity and linearity etc., compactness and cost effectiveness). This experimental study is used to validate Support Vector Machine Regression and Nonlinear Regression model and realized by MATLAB 2020b software. A set-up to run the tests is designed and fabricated and shown in Figure 1 with the help of the photograph. It has following sections: (a) Mechanical Actuation System—It has two guide rods, with two linear bearings on them to actuate the SMA spring biased with an antagonistic tensile passive steel spring. This helps obstacle free movement which is measured with the help of a flap placed between two springs and Keyence—made contactless laser displacement sensor. A force sensor is also connected between the fixed frame and the SMA spring. The complete assembly is fixed in an acrylic frame. (b) Electronic Actuation System—This system consists of on Metal-Oxide-Semiconductor Field-Effect Transistor (MOSFET, TIP-122 ST Microelectronics) with gate resistance (1.5 kΩ and ¼ watt) to limit the base current; a source with a rheostat (4 Ω and 8.5 A) and drain is connected to the ground. The SMA spring is connected between the rheostat and the source of power transistor. The current sensor is connected between the ammeter and the rheostat so that it can display the current flowing through the SMA spring. (c) Power Supply—Different power supply systems are required for working of different auxiliary devices and the complete actuation systems. (i) DC regulated power supply—this is required for relay circuit, excitations for current sensor, transistor circuit, and as an input signal to op amp circuits. (ii) Dual Power Supply—Dual power supply provides +/− 15 V and 0.5 A current. This is important for op amp-based amplification circuits to boost physical signals like temperature signal and displacement signal. (iii) AC Power supply is required for bigger auxiliary devices. (d) Instrumentation and Data Acquisition (DAQ) System—These includes current sensor, temperature sensor, miniature force sensor, laser displacement sensor, voltages across SMA spring and rheostat.

Voltage signals from different sensors are converted into proper level (0 to 10 V) through signal conditioning, so that it is compatible with the data acquisition system and stored in the personal computer's memory. Figure 1 also shows the DAQ card used for data acquisition and forwarding it to the computer memory. (e) Shape memory alloy spring and passive steel spring—The SMA spring is manufactured by Dynalloy Inc. (1562 Reynolds Avenue (949) 502-8548 office, Irvine, CA 92614 USA) and their technical specifications are given in Table 1. Other details of the passive steel spring are shown in Table 2. During activation/heating of the SMA spring, the biased tensile spring expands and stores the mechanical energy. During deactivation/cooling, the bias spring will use the stored energy to pull the SMA spring back to its pre-stress/deform state.

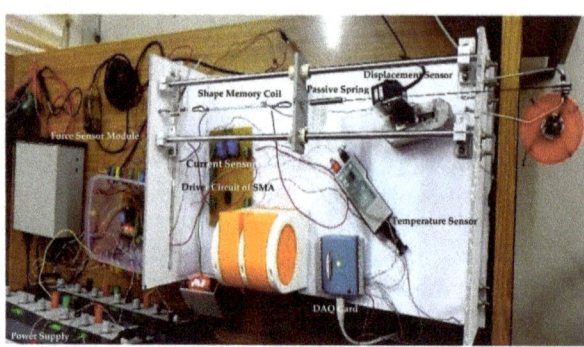

Figure 1. Experimental setup.

Table 1. Technical specifications of the passive steel spring.

Physical Properties	Value
Hardness (max.)	220 HV
Yield stress (min.)	290 MN/m^2
Tensile strength	640 MN/m^2
Spring rate (Stiffness constant)	130 N/m

2.2. Experimentation

The experimental modeling and analysis of self-sensing of the stiffness in the Shape Memory Coil during variable stiffness actuation is performed in the following ways. In the first set of experiments, activation currents (0.8 A, 1.0 A and 1.2 A) are varied by D.C. regulated power supply and by keeping voltage constant. Then different sensor voltages, the voltage across rheostat and voltage across the Shape Memory Coil are recorded in the memory of personal computer via DAQ card through repetitive cycle of switching of the power transistor. This procedure is repeated for aforementioned activation currents by keeping the switching frequency, duty cycle and pre-stress constant. The recorded information is used to predict stiffness by nonlinear regression modeling and validation. It is presented in detail in Section 4.

The recorded instantaneous value is used to determine the resistance and stiffness properties of SMC by use of Equations (6) and (7) for the aforementioned activation currents. In the second set of experiments, the switching frequency of the power transistor is changed e.g., 10 mHz, 20 mHz and 30 mHz by ensuring that all other parameters such as activation current, pre-stress on the SMC and duty cycle of the switching frequency are constant. The instantaneous values of the SMA spring's properties in terms of voltages is continuously recorded in the memory of personal computer via DAQ card. These recorded voltages are converted into proper units of the properties of SMC such as force, displacement, temperature, resistance, and stiffness.

Also, the experimental modeling and validations are explained in detail in Section 4. In the third set of experiments, the pre-stress (100 g, 150 g and 200 g) on SMC is varied by applying more tension with the help of a tensile passive steel spring. All other parameters are kept constant mentioned in the earlier set of experimentation. Similarly, the properties of SMC in terms of voltages are recorded by different sensors and described in detail in Section 4. Some of the properties of SMC e.g., stiffness and resistance are derived with help of Equations (6) and (7), respectively. In the fourth set of experiments, the duty cycle (40%, 50%, and 60%) of switching frequency is varied by adjusting the knob of the function generator such that activation and deactivation of SMC occur smoothly with help of passive bias tensile spring and explained in detail in Section 4. Basically, SMA works in three different modes of operations as actuators: (i) Free recovery mode means a constant force and variable contraction of SMC. (ii) Constraint recovery mode means a variable force and fixed contraction of SMC. (iii) Work production mode means both force and contraction of SMC changing. The work production mode is the most popular and applicable to practical engineering applications. It is a controllable actuator where both force and displacement vary. The first mode of operation is free recovery where force is constant, and stiffness is a function of displacement and varies. In the second mode, displacement is constant in which stiffness is a function of force and varies [15]. The inferior vena cava filter and eyeglass frame are designed in the free recovery mode of SMA operation. Fasteners, connectors, and hydraulic coupling uses constrained recovery mode in the SMA operation. Circuit breakers, heat engine and actuators are a few applications of the work production mode in the SMA operation [15]. In the experiment, the variable stiffness actuation of the SMA coil is controlled by using currents of 0.8 A, 1.0 A, and 1.2 A, and the corresponding forces, displacements, currents, and voltages are monitored. The data are displayed to investigate the system characteristics after preprocessing.

Table 2. Specifications of the SMC.

Physical Properties	Range/Value
Melting point	1310 °C
Electrical resistivity	76×10^{-5} Ω m
Modulus of elasticity	28–41 GPa
Latent heat of transformation	5.78 kCal/kg
Thermal conductivity	18.0 W/m °C
Thermal expansion coefficient	Martensite 6.6×10^{-6}/°C Austenite 11.0×10^{-6}/°C
Poisson ratio	0.33
Electrical resistivity	Martensite 80×10^{-8} Ω cm Austenite 100×10^{-8} Ω cm
Specific heat, C_p	1.84 J or 0.44 kCal/kg °C
Convective heat transfer coefficient, h	54.50
Transformation temperatures:	
Ingot austenite finish (A_f)	75 °C to 110 °C
Finished product A_f	50 °C to 80 °C
Mechanical properties	
Ultimate tensile strength	>1070 MPa
Total elongation	≥10%
Loading plateau stress @ 3%	≥100 MPa
Shape memory strain	≤8.0%
Geometrical parameters	
Wire diameter	5.0×10^{-4} m
No. of coils	45
Coil diameter	3.0×10^{-3} m
Volume	81.67×10^{-8} m^2

3. Facility and Experimentation

3.1. Principle of Self Sensing of Variable Stiffness Actuation by Support Vector Machine Regression

The regression is statistical tool to model and analyze the relation between one or more than one independent variable and a dependent variable to produce a particular outcome. In other words, the basic idea is to approximate the functional relation between set of independent variable and dependent variable by minimizing risk function which will use prediction error. Kernel: A lower dimensional data set is mapped into a higher dimensional data set using the Kernel function. In essence, a hyperplane is a line that will enable us to estimate a continuous value or aim. Boundary Line: In SVM, a margin is created by two lines other than the hyperplane. The Support Vectors may be on or outside the boundary lines. The experimental data recorded for resistance and stiffness of shape memory coil are denoted as X_i and Y_i.

$$\{(X_1, Y_1), (X_2, Y_2), (X_3, Y_3), \ldots \ldots \ldots (X_n, Y_n)\} \in R^N \times R \tag{1}$$

where, i is varying from 0 to n and n is number of training data points. The goal is to find the function which map the relation between X_i and Y_i. The Support Vector Regressor algorithm approximate the function as,

$$f(x) = <w, \varphi(x)> + b \text{ and } w \in R^N, b \in R \tag{2}$$

The one dimensional and multidimensional SVR problem is defined as

$$f(x) = \sum_{j=1}^{M} w_j * x_j + b \text{ and } w \in R^M, b \in R \tag{3}$$

$$f(x) = \binom{w}{b}\binom{x}{1} = w^T x + b; \ x, w \in R^{M+1} \tag{4}$$

where, w is weight vector, b is bias and $\varphi(x)$ is high dimensional data space. The weight vector and bias can be determined from risk function and as,

$$R(C) = \frac{1}{2}|w|^2 + C\frac{1}{2}\sum_{i=1}^{n} L_\varepsilon(f(X_i), Y_i) \tag{5}$$

The $\frac{1}{2}|w|^2$ control the function capacity and $C\frac{1}{2}\sum_{i=1}^{n} L_\varepsilon(f(X_i), Y_i)$ is the error. C is regularization constant. The insensitive loss function is defined as,

$$L_\varepsilon(f(X_i), Y_i) = \begin{cases} |f(X_i), -Y_i| - \varepsilon. & \text{when } |f(X_i), -Y_i| \geq \varepsilon \\ 0, & \text{and otherwise} \end{cases} \tag{6}$$

where, ε is the boundary line [18].

$$f(X_i), = \varphi(x_i)^T w + b \tag{7}$$

$\varphi(x)$ is high dimensional data space.

3.2. Principle of Self-Sensing of Variable Stiffness Actuation by Nonlinear Regression

Most self-sensing actuation model literature have related SMA in terms of the displacement/strain with self-sensed electrical resistance. To represent the stiffness of SMA in terms of its electrical resistance, there is a need to establish an appropriate and reliable stiffness-resistance model. To find the appropriate mathematical model that expresses the relationship between dependent variable (stiffness) and the independent variable (resistance), a data driven model is used; it is a parallel to mathematical model with self-sensing characteristics i.e., sensing under actuation. So, the data driven model is a function of the independent variable involving one or more coefficients. The nonlinear regression model with continuous one-to-one mapping is efficient to describe the relation between the dependent variable (stiffness) and independent variable (resistance). The Nonlinear Regression model is preferred as the modeling of the self-sensing actuation phenomenon (the relation of change in electrical resistance to the change in stiffness during the nonlinear thermo-mechanical phase transformation) is not as complex as that of modeling the basic phenomenon of SMA, the thermo-mechanical phase transformation. Also, the Nonlinear Regression model can be used to approximate complex nonlinear phenomena and then the relationship is curvilinear. The jth order polynomial model in one variable is given by,

$$k = \beta_0 + \beta_1 R_{sma} + \beta_2 R_{sma}^2 + \ldots + \beta_j R_{sma}^j + \varepsilon \qquad (8)$$

where, R_{sma} is resistance of SMA spring, $\beta_0, \beta_1, \beta_2, \ldots, \beta_i$, and R_{sma} $R_{sma}2$ $R_{sma}3 \ldots R_{sma} \ldots R_{sma}i$, $i = 1, 2, 3, \ldots, j$ are the effect parameters and ε an error.

The nonlinear regression of sufficiently high degree can always be found that provides a good fit for data. A good strategy should be used to choose the order of an approximate polynomial; keep the order increasing until t-test for the highest order term is non-significant. It is called the forward selection procedure to fit the model with experimental data. Also, goodness of fit statistics is used to find the best polynomial. MATLAB function "polyfit" is used to obtain coefficients of the polynomials [3]. Data from the measurement of the force, displacement and voltage sensors is saved in an Excel.csv file and used whenever required for training and testing the model. In the first step, characteristics must be represented as predicted data, response data, and weights. In the second step, nature i.e., shape and specificity of the self-sensing characteristic of the appropriate parameter polynomial model is selected. After fitting the data into a model, its goodness of fit is determined by adopting any of the following two ways: (i) Graphical (ii) Numerical. The plotting residuals and prediction bound aid visual interpretation. Graphical measures allow viewing the entire data set at once, and they easily display a wide range of relationships between the model and data. Numerical measures are more narrowly focused on a particular aspect of the data and often try to compress that information into a single number. In practice, to find the best fit of the sensor's characteristics, the above-mentioned methods are used on extensive experimental data and analyzed [17]. Figure 2 shows the trial-and-error procedure to find the correct polynomial model in comparison with the experimental sensor's characteristics; it can be seen that the third-order and above models match the experimental data.

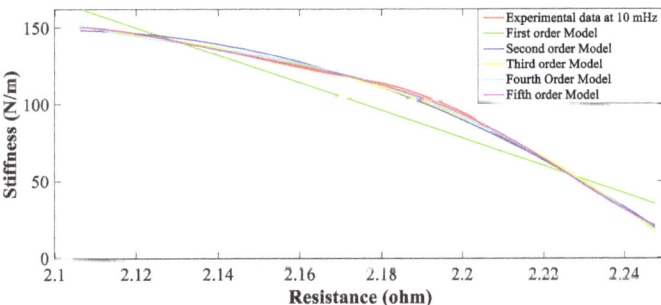

Figure 2. Polynomial model and experimental self-sensing variable stiffness actuation characteristics.

4. Result and Discussion of Self-Sensing Variable Stiffness Actuation

The influence of different factors such as activation current, excitation frequency, duty cycle, and pre-stress on self-sensing characteristics are observed and presented in this section. The influence of different factors such as activation current, excitation frequency, duty cycle, and pre-stress on self-sensing characteristics are observed and presented in this section. The SMA's electrical resistance is sensitive to compositions, transformation path and heat treatment [1]. During phase transformation, the crystallographic structure of SMA changes due to heating and cooling. As a result, SMA's electrical resistance changes. This resistance change is useful to measure SMA's stiffness without any physical sensor. Furthermore, it is possible to measure stiffness of the SMA based structure. Table 3 has useful information about SMA material. It is provided by the manufacturer and that the resistance of the SMA wire depends on its length and diameter. It also says that resistance per meter decreases with an increase in wire diameter. The basic relation used to calculate resistance [3,5] and stiffness of the SMC actuator are as follows.

$$R_{SMA} = \frac{V_{SMA}}{V_S - V_{SMA}} * R \quad (9)$$

$$k = \frac{d^4 G}{8\, n\, D^3} \quad (10)$$

where, R_{SMA} is the resistance of the SMA spring (Ω), V_{SMA} is the voltage of the SMA spring (V), R is the known resistance (Ω), V_S is the bias voltage of the MOSFET (V),

k is the instantaneous stiffness of the SMA spring (N/m), G is the instantaneous shear modulus of the SMC (N/m^2), d is the wire diameter of the SMC (m), and D is the coil diameter of the SMC (m). The instantaneous value of G is calculated from force and displacement measurements using transducers.

The first step in the design process is to choose the smallest wire diameter, or "d". The force-displacement relationship and cooling performance associated to the actuation frequency are most sensitively influenced by the wire diameter "d", which is a dominant design parameter of the SMA coil spring actuator. The SMA coil spring actuator has the smallest material mass and the quickest cooling time when the wire diameter is the smallest.

Iterative calculations are used to determine the coil diameter "D". When the shear strain reaches the predetermined value, which is adjusted to be slightly greater than the wire diameter "d", the force is calculated. If "D" is tiny, the shear stain does not reach its maximum value before the force surpasses the intended value. If so, the calculation is redone with a larger "D" The iteration ends and the "D" value at the last step is the maximum coil diameter if the force reaches the required value at the maximum shear strain while "D" is growing. With the desired stroke and the single coil stroke at the necessary loading condition, the coil number "n" is calculated. The displacement gap between the martensite and austenite models is used to determine the single coil stroke. The desired actuation stroke value divided by the single coil stroke yields the coil number "n".

Table 3. General properties of SMA [1].

Wire Diameter (μm)	100	125	200
Linear Resistance (Ω/m)	126	75	29
Maximum allowable force (N)	4.601	7.220	18.247
Nominal force (N)	0.275	0.422	1.079

So, the initial value of displacement of SMC is assumed to be zero and it is set to zero in the transducers and recorded in the personal computer. This modeling is aimed at the self-sensing phenomenon when the SMA is under variable stiffness actuation i.e., not particularly on the modeling of the basic actuation or shape memory effect or phase transformation of SMA. Moreover, the study is based on the SMA being activated by joule heating, whereby it is controlled by different electrical parameters such as current, frequency and duty cycle and, pre-stress. The change in resistance corresponding to the change in stiffness is determined during the heating phase, and the relation is extracted as a nonlinear regression model and validated by different metrics through experimentation. The model is valid for the joule heating current of 0.7 A to 1.2 A. Figure 3 shows the stiffness characteristics at 0.8 A, 1.0 A and 1.2 A which is when the phase change starts before which the SMA does not display any linear response. But then after 1.5 A, the response is more linear in characteristic as seen in Figure 3 and also at a current 1.0 A and 1.2 A, respectively. The model and experimental response are compared in the heating cycle when work is completed, specifically between 0.7 A and 1.2 A also, wherein a large change in stiffness and resistance is revealed.

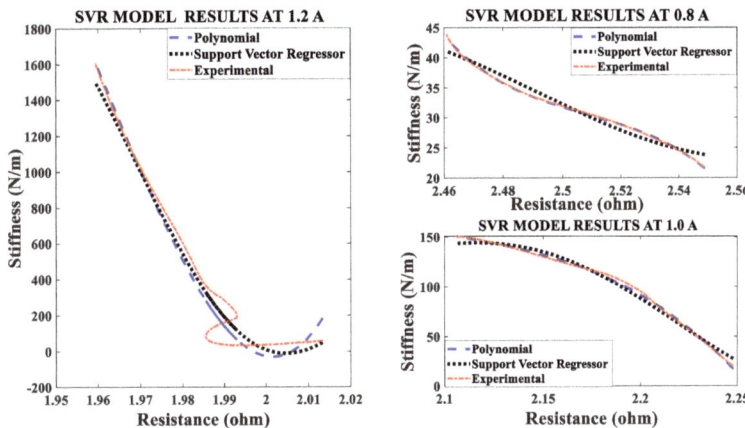

Figure 3. Comparison of models of stiffness sensing characteristics at different currents.

4.1. The Effect of Different Activation Currents

In the first set of experiments, the SMA spring is electrically heated by a 1/100 Hz square wave signal with a constant duty cycle and constant pre-stress. The current of the heating signal is varied, and the data recorded. The current/electrical power affects both the stiffness and resistance of the SMA spring actuator. The effect of changing current is clearly seen in Figure 3. Stiffness-resistance heating characteristics are modeled by the SVR and Nonlinear regression. Figure 3 reveal, that as electrical current increases, the slope of the curve increases, and the experimental characteristics overlap the modeled characteristics. The implementation of both models is done in MATLAB by "polyfit", "polyval" and other built-in functions.

The mathematical Nonlinear regression model between stiffness and resistance during the austenite phase is estimated from the experimental data.

$$k = -1.6446 * R_{SMA}^3 + 2.7072 * R_{SMA}^2 - 2.0349 * R_{SMA} + 0.9655 \qquad (11)$$

$$k = -0.5627 * R_{SMA}^3 - 0.0684 * R_{SMA}^2 - 0.3944 * R_{SMA} + 1.0032 \qquad (12)$$

$$k = 1.1301 * R_{SMA}^3 - 0.0543 * R_{SMA}^2 - 1.9872 * R_{SMA} + 1.0067 \qquad (13)$$

where, k is the instantaneous stiffness in N/m and "$RSMA$" is the resistance in ohm of the SMA spring actuator. Three cases are considered to present the data uniformly corresponding to each effect in parameter variations like current, frequency, duty cycle and pre-stress. The Nonlinear Regression model is used to represent self-sensing actuation in particular to relate stiffness with electrical resistance. The big and unusual coefficient of the nonlinear regression model can be reduced by normalizing stiffness and resistance data. The modeled and experimental self-sensing of stiffness of the Shape Memory Coil during variable stiffness actuation agree in terms of quality as Figure 3 has performance metrics such as goodness factor, mean squared error, correlation matrix and root mean square error within the specified range. The root mean square error (RMSE) should be less than 0.80. The goodness factor is out of range in Figure 3 as nonlinearity is present for the phase conversion which has not yet started.

The values of metrics of the model comparison for Figure 3 is mentioned in Table 4; there is large difference in stiffness for the three (maximum values are 75, 145 and 1500 N/m) cases. Table 5 gives the Correlation matrix which displays the correlation coefficients for matching the stiffness (model and experimental) at different independent variables, and the activation current. The matrix depicts the correlation between the possible pairs of values in the table; this tool helps to summarize the dataset, to identify and visualize the match of patterns in the data. From the matrix tables it is observed that, the characteristics at 0.8 A do not match as they are more non-linear than that for the other two higher activation currents.

Table 4. Metrics of inferential models at different currents.

Metrics	Current (A) / Type of Inferential Model	0.8 A	1.0 A	1.2 A
MSE	Polynomial Model	8.8421×10^{-5}	1.5728×10^{-4}	0.0043
RMSE		0.0094	0.0125	0.0657
Goodness of Fit (R-squared) (%)		99.8991	99.8731	94.9956
MSE	Support Vector Regression	0.0025	0.0012	0.0051
RMSE		0.0500	0.0345	0.0717
Goodness of Fit (R-squared) (%)		97.1421	99.0424	94.0439

Table 5. Correlation Coefficient between observed and predicted stiffness at different currents.

Activation Current (A)	0.8		1.0		1.2	
Correlation Coefficient of Polynomial Model	1.0000	0.9995	1.0000	0.9994	1.0000	0.9747
	0.9995	1.0000	0.9994	1.0000	0.9747	1.0000
Correlation Coefficient of Support Vector Regression	1.0000	0.9865	1.0000	0.9961	1.0000	0.9731
	0.9865	1.0000	0.9961	1.0000	0.9731	1.0000

4.2. The Effect of Different Excitation Frequencies

In the second set of experiments, the Shape Memory Coil is electrically heated over a fixed current of 1.2 A of different frequencies (10 mHz, 20 mHz, and 30 mHz) of square wave signal with fixed duty cycle and pre-stress (pre-tension). The self-sensing of stiffness is modeled during the heating cycle only. Both the curves almost agree with each other (modeled and experimental). Figure 4 show the characteristics modeled and experimental plots at different frequencies. The effect of frequencies on stiffness is inversely proportional i.e., stiffness decreases when resistance increase with an increase in frequency. The quadratic mathematical models of stiffness at different frequencies are as follows:

$$k = 1.1074 * R_{SMA}^2 - 1.9230 * R_{SMA} + 0.8835 \tag{14}$$

$$k = 1.5465 * R_{SMA}^2 - 2.4596 * R_{SMA} + 0.9701 \tag{15}$$

$$k = -0.5693 * R_{SMA}^2 - 0.2908 * R_{SMA} + 0.9574 \tag{16}$$

The experimental results validated the self-sensing of stiffness of the SMC actuator by measurement of resistance during the heating cycle (austenite phase). Figure 4 reveals the linear relationship between these two properties of the SMA. Also, the resistance change of the SMA spring actuator is higher at a lower frequency and lower at higher frequency over 0 to 1.2 A of electrical power.

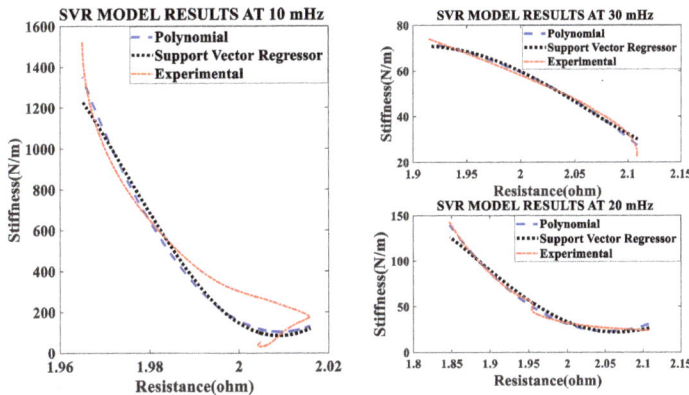

Figure 4. Comparison of models of self-sensing stiffness characteristics with experimental result at different excitation frequencies.

The modeled and experimental self-sensing of stiffness of the SMC during variable stiffness actuation agree in terms of quality because Figure 4 has the performance metrics such as goodness factor, standard deviation, correlation matrix and root mean square error within the specified range, as seen from Table 6. Also, Table 7 provides the correlation matrix which validates the match for the range of frequency (10 mHz to 30 mHz) though the study is conducted until 0.6 Hz.

Table 6. Metrics of inferential models at different frequencies.

Metrics \ Frequency (mHz)	Type of Inferential Model	10 mHz	20 mHz	30 mHz
MSE	Polynomial Model	0.0012	5.2667×10^{-4}	0.0026
RMSE		0.0340	0.0229	0.0508
Goodness of Fit (R-squared) (%)		98.6401	99.3929	96.9936
MSE	Support Vector Regression	0.0025	0.0022	0.0033
RMSE		0.0496	0.0471	0.9699
Goodness of Fit (R-squared) (%)		97.1139	97.4384	96.1031

Table 7. Correlation Coefficient between observed and predicted stiffness at different frequencies.

Frequency (mHz)	10		20		30	
Correlation Coefficient of Polynomial Model	1.0000	0.9932	1.0000	0.9970	1.0000	0.9849
	0.9932	1.0000	0.9970	1.0000	0.9849	1.0000
Correlation Coefficient of Support Vector Regression	1.0000	0.9868	1.0000	0.9894	1.0000	0.9818
	0.9868	1.0000	0.9894	1.0000	0.9818	1.0000

4.3. The Effect of Different Duty Cycles

An SVR and Nonlinear regression model is developed to understand the effect of duty cycle on stiffness-resistance characteristics. The comparison of experimental and curve-fitted model is simulated by the MATLAB® program, the characteristics for different duty cycles (40%, 50% and 60%), at a constant current of 1.5 A and constant frequency of 20 mHz showed that they almost agree with each other. The nonlinear regression model of stiffness at different duty cycles with resistance change as independent variable are as follows:

$$k = 0.5778 * R_{SMA}^2 - 1.5332 * R_{SMA} + 0.9982 \quad (17)$$

$$k = 0.3808 * R_{SMA}^2 - 1.3471 * R_{SMA} + 1.0264 \quad (18)$$

$$k = -0.2699 * R_{SMA}^2 - 0.7399 * R_{SMA} + 1.0239 \quad (19)$$

The effect of duty cycle on stiffness-resistance characteristics are linear and useful in controlling stiffness effectively. The comparison between the experimental and modeled characteristics at different duty cycles are presented in Figure 5 and mathematically represented by quadratic (second-order polynomial) Equations (17)–(19). The modeled and the experimental self-sensing of stiffness of the SMC during variable stiffness actuation agree in terms of quality as Figure 5 contains performance metrics such as goodness factor, mean squared error, correlation matrix and root mean square error within the specified range, as seen in Table 8. Table 9 also gives the correlation matrix which validates the match for a range of duty cycle (40% to 60%), though the study is conducted from 20% to 80%.

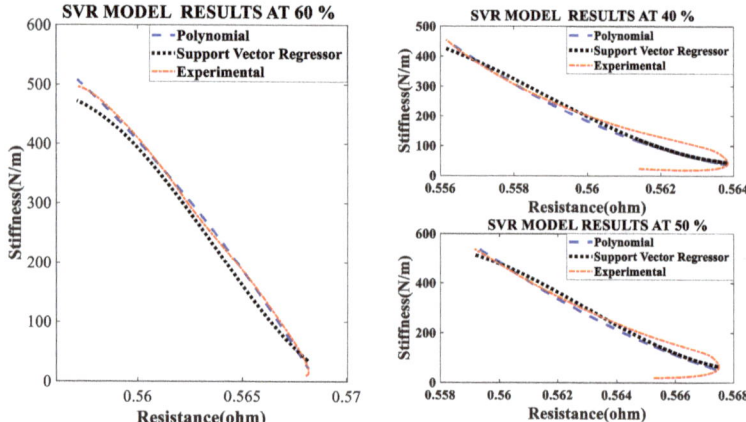

Figure 5. Comparison of models of self-sensing stiffness characteristics with experimental results at different duty cycles.

Table 8. Metrics of Inferential models at different duty cycles.

Metrics \ Duty Cycle (%)	Type of Inferential Model	40 (%)	50 (%)	60 (%)
MSE	Polynomial Model	0.0052	0.0066	1.5130×10^{-4}
RMSE		0.0722	0.0811	0.0123
Goodness of Fit (R-squared) (%)		94.4167	92.4220	99.8835
MSE	Support Vector Regression	0.0053	0.0067	0.0016
RMSE		0.0731	0.0067	0.0396
Goodness of Fit (R-squared) (%)		94.2709	92.2769	98.7947

Table 9. Correlation coefficient at different duty cycles.

Duty Cycle (%)	40		50		60	
Correlation Coefficient of Polynomial Model	1.0000	0.9717	1.0000	0.9614	1.0000	0.9994
	0.9717	1.0000	0.9614	1.0000	0.9994	1.0000
Correlation Coefficient of Support Vector Regression	1.0000	0.9718	1.0000	0.9632	1.0000	0.9980
	0.9718	1.0000	0.9632	1.0000	0.9980	1.0000

4.4. The Effect of Different Pre-Stresses (Pre-Tension)

The effect of pre-stress on stiffness-resistance characteristics is developed as mathematical models for different pre-stresses (100 g, 150 g and 200 g) at a constant current of 1.2 A and constant frequency of 10 mHz. The nonlinear regression model of stiffness at different duty cycles with resistance change as independent variable are as follows:

$$k = -2.9194 * R_{SMA}^3 + 5.3974 * R_{SMA}^2 - 3.3947 * R_{SMA} + 0.8517 \tag{20}$$

$$k = -2.4860 * R_{SMA}^3 + 4.6766 * R_{SMA}^2 - 3.0950 * R_{SMA} + 0.8585 \tag{21}$$

$$k = -0.9385 * R_{SMA}^3 + 1.5918 * R_{SMA}^2 - 1.5918 * R_{SMA} + 1.0084 \tag{22}$$

The comparison between experimental and modeled characteristics at different pre-stresses found in Figure 6 and mathematically represented by third order polynomial Equations (20)–(22). The effect of pre-stress on stiffness-resistance characteristics is highly nonlinear and difficult to model in comparison with those on the effect of current, frequency and duty cycle. Figure 6 reveals this and it is found from the correlation matrix that stiffness and resistance of the SMA spring at different stresses do not have strong statistical correlation. Table 10 validates the two models, compares the two models with each other and gives the information about the accuracy of prediction by using experimental and predicted data with the help of different metrics. There is a perfect correlation of each variable with itself as seen from Table 11.

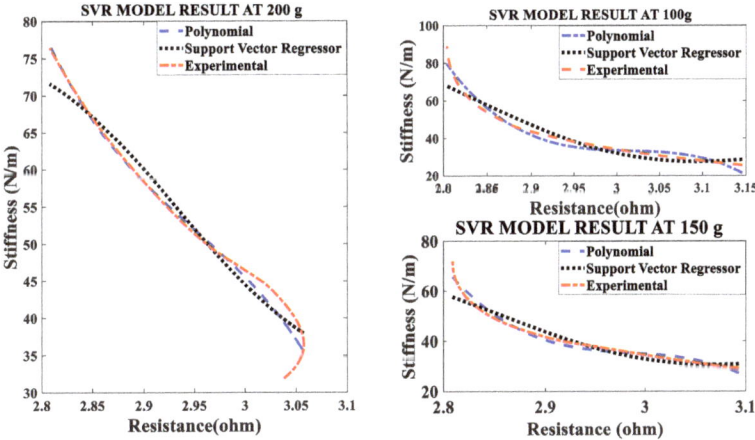

Figure 6. Comparison of Models of Self-sensing Stiffness characteristics with experimental results at different pre-stresses.

Table 10. Metrics of inferential models at different pre-stresses.

Metrics \ Pre-Stress (g)	Type of Inferential Model	100 g	150 g	200 g
MSE	Polynomial Model	0.0022	0.0018	0.0025
RMSE		0.0464	0.0421	0.0501
Goodness of Fit (R-squared) (%)		97.4866	97.9452	97.0727
MSE	Support Vector Regression	0.0100	0.0093	0.0040
RMSE		0.0998	0.0966	0.0634
Goodness of Fit (R-squared) (%)		88.3812	89.1636	95.3135

Table 11. Correlation coefficient at different pre-stresses.

Pre-Stress	100 g		150 g		200 g	
Correlation Coefficient of Polynomial Model	1.0000	0.9874	1.0000	0.9897	1.0000	0.9583
	0.9874	1.0000	0.9897	1.0000	0.9583	1.0000
Correlation Coefficient of Support Vector Regression	1.0000	0.9532	1.0000	0.9583	1.0000	0.9791
	0.9532	1.0000	0.9583	1.0000	0.9791	1.0000

5. Investigation of Stiffness Characteristics of the SMC Actuator

5.1. Effect of Current on Stiffness-Resistance Characteristics

With the help of four sets of experiments, the stiffness-resistance characteristics of the SMC actuator are analyzed to explore its self-sensing capability. Data recorded from the first set of experiments are used to plot and analyze. Resistance response to the heating cycle is plotted for 50 s; it found that as activation current increased, resistance decreased and that the change of resistance decreased over a period of time as shown in Figure 7. Stiffness response to different activation currents found that at 1.2 A, stiffness increased very rapidly in comparison to the other two activation currents. Excitation frequency is chosen as 10 mHz, as enough time is available to relax/deform the SMA spring and avoid residual strain. As excitation frequency increased, the time to complete the cycle is reduced e.g., two heating-cooling cycles occurred at 10 mHz and 6 cycles at 50 mHz. Data of force, displacement, the voltage across fixed resistance and the SMA spring are recorded for 3 min and are also saved in computer memory via 1408FS plus DAQ card with a sampling frequency of 2 Hz. At 0.8 A stiffness is less in value, compared to the other two activation currents (1.0 A and 1.2 A) as the SMA spring does not completely transform from martensite phase to the austenite phase. Corresponding resistance (Ω) is recorded in terms of its voltage and plotted in Figure 7; at 0.8 A. It is observed that resistance change is larger than that at 1.2 A. Responses for the three different currents are plotted and shown in Figures 8 and 9. Figure 8 shows stiffness variations at different currents (0.8 A, 1.0 A and 1.2 A). Figure 9 shows a linear relation between stiffness and resistance. The minimum and maximum values of resistance at these activation currents and their respective stiffness values are shown in Table 12.

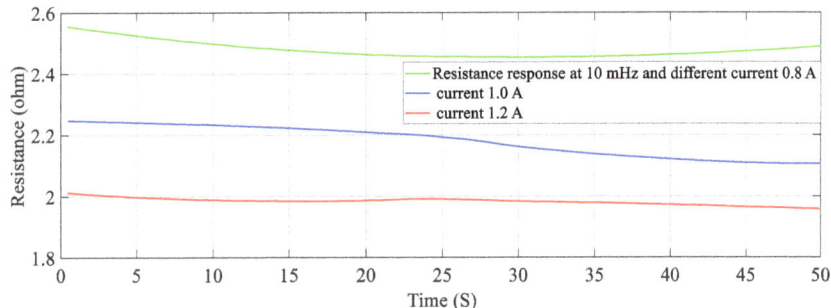

Figure 7. Resistance of SMA spring actuator at different current.

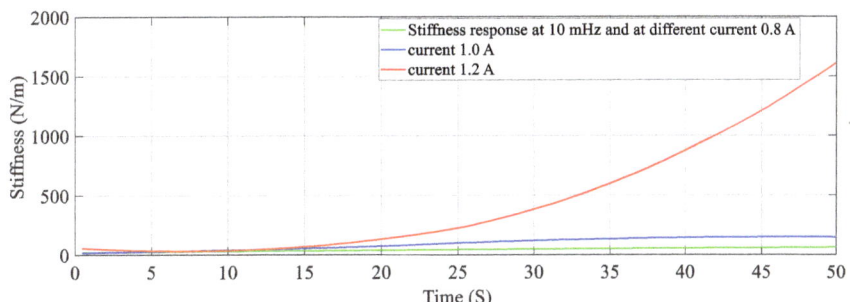

Figure 8. Stiffness of the SMA spring actuator at different currents.

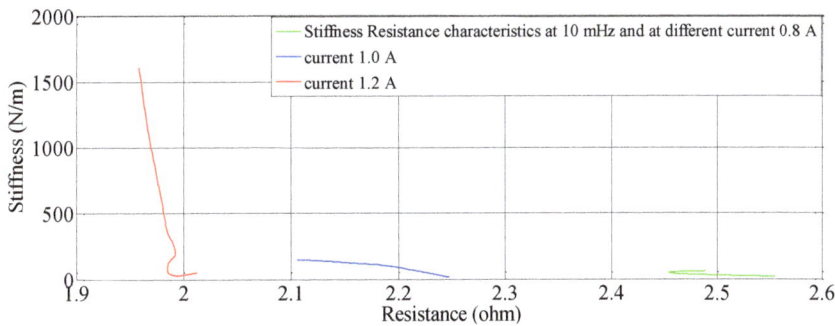

Figure 9. Stiffness − Resistance characteristics of the SMA spring actuator at different currents.

Table 12. Resistance and Stiffness at different currents.

Current (A)	Resistance Change (Ω)		Stiffness Change (N/m)		Number of Cycles
	Min.	Max.	Min.	Max.	
0.8	2.4426	2.5461	21.7310	62.8684	02
1.0	2.1310	2.2530	21.7521	156.2679	02
1.2	1.9454	2.0446	23.4013	2130.4059	02

5.2. Effect of Frequency on Stiffness—Resistance Characteristics

Data recorded from the second set of experiments are used to plot and analyze. Self-sensing actuation characteristics of the SMA spring actuator is obtained for varied frequencies from 10 mHz to 30 mHz keeping activation current constant at 1.2 A; Stiffness is determined and plotted as shown in Figures 10–12. When the excitation frequency of PWM signal is increased beyond 50 mHz, the number of cycles is reduced to less than one, also the heating and cooling cycle frequency (mechanical cycle) did not match the excitation frequency (electrical cycle), subsequently, the SMA spring would not completely contract or deform. Some significant observations are arrived at from these plots: (i) The excitation frequency has a significant effect on stiffness and resistance of Shape memory Spring: At a higher frequency, resistance change is higher and at a lower frequency, the resistance change is lower. (ii) The effect of frequency on stiffness change of the SMA spring actuator is converse to resistance change. (iii) Overall linear relationship exists between resistance and stiffness. (iv) The Resistance and Stiffness change from minimum to maximum values at different frequencies is in Table 13.

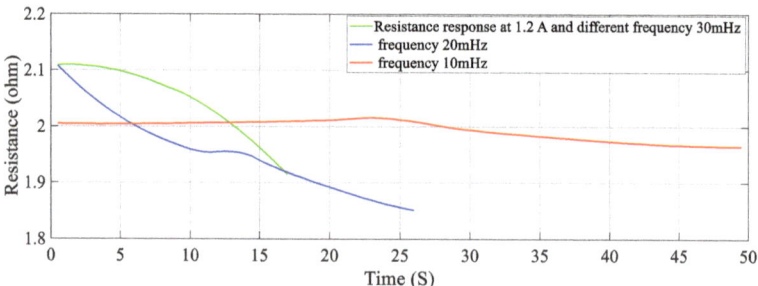

Figure 10. Effect of frequency on Resistance of the Shape memory Spring.

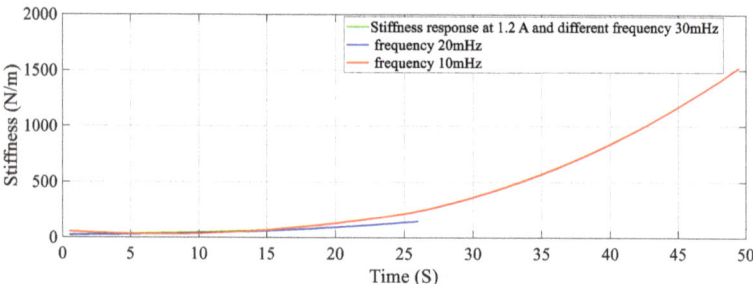

Figure 11. Effect of frequency on Stiffness of the Shape memory spring.

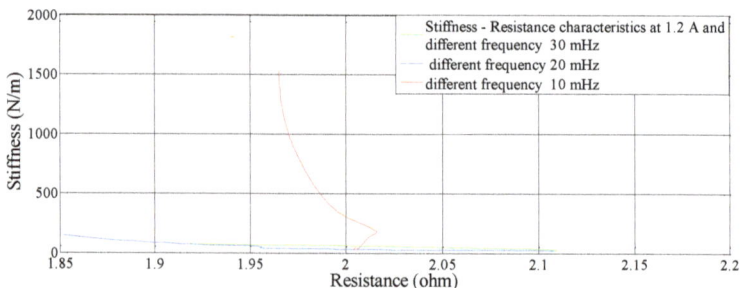

Figure 12. Effect of different frequency on Stiffness − Resistance Characteristics of the Shape Memory spring actuator.

Table 13. Stiffness and resistance at different frequencies.

Frequency (mHz)	Resistance Change in (Ω)		Stiffness Change in (N/m)		Number of Cycles
	Min.	Max.	Min.	Max.	
10	1.94	2.04	23.25	2130.90	02
20	1.83	2.12	22.12	144.44	04
30	1.89	2.11	21.91	79.45	06

5.3. Effect of Pre-Stress on Stiffness—Resistance Characteristics

At a constant current (1.2 A) passing through the SMA spring and constant frequency (10 mHz) of excitation current, stiffness is determined for pre-stress which is varied from 100 g to 200 g. An increase in pre-stress beyond 200 g would not allow complete contraction (bias force is higher) and would not completely deform below 100 g for the requirement of restraining/pulling force [15]. It is learnt from Figures 13 and 14 that stiffness increased, and resistance decreased with an increase in pre-stress. Figure 15 provides information about the stiffness sensing characteristics at different pre-stresses, which reveal a large change in stiffness at a lower value of resistance of the SMA spring actuator.

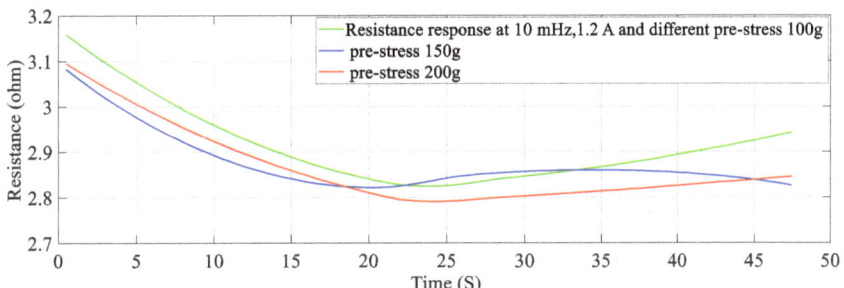

Figure 13. Resistance response at different Pre-Stresses.

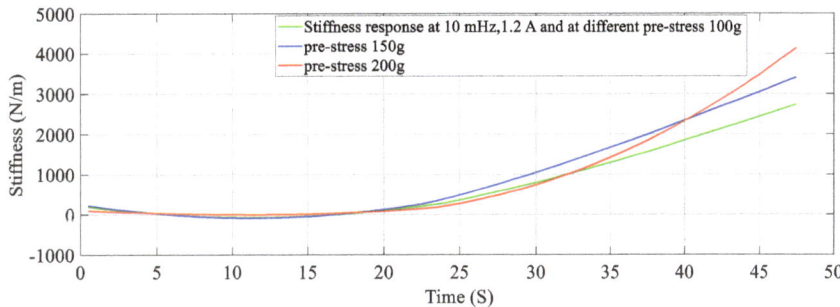

Figure 14. Stiffness response at different Pre−Stress.

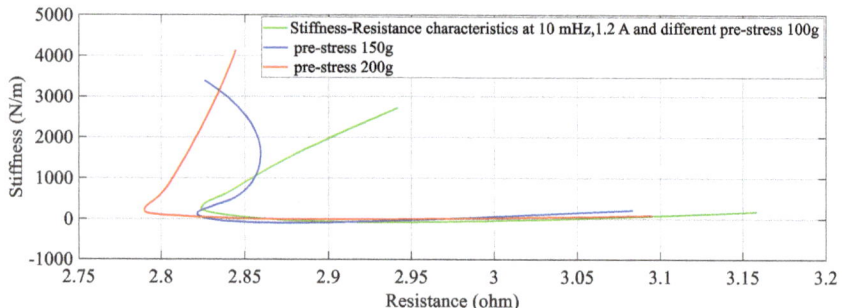

Figure 15. Stiffness-Resistance characteristics at different Pre-Stresses.

5.4. Effect of Duty Cycle on Stiffness—Resistance Characteristics

Similarly, for different duty cycles (40%, 50%, and 60%) at 1.5 A and 20 mHz, the resistance response, stiffness response and stiffness—Resistance characteristics of the SMA spring actuator are obtained and presented in Figures 16–18 respectively. Resistance values are smaller in comparison to the effect of current, frequency and pre-stress. The change in resistance is higher for higher duty cycles and lower for lower-duty cycles. Change in stiffness is also higher for a higher duty cycle and lower for a lower duty cycle; stiffness is higher in comparison with a lower duty cycle due to the availability of minimal time to completely heat the SMA spring. Figure 16 presents the resistance variation due to changes in duty cycles and Figure 17 corresponds to the stiffness variations. As the duty cycle increased, stiffness also increased some extent. Figure 18 shows the characteristics at different duty cycles, indicating a large change in stiffness with a large change in the resistance of the SMA spring actuator at a higher duty cycle. It also, proved that at higher stiffness, resistance is also higher but within the specified limit of duty cycle. Table 14 summarizes stiffness and resistances at different pre-stresses and their effect. Table 15 depicts the effect of duty cycle on stiffness and resistance, which is more on stiffness and less on resistance.

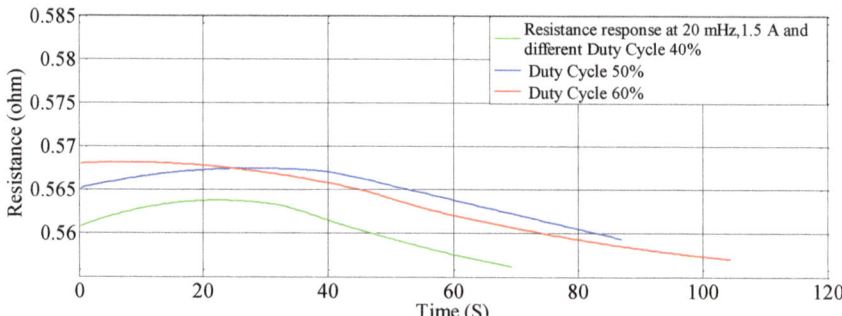

Figure 16. Resistance response at different duty cycles.

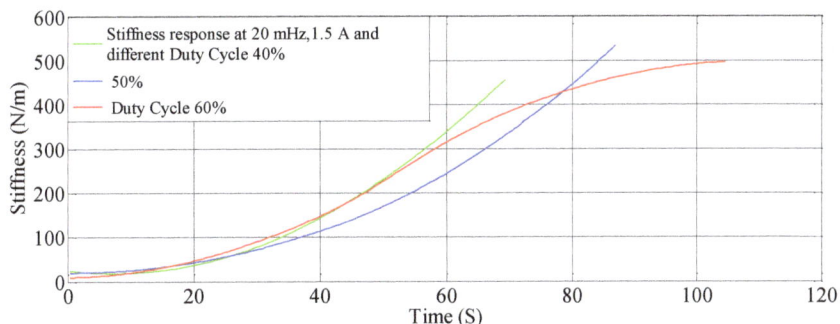

Figure 17. Stiffness response at different duty cycles.

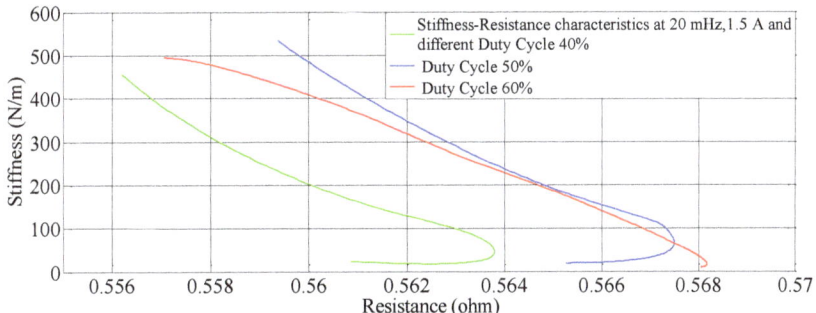

Figure 18. Effect of duty cycles on the Stiffness—Resistance characteristics.

Table 14. Resistance and Stiffness Values at different Pre−Stresses.

Pre-Stress (g)	Resistance (Ω)		Stiffness (N/m)		Number of Cycles
	Min.	Max.	Min.	Max.	
100	2.80	3.15	24.24	2248.97	02
150	2.76	3.12	31.66	2912.84	02
200	2.70	3.05	30.79	3251.99	02

Table 15. Resistance and Stiffness at different Duty Cycles.

Duty Cycle (%)	Resistance (Ω)		Stiffness (N/m)		Number of Cycles
	Min.	Max.	Min.	Max.	
40	0.55	0.56	16.90	423.99	03
50	0.55	0.57	19.71	574.25	03
60	0.55	0.57	16.79	495.21	03

Experimental data is collected for repeated cycles (3 consecutive cycles), and the responses are similar/not with much deviation. One set of data is used for the plotting and analysis of the stiffness-resistance characteristics, the usable form of the data is through the use of an average function and normalization; the other set of data are used for the validation. The highest change in resistance corresponding to the change of stiffness with regard to the effect of the influencing factors like activation current, excitation frequency, pre-stress and duty cycle are presented in Table 16. It is observed that a change in resistance of the SMA spring in the configuration switches is the highest (0.3516 Ω) during the change in pre-stress and stayed the lowest (0.0160 Ω) during the change in duty cycle. The purpose of this study is to use the suggested technique during control of actuation in the SMA spring by using an appropriate controller. The polynomial models are appropriate to the relevance to the factor of consideration and are able to accurately predict the stiffness equivalent to that obtained through experimentation by the measurement of change in electrical resistance. The level of predictability is high for the factor's activation current, excitation frequency and duty cycle but low for pre-stress and low value of current (0.8 A) due to nonlinear characteristics of self-sensing of the SMA spring; the statistical analysis is presented in Tables 4–11. Table 17 attests that the polynomial model, predicted accurately at different activation currents, excitation frequencies and duty cycle but at the pre-stress.

Table 16. Resistance and stiffness values at different Influencing factors.

Parameters	Shape Memory Coil Resistance Change (Ω)	Shape Memory Coil Stiffness Change (N/m)
Activation Current (A)	0.12	134.51
Excitation Frequency (Hz)	0.29	122.32
Pre-stress (g)	0.35	3220.20
Duty Cycle (%)	0.01	478.42

Table 17. Performance of SVR and nonlinear regression model prediction.

Parameter	Average Goodness of Fit (SVM Regression)	Average Goodness of Fit (Nonlinear Regression)
Different Activation Currents	96.74	98.25
Different Excitation Frequencies	96.88	98.34
Different Duty Cycles	95.11	95.57
Different Pre-stress	90.95	97.50

6. Conclusions

In this work, an experimental facility is developed to determine the electrical resistance of the Shape Memory Coil (SMC) actuator that is biased by a tensile steel spring under self-sensing variable stiffness actuation. The SVM regression model is constructed based on experimental data (Expert Knowledge) and provided excellent performances. The performance of the SVM regressor model is verified by a correlation coefficient, mean square error (MSE), root mean square error (RMSE) and goodness of fit (R^2). The developed SVM model showed an excellent result of prediction in comparison with the nonlinear regression model and experimental data. The experimental analysis has proved that the stiffness of the SMA is sensed from its resistance change. While the stiffness is changed due to different activation currents/joule heating, excitation frequencies, pre-stresses and duty cycles, the stiffness of the SMC is successfully determined as the variable stiffness actuator. Among many new findings from this work, the most interesting result is that the stiffness of the SMA spring can be measured without knowing the activation current and initial geometry or configurations of the SMC. This is possible from the realization of both SVR and nonlinear regression models of the stiffness using the electrical resistance of the SMC during austenite phase transformation. The responses achieved from two models are compared to the experimental response showing both models would harness the self-sensing capability of the SMC actuator. In addition, it has found from this work that the effect of frequency and duty cycle is more linear when compared to the other two parameters of current and pre-stresses. It has been concluded from this work that from the practical view of point, the self-sensing of stiffness of SMC can reduce the number of sensors for making application systems associated with shape memory alloys. For example, one stiffness sensor can use for two sensors of force and displacement. Therefore, it is self-explanatory justifying that the self-sensing technique gives birth to sensor-less control systems which are relatively cost effective, and hence the overall system becomes compact in comparison with traditional control systems having dedicated many sensors. Therefore, it is expected that the proposed self-sensing variable stiffness actuation method can be applicable to many control systems including the grasping force of robot grippers, surgical SMA wire of biomedical sciences, vibration and dynamic motion control of flexible structures in aeronautical fields such as morphing control and health monitoring control system using SMA wires Associated magnetic coils. It is finally remarked that some benefits achieved from this work will be demonstrated by applying to robot gripper systems in near future.

Author Contributions: B.B.S. and D.K. contributed equally to carry out the research work under the title "Self-Sensing of variable stiffness actuation of Shape Memory Coil by an Inferential Soft Sensor". They conceived and designed the analysis of self-sensing variable stiffness actuation by support vector regression and nonlinear regression method. S.-B.C. contributed to clearly addressing the technical novelty of this work, and he carefully checked and revised all equations and figures to improve the article quality. All authors have read and agreed to the published version of the manuscript.

Funding: This research received no external funding.

Institutional Review Board Statement: Not applicable.

Informed Consent Statement: Not applicable.

Data Availability Statement: The raw/processed data required to reproduce these findings cannot be shared at this time as the data also form part of an ongoing study. In the future, however, the raw data required to reproduce these findings will be available from the corresponding authors.

Conflicts of Interest: The authors declare no conflict of interest. The authors also declare that they have no known competing financial interests or personal relationships that could have appeared to influence the work reported in this paper.

References

1. Ikuta, K. Micro/Miniature Shape Memory Alloy Actuator. In Proceedings of the IEEE International Conference on Robotics and Automation, Cincinnati, OH, USA, 13–18 May 1990; pp. 2156–2161.
2. Ma, N.; Song, G.; Lee, H.-J. Position control of shape memory alloy actuators with internal electrical resistance feedback using neural networks. *Smart Mater. Struct.* **2004**, *13*, 777–783. [CrossRef]
3. Gurang, H.; Banerjee, A. Self-sensing shape memory alloy wire actuator based on unscented Kalman filter. *Sens. Actuators A Phys.* **2016**, *251*, 258–265. [CrossRef]
4. Lan, C.-C.; Fan, C.-H. An accurate self-sensing method for the control of shape memory alloy actuated flexures. *Sens. Actuators A Phys.* **2010**, *163*, 323–332. [CrossRef]
5. Liu, S.-H.; Huang, T.-S.; Yen, J.-Y. Tracking Control of shape-memory-alloy actuators based on self-sensing feedback and inverse hysteresis compensation. *Sensors* **2009**, *10*, 112–127, ISSN 1424-8220. [CrossRef] [PubMed]
6. Wang, T.-M.; Shi, Z.-Y.; Liu, D.; Ma, C.; Zhang, Z.-H. An accurately controlled Antagonistic shape memory alloy actuators with self-sensing. *Sensors* **2012**, *12*, 7682–7700, ISSN 1424-8220. [CrossRef]
7. Asua, E.; Feutchwanger, J.; García-Arribas, A.; Etxebarria, V. Sensorless control of SMA-based actuators using. *J. Intell. Mater. Syst. Struct.* **2010**, *21*, 1809–1818. [CrossRef]
8. Narayanan, P.; Elahinia, M. Control of a shape memory alloy-actuated rotary manipulator using an artificial neural network-based self-sensing technique. *J. Intell. Mater. Syst. Struct.* **2016**, *27*, 1885–1894. [CrossRef]
9. Gurley, A.; Lambert, T.R.; Beale, D.; Broughton, R. Dual measurement Self–sensing Technique of NiTi Actuators for use in Robust Control. *Smart Mater. Struct.* **2017**, *26*, 105050. [CrossRef]
10. Suzuki, Y.; Kagawa, Y. Dynamic tracking control of an SMA wire actuator based on model matching. *Smart Mater. Struct.* **2019**, *292*, 129–136. [CrossRef]
11. Finio, B. Available online: www.sciencebuddies.com (accessed on 7 August 2018).
12. Available online: www.dynalloy.com (accessed on 30 June 2017).
13. Kumon, M.; Mizumoto, I.; Iwai, Z. Shape Memory Alloy Actuator with Simple Adaptive Control. In Proceedings of the 2nd International Conference on Innovative Computing, Information and Control, Kumamoto, Japan, 5–7 September 2007.
14. Sul, B.B.; Dhanalakshmi, K. Self-sensing characteristics and analysis of the stiffness of the SMA spring actuator. In Proceedings of the 8th IEEE India International Conference on Power Electronics (IICPE), Jaipur, India, 13–15 December 2018.
15. Sul, B.B.; Dhanalakshmi, K. Modified sigmoid based model and experimental analysis of SMA spring as variable stiffness actuator. *Smart Struct. Syst.* **2019**, *24*, 361–377.
16. Sul, B.B.; Subudhi, C.S.; Dhanalakshmi, K. Neural Network based Displacement Modeling of Shape Memory Alloy Spring Actuator. In Proceedings of the IEEE Sensors International Conference, New Delhi, India, 29–31 October 2018.
17. Marinova, B.; Nikol, G.T.; Todorov, M.H. Curve Fitting of Sensor's Characteristics. *J. Electron.* **2009**, 188–191. Available online: http://ecad.tu-sofia.bg/et/2009/ET_2009/AEM2009_1/Electronic%20Systems%20in%20Measurement%20and%20Control/188-Paper-B_Nikolova2.pdf (accessed on 30 June 2017).
18. Ranković, V.; Grujović, N.; Divac, D.; Milivojević, N. Development of support vector regression identification model for prediction of dam structural behaviour. *Struct. Saf.* **2014**, *48*, 33–39. [CrossRef]

19. Chitralekha, S.B.; Sirish, L.S. Application of support vector regression for developing soft sensors for nonlinear processes. *Can. J. Chem. Eng.* **2010**, *88*, 696–709. [CrossRef]
20. Kaneko, H.; Funatsu, K. Adaptive soft sensor model using online support vector regression with time variable and discussion of appropriate parameter settings. *Procedia Comput. Sci.* **2013**, *22*, 580–589. [CrossRef]
21. Mozhi, G.T.; Sundareswari, M.B.; Kaliaperumal, D. The influencing parameters of variable stiffness actuation of shape memory spring for self-sensing. In Proceedings of the 2020 IEEE 15th International Conference on Industrial and Information Systems (ICIIS), Ropar, India, 26–28 November 2020; pp. 306–311.
22. Rodríguez, A.G.; Chacón, J.M.; Donoso, A.; Gonzalez Rodriguez, A.G. Design of an adjustable-stiffness spring: Mathematical modeling and simulation, fabrication and experimental validation. *Mech. Mach. Theory* **2011**, *46*, 1970–1979. [CrossRef]
23. Morishima, T. Variable Stiffness Actuator. USA Patent Application No. 15/658684, 27 November 2017.
24. Nalini, D.; Ruth, D.J.S.; Dhanalakshmi, K. Investigation of functional characteristics of a synergistically configured parallel-type shape memory alloy variable stiffness actuator. *J. Intell. Mater. Syst. Struct.* **2019**, *30*, 1772–1788. [CrossRef]
25. Olivier, S.; Flayols, T. An overview of humanoid robots technologies. *Biomech. Anthr. Syst.* **2019**, *124*, 281–310.
26. Sun, Y.; Tang, P.; Dong, D.; Zheng, J.; Chen, X.; Bai, L. Modeling and experimental evaluation of a pneumatic variable stiffness actuator. *IEEE/ASME Trans. Mechatron.* **2021**, *27*, 2462–2473. [CrossRef]
27. Xu, Y.; Guo, K.; Sun, J.; Li, J. Design and analysis of a linear digital variable stiffness actuator. *IEEE Access* **2021**, *9*, 13992–14004. [CrossRef]
28. Din, I.U.; Aslam, N.; Medhin, Y.; Sikandar Bathusha, M.S.; Irfan, M.S.; Umer, R.; Khan, K.A. Electromechanical behavior of self-sensing composite sandwich structures for next generation more electric aerostructures. *Compos. Struct.* **2021**, *300*, 116961.
29. Koh, J.-S. Design of Shape Memory Alloy Coil Spring Actuator for Improving Performance in Cyclic Actuation. *Materials* **2018**, *11*, 2324. [CrossRef]
30. Xie, M.; Zhu, M.; Yang, Z.; Okada, S.; Kawamura, S. Flexible self-powered multifunctional sensor for stiffness-tunable soft robotic gripper by multimaterial 3D printing. *Nano Energy* **2020**, *79*, 105438. [CrossRef]

Disclaimer/Publisher's Note: The statements, opinions and data contained in all publications are solely those of the individual author(s) and contributor(s) and not of MDPI and/or the editor(s). MDPI and/or the editor(s) disclaim responsibility for any injury to people or property resulting from any ideas, methods, instructions or products referred to in the content.

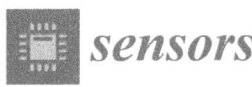

Article

A Soft Sensor Model of Sintering Process Quality Index Based on Multi-Source Data Fusion

Yuxuan Li [1,2], Weihao Jiang [1], Zhihui Shi [1] and Chunjie Yang [2,*]

[1] Hikvision Research Institute, Hangzhou 310051, China; yuxuanli@zju.edu.cn (Y.L.)
[2] State Key Laboratory of Industrial Control Technology, College of Control Science and Engineering, Zhejiang University, Hangzhou 310027, China
* Correspondence: cjyang999@zju.edu.cn

Abstract: In complex industrial processes such as sintering, key quality variables are difficult to measure online and it takes a long time to obtain quality variables through offline testing. Moreover, due to the limitations of testing frequency, quality variable data are too scarce. To solve this problem, this paper proposes a sintering quality prediction model based on multi-source data fusion and introduces video data collected by industrial cameras. Firstly, video information of the end of the sintering machine is obtained via the keyframe extraction method based on the feature height. Secondly, using the shallow layer feature construction method based on sinter stratification and the deep layer feature extraction method based on ResNet, the feature information of the image is extracted at multi-scale of the deep layer and the shallow layer. Then, combining industrial time series data, a sintering quality soft sensor model based on multi-source data fusion is proposed, which makes full use of multi-source data from various sources. The experimental results show that the method effectively improves the accuracy of the sinter quality prediction model.

Keywords: multi-source data fusion; sintering quality prediction; image feature extraction; keyframe extraction

1. Introduction

In the process industry such as the sintering process, process monitoring is mainly based on conventional sensors which measure the temperature, pressure, flow and other data of the process. The measurement of quality indicators is generally offline testing and it is difficult to achieve online analysis. At present, some online sensors that meet the needs have been developed and applied to some processes with relatively simple reaction mechanisms.

The most important quality index of the sinter is the FeO content of the sinter, which can reflect the reducibility and strength of the sinter. The reducibility of iron ore raw material is an important index for the later blast furnace ironmaking, which determines the furnace conditions and the adjustment of various parameters.

With the increase in FeO content, the output of molten iron in the blast furnace will decrease. However, we cannot simply pursue low FeO content, because FeO content also determines the strength of the sinter. The low content will reduce the strength of the sinter, damage the morphology and increase the proportion of powder. This will hinder the rise of gas flow in the furnace body of the blast furnace, affect the permeability of the material column, make it difficult for the furnace to run smoothly and reduce the output [1].

The common detection method is offline laboratory tests. The operator takes the sintered sample on the conveyor belt and sends it to the chemical composition analysis room. Potassium dichromate titration is often used for offline laboratories and the operation is cumbersome. This method necessitates grinding the sample. If the sample is difficult to dissolve, the analysis results will be poor. However, in general, the method has high accuracy and is the common chemical analysis method for FeO of sinter in iron and steel enterprises [2]. Another test method is X-ray diffraction, which is still an offline detection method. The ore sample to be measured and the supporting internal standard reagents need to be dried in an oven at 105 °C for 2 h and cooled to room temperature before they can be taken. The powder must then be carefully ground to a uniform and consistent level; otherwise, errors may be introduced [3].

The above offline tests are relatively accurate; however, they are time-consuming, often taking three or four hours to produce a result, and the labor and material costs of the tests are high. Whereas the process of sintering ore from batching to completion of sintering takes about one hour, the test results obtained after three or four hours have a significant lag. If the test results do not meet the process requirements, only the current working condition parameter settings can be adjusted to compensate. This is a great challenge for line operators who want to obtain the control objective of consistently good sinter quality.

Therefore, it is urgent to develop online measurement means of sintering quality indicators. Moreover, sophisticated online measurement means are the basis for building an automatic control system for sinter production. At present, online measurement means mainly include magnetic analyzers and online measurement devices. Shougang Group introduced the magnetic analyzer of the Belgium company to detect via cutting the magnetic induction line when the iron ore passes and causing the change of magnetic field current [4]. However, this method has strict requirements for samples and it also needs regular calibration and calibration by the instrument side. Shougang Group reported that the measurement accuracy of the magnetic induction coil was poor because the particles of the measured sinter samples were too small and there were many powder particles and the problem could not be solved by the equipment manufacturer's personnel again.

As more and more industrial data can be recorded with the use of automated systems in factories, data-driven soft measurement methods are emerging as viable solutions for industrial measurements. Li et al. used LSTM neural networks with self-encoders to construct a prediction model for FeO content [5,6]. Yan et al. proposed a denoised self-encoder framework for predicting sintering endpoints [7]. Yang et al. used a hidden variable model to model sinter quality index [8].

With the development of industrial cameras and image algorithms in recent years, image-based online soft sensors in the field of industrial inspection have gradually gained the attention of academia and industry [9]. Usantiaga proposed a temperature measurement system for the sinter cooling process based on infrared thermal imaging technology [10]. Jiang combined the mechanism with the image characteristics acquired via the infrared imager and proposed a method for measuring the polymorph of FeO content in sinter based on the heterogeneous characteristics of infrared thermal images [11]. However, this method uses the fuzzy classification labels obtained via mechanism analysis and the label accuracy required via regression analysis is insufficient. In addition, the above study used BP neural networks as regressors, which made it difficult to obtain time-series information. And the shallow feature extractor used in this study, cannot obtain deep feature information of the image. In recent years, deep learning methods have been increasingly applied in the image field, such as deep convolutional network models such as ResNet [12,13], achieving better results than shallow networks. This is also one of the motivations for the research in this paper.

This paper combines the low-resolution images of a thermal imaging camera with the high-resolution images of an industrial camera to achieve more accurate access to critical information. Because there are too few assay labels, it is difficult to detect in real time, and more quality variable labels need to be predicted. The work in this paper relies on experts to calibrate a batch of label data and obtains a better database. On this basis, a sintering quality prediction model based on multi-source data fusion is proposed and video data collected via industrial cameras and thermal imagers are introduced. Firstly, the keyframe information of the tail video of the sintering machine is obtained via the keyframe extraction method based on the feature height. Secondly, using the shallow layer feature construction method based on sinter layering and the deep layer feature extraction method based on ResNet, the feature information of the image is extracted from both the deep layer and the shallow layer. Then, the industrial time series data information is fused and the sintering quality prediction model based on multi-source data fusion is designed, which fully extracts the heterogeneous data information from multiple sources. Finally, the method is applied in a practical industrial case. The experimental results show that the model can effectively improve the accuracy of the sinter quality prediction model.

The main contributions of this paper are as follows:
1. Obtaining shallow features based on industrial mechanics with thermal and visible images.
2. Extracting deep features based on the ResNet model and constructing a multi-scale feature extraction model.
3. Fusing time series data to construct a novel soft measurement model based on multi-source data fusion for FeO content of sintered ore.

The remainder of this paper is organized as follows. In Section 2, the characteristics of the sintering process and quality variables are analyzed. The method and model proposed in this paper are introduced in Section 3. Then, the proposed method is verified via the actual production process data in Section 4. Section 5 summarizes the full text and puts forward the new prospect and future work direction.

2. Characteristics of Multi-Source Data in Sintering

2.1. Description of the Sintering Process and Test Data

A sintering process is shown in Figure 1. Before the sintered ore is fed into the blast furnace, it is divided into several processes: proportioning, mixing, sintering, crushing, screening and cooling. There are many different types of raw materials used for sinter production. There are more than 10 different bins, consisting mainly of iron ore fines, fuels, fluxes and some additional raw materials. A reasonable material ratio should be developed based on the different compositions of the raw materials, the quality requirements of the sinter ore and the quality requirements of the blast furnace ironmaking. The sintering ore mixing process requires full mixing of the components to obtain a mixture with a uniform and stable chemical composition, while adding water to obtain a good granularity and the necessary material temperature and to improve permeability. The mixture is fed into the belt sintering machine for production and after the sintering is completed, crushing, screening and cooling are required. The finished sintered ore obtained is sent to the ironmaking plant as raw material for blast furnace ironmaking. The sintering data collected contain operational variables, condition variables and quality variables. The quality variables depend on manual testing.

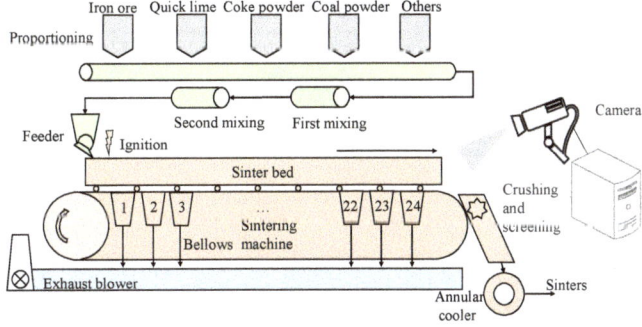

Figure 1. Schematic diagram of image acquisition system of sintering process.

2.2. Sintering Image Data Acquisition

Due to the scarcity of laboratory data, the sintering process information is not perfect. To better obtain information on the sintering process, an industrial camera and a thermal camera were set up at the observation port at the end of the sintering machine. A schematic diagram of the sintering machine image acquisition is shown in Figure 1. The industrial visible light camera has a resolution of 1920 × 1080 and the captured images are shown in Figure 2. The thermal imager has a resolution of 640 × 480 and the captured image is shown in Figure 3.

The captured information is uploaded to the database for storage via the industrial fieldbus. Live video information is displayed on a display screen in the central control room for the controller to view or can be downloaded to a cloud server via a remote connection.

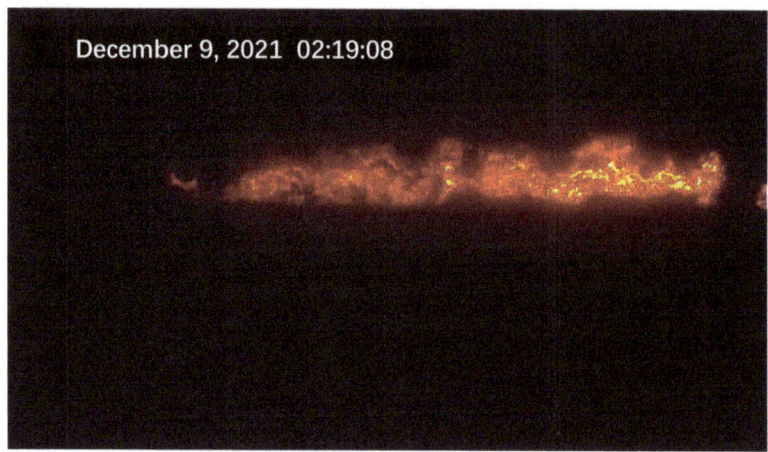

Figure 2. The visible light image acquired via the sintering system.

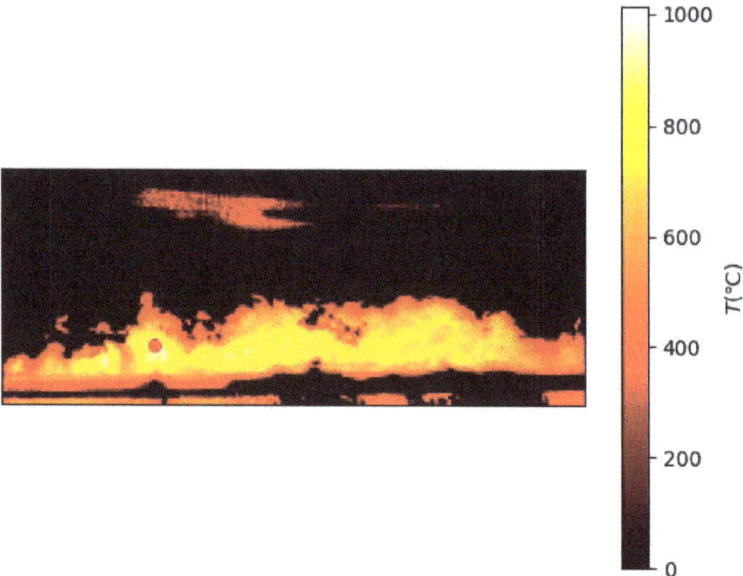

Figure 3. Thermal image acquired via the sintering system.

2.3. Analysis of Sintering Image Data

At present, most of the quality indexes of sinter are obtained via laboratory analysis. In the process of sinter production, due to the lag of laboratory analysis, the actual working conditions often depend on expert experience to judge. During the sintering process, the internal state of the sinter is not visible and only the topmost surface is exposed. However, the topmost part is the part that is ignited and sintered first. Therefore, on the sintering machine with a length of 90 m, most of the length is in a sintered and finished state. Only the flatness information about the ore laying can be observed from the top and the key sintering state information cannot be obtained. Fortunately, once sintering is complete, the sintered ore reaches the end of the trolley and falls naturally into the collection bin. After the last piece of sintered ore has fallen and before the next piece of sintered ore falls, we can observe the flame information in the sinter section. There is a flame viewing port at the end of the sintering machine. Experts with rich production experience can analyze the range of the FeO quality index of the sinter at the moment by observing the flame red layer data at the end of the sintering machine. Through such manual judgment, it is possible to rely on expert experience to help judge and control the process in the absence of sufficient test indicators. However, there are still significant limitations to this method, with the subjective errors of manual judgement being high and subject to the harsh conditions of the industrial site. In harsh conditions such as high temperatures, loud noises, vibrations and dust, it is difficult for workers to carry out observations for long periods of time, making it difficult to replace conventional observation with fire observation as an aid. Therefore, in the actual production process, it is necessary to develop stable measurement means to replace expert manual observation. Experts can make judgements by observing flame images. Therefore, in this experiment a camera is set up to capture the images and learn information and it is feasible to gauge experts' levels of experience and knowledge through soft measurements.

Due to the different sintering states of raw materials in different directions and different temperatures, the flame colors presented by them are also different. The surface of the black part is sintered and the temperature is reduced to below 300 °C, resulting in dim color and unclear observation. The red fire layer is the burning part of the sinter. It is generally located in the lower part of the sinter, mainly in red, and the temperature is about 600 °C. The stomatal layer is the brightest part of the image. Because the temperature exceeds 800 °C, it appears yellow and white in the image. The sinter will fall periodically at the tail of the sintering machine. When a batch of sintered ore reaches the last wind box at the end of the sintering machine, it will break and fall with the rest of the ore still on the trolley due to the loss of the support of the trolley. At the moment of falling, the flame information of the fault is very clear. After a short time, the falling of ore will raise a large amount of dust and cause vibration at the same time, making the image captured via the camera blurred and accompanied by shaking. It is difficult to obtain accurate flame information from the image at this time. Therefore, the system needs to screen out the clear images at the moment of falling as the analysis sample set. Experienced workers can judge the FeO content of the sinter at this time by observing the section.

3. The Soft Sensor Model Based on Multi-Source Data Fusion

3.1. Keyframe Extraction from Video Image of Sintering Machine Tail

In this experiment, the monitoring video is obtained from the sintering monitoring system for preprocessing. Since the original color image is three-channel RGB data with a data dimension of 16.77 million, the processing is relatively complicated and the calculation pressure is relatively large, so it is grayed first. The grayscale calculation formula is as follows:

$$Gray = Blue \times 0.114 + Green \times 0.587 + Red \times 0.299 \tag{1}$$

where *red*, *green* and *blue*, respectively, represent the values of red, green and blue channels and gray is the gray value.

According to the monitoring video, the falling of sinter is a periodic process. When a batch of ore arrives at the tail, the front part breaks and falls, exposing the red fire layer of the section. The image at this time is the keyframe required for the experiment. After that, this batch of ore will continue to fall and its shape will change in the air and at the same time it will raise smoke and dust, which is unfavorable for observing its sintering characteristics.

Therefore, we need to obtain these keyframes in the video as our input. The inter-frame difference method is often used for the algorithm of acquiring the keyframe of the target motion when video monitoring the moving target [14]. The algorithm performs differential processing on continuous images in continuous time. The difference in the grayscale is calculated by subtracting the pixel values of different frames. Then, the threshold value of the gray difference is set. When the value exceeds the threshold value, this frame is selected as the keyframe, indicating that the monitoring target has changed greatly from the previous time at this frame time. When the inter-frame difference method is used to monitor the red layer at the tail of the sintering machine, the brightness difference between different frames can be used as the threshold control to select the keyframe. Since the falling of sinter is a periodic process, when the current ore falls to the bottom and the new batch of ore has not yet broken down, the brightness of the image is the lowest. After a new batch of ore appears, the image information will increase rapidly. Through this characteristic, the sinter keyframe extracted based on the inter-frame difference intensity is the required cross-sectional image. For each frame, the difference is made with the previous frame to obtain the different strengths between the frames and the drawing is as shown in Figure 4. After smoothing, each extreme point can be extracted as our keyframe and the result is shown in Figure 5.

However, the accuracy of the inter-frame differencing algorithm depends on the choice of threshold values. In addition, there are some abnormal states during the falling process of the sinter. The sinter disintegrates in the air due to collision and other reasons, resulting in sudden changes in image intensity. As shown in Figure 6, abnormal frames are extracted and need to be manually removed during calculation.

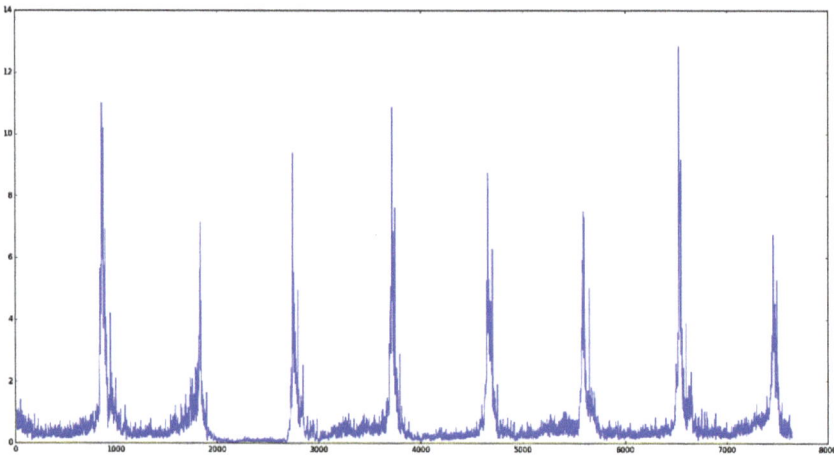

Figure 4. Graph of raw inter-frame difference intensity.

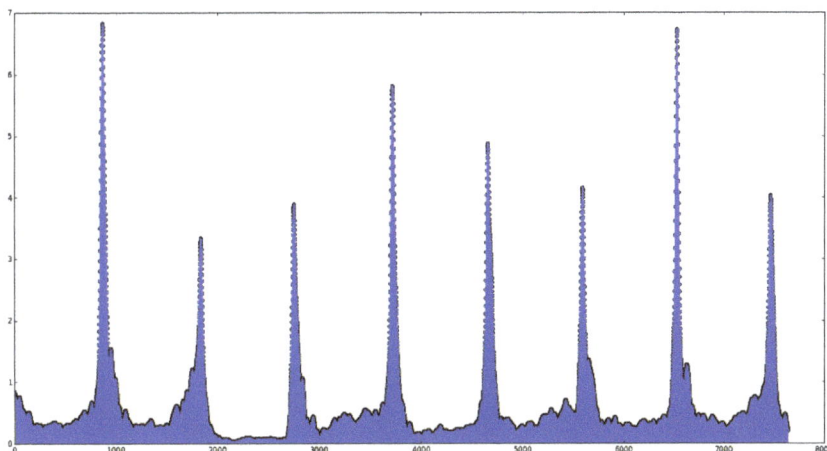

Figure 5. Graph of smmoothed inter-frame difference intensity.

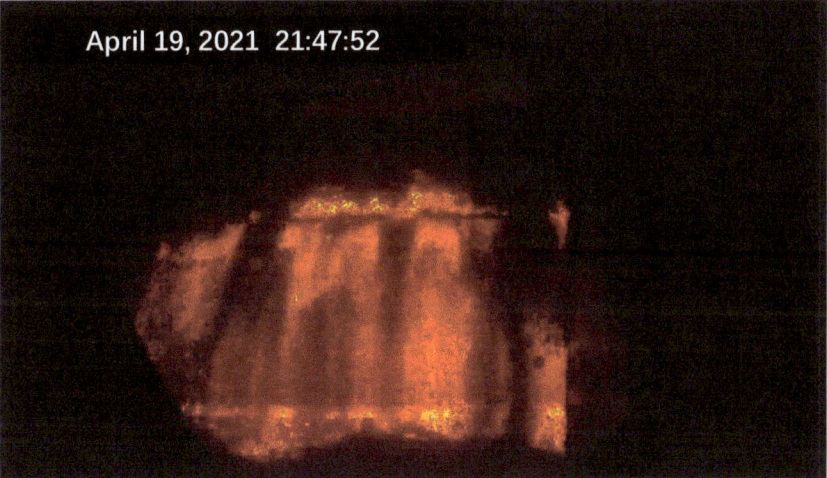

Figure 6. Abnormal frames extracted via the inter-frame difference algorithm.

Because of the limitation of the algorithm based on inter-frame difference, a more intuitive keyframe extraction algorithm based on feature height is proposed in this experiment.

First, mask segmentation based on the gray threshold is performed on the image that has been converted to gray level by mask and the segmented image is the red fire layer area to be monitored. Next, the contour of the red fire layer is obtained by using the findcontours algorithm. According to the contour, the circumscribed rectangle is fitted to represent the current sintering red layer. The center of gravity of this rectangle is the feature height. The feature height of the video collected in this experiment is shown in Figure 7 and the periodic feature height fluctuation diagram obtained after smoothing is shown in Figure 8.

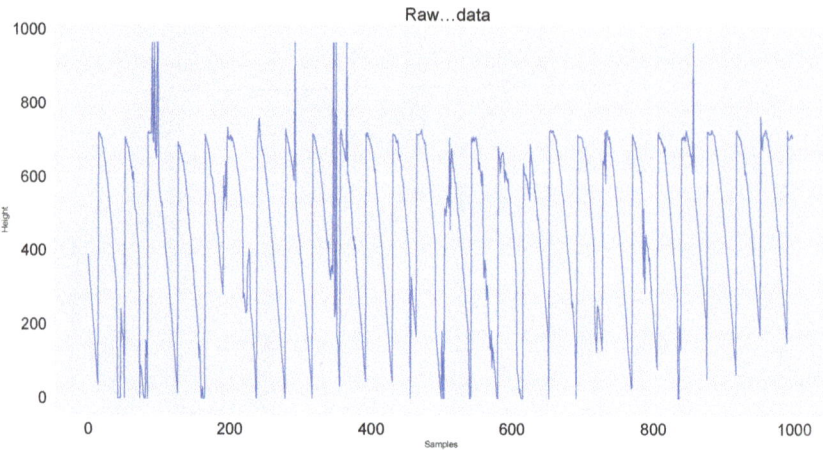

Figure 7. Plot of feature height.

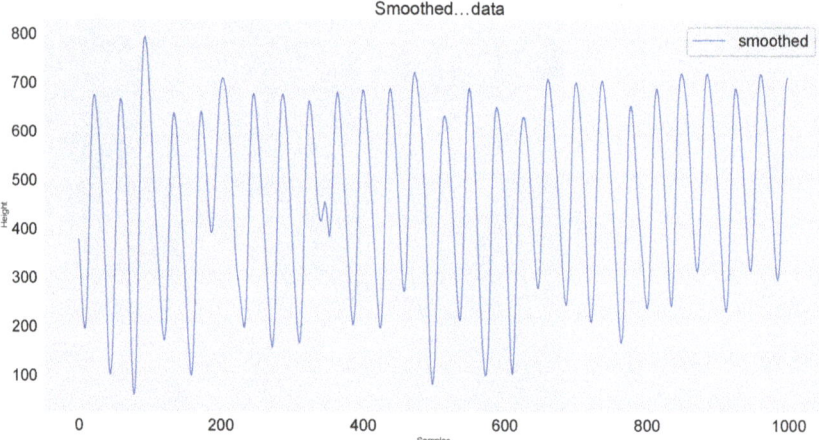

Figure 8. Plot of smoothing feature height.

Because the sinter falls periodically, the characteristic height of the red layer of the sinter section is at the highest point when the red fire layer we need has just appeared. Therefore, according to the peaks extremum algorithm, the maximum value of the feature height is obtained and its abscissa is the index of the required keyframe, that is, the image keyframes when the red fire layer has just appeared. The keyframe is extracted via the algorithm based on the characteristic height of the red layer of the sinter and then saved, as shown in Figure 9. The inter-frame intensity difference method of keyframe extraction is disturbed by anomalous image intensity variations, as shown in Figure 6. The feature height method, designed in this paper, is a combination of specific processes where the intensity changes abruptly, but the feature height does not change abruptly, so keyframes are extracted more accurately.

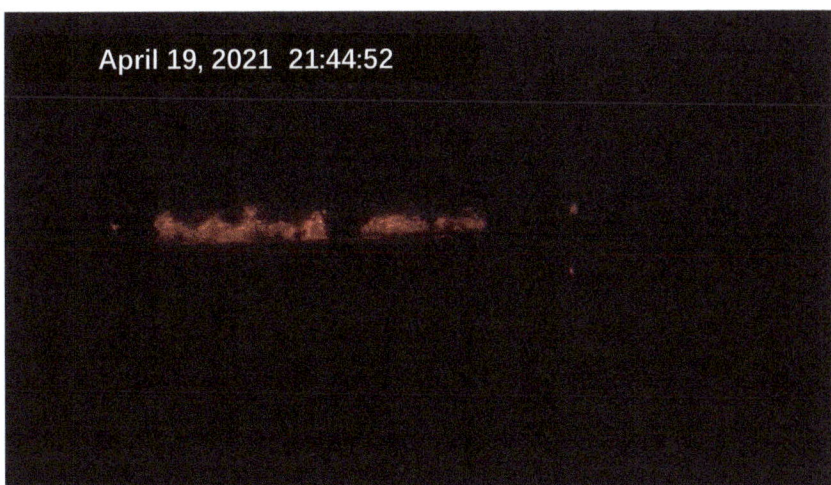

Figure 9. Keyframes extracted via the characteristic height algorithm.

3.2. Construction and Extraction of Image Shallow Features

Using the video keyframe extraction algorithm for the red layer at the end of the sinter in the previous section, several image keyframes were obtained for this experiment. For each keyframe image, the sintered red layer appears at the same position at the top. This location is our region of interest (ROI). First, we fix the region and calculate the area of the region as a fixed observation window. Again, the keyframe is segmented by using a mask based on a grey threshold. Based on practical industrial experience and mechanisms, sintered ore has different sintering states and corresponding temperatures. Assisted by an infrared thermal imager for temperature measurement, the layered temperature is converted into an image threshold. Four different thresholds are chosen, as shown in Table 1.

Table 1. Image threshold selection table.

Threshold	Meaning	Temperature (°C)
100	Gas hole layer	800
40	Red fire layer	600
20	Dark fire layer	400
10	Sintering finished layer	200

According to the threshold segmentation, four regions are obtained and then their contours are obtained respectively and the area around each contour is calculated as a feature. To better extract the feature information of the image, the area ratio of the area surrounded by each contour to the ROI is further calculated. The proportion information represents the information of the red fire layer and reflects the distribution characteristics and temperature characteristics of the sintering fault, to calculate the shallow layer characteristic information of the ROI area. The shallow layer features and time series data features of the red layer image at the tail of the sintering machine are extracted and the correlation is shown in Figure 10. Features 0, 1, 2 and 3 in the figure are shallow features, while the remaining features are features of industrial time series data. The shallow features are concatenated with the time series data features for fusion.

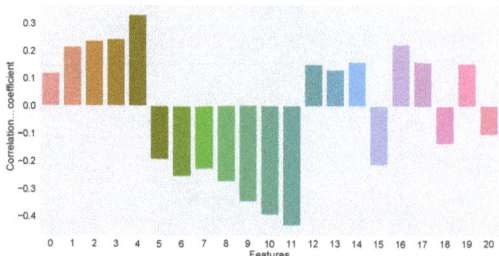

Figure 10. Correlation between shallow features of sintering machine tail image and time series data features.

3.3. Deep Feature Extraction Based on ResNet

Convolutional neural network (CNN) is a neural network modeled on human visual mechanisms. When humans first saw an image, they could not judge the whole image. Instead, different nerve cell receptive fields transformed the image into different features for recognition. Similar to the receptive field in human visual cortex cells, CNN extracts the features of images through convolution kernels. The convolution kernel successively crosses the picture with the set convolution step in order and calculates the convolution results of the elements of the picture in the receptive field. As a computer, the ability to recognize images is not as good as human beings. After an image is simply rotated, the matrix information stored in the computer is completely different. Therefore, the convolution kernel is designed to extract features for computer image recognition by imitating the human visual perception field. After convolution, multi-level features such as color and contour can be extracted from the original image to help identify the image [15]. For images that cannot be recognized via single-layer convolution, multi-layer convolution needs to be stacked to extract deep features. However, after convolution, the dimension of the original image will be increased. Simply stacking convolution layers will cause the dimension to be too high and it is difficult to train the depth network. Therefore, it is necessary to perform a pooling operation after convolution. The structure is shown in Figure 11. By calculating the mean value or the maximum value of the rectangular window of the specified size to replace the original rectangle, dimension reduction can be completed and the function of nonlinear mapping can be achieved. The stacking of convolution and pooling layers has a good effect within 20 layers. However, after increasing the number of layers of the network, the performance of the model does not improve, but will decline. when the network depth is increased, the network performance will neither improve nor even deteriorate [16].

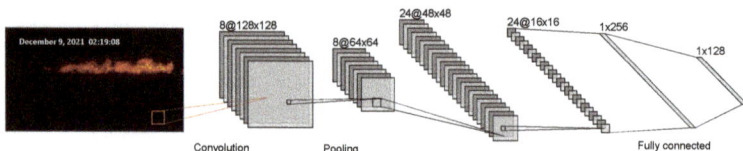

Figure 11. Schematic diagram of CNN structure for identifying numbers.

To solve this problem, He et al. proposed a deep residual network (ResNet), which sets a residual connection between every two layers [12]. Similar to the circuit short-circuit mechanism, the residual connection method constructs an identity map, which enables the network to have the ability of layer hopping transmission. When the number of stacked layers is too deep, the weight of training can select layer hopping connection, as shown in Figure 12. The original function mapping is expressed as $\mathcal{H}(x)$. Here, we build another map $\mathcal{F}(x) = \mathcal{H}(x) - x$ that is used to fit stacked networks. At this time, the original mapping is transformed into $\mathcal{H}(x) = \mathcal{F}(x) + x$, which can be achieved by a short circuit connection. Such processing does not increase the number of additional parameters, nor does it increase the computational complexity, and it is still easy to train.

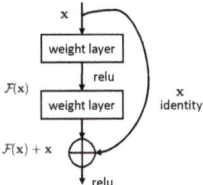

Figure 12. Schematic diagram of residual connection structure.

The network achieved good results in Imagenet image recognition. For the deep stacked network, the residual connection block set between every two layers can be expressed as:

$$y = \mathcal{F}(x, \{W_i\}) + x. \tag{2}$$

x, y are the input vector and output vector of the residual layer, respectively. $\mathcal{F}(x, \{W_i\})$ is a representation of the residual map that needs to be learned.

The trained network classifier ResNet-50 is used in this experiment and the 1000 output of its classification is used as the deep feature fixed extractor of the experiment. A total of 1000 deep-seated features were obtained through the ResNet model and their correlation was analyzed, as shown in Figure 13. The features were selected with the correlation coefficient greater than 0.25 as the deep features of the red layer image at the tail of the sintering machine, as shown in Figure 14.

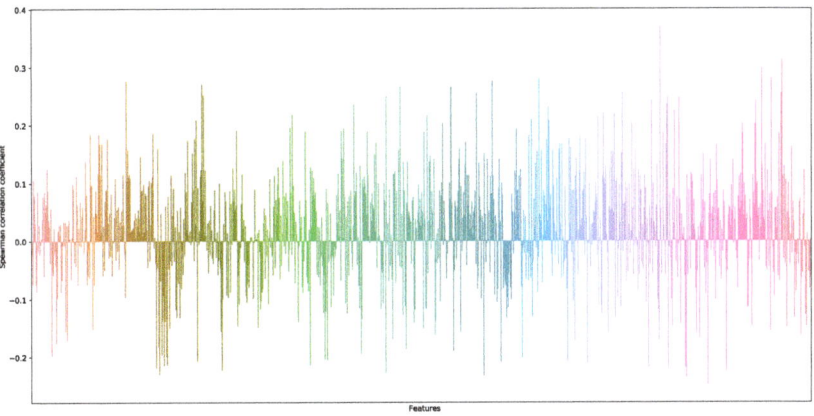

Figure 13. Schematic diagram of deep feature correlation extracted via ResNet model.

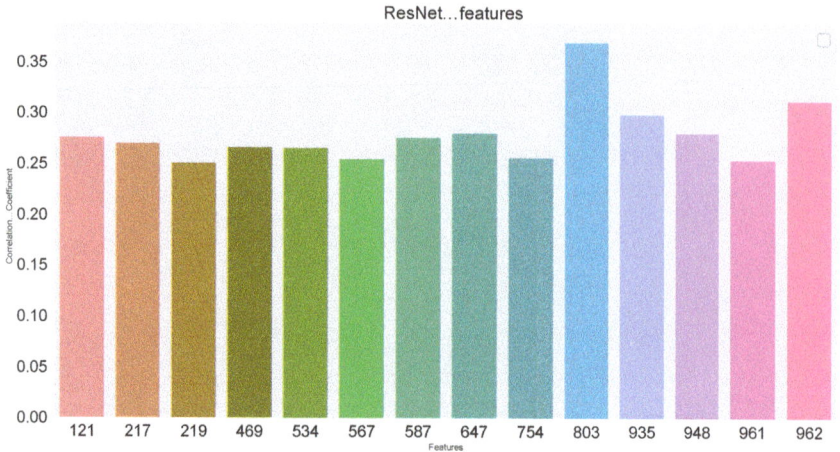

Figure 14. Schematic diagram of selected deep feature correlation.

3.4. Prediction Method of Sintering Multi-Source Data Fusion

Because the data information from many different sources can not be directly extracted and utilized, we propose a prediction method of the sintering process based on multi-source data fusion. The shallow features obtained via keyframe extraction, threshold segmentation, edge detection and feature construction and the deep features obtained via ResNet model are connected to obtain our deep and shallow fused image features. The time series data information from the process is processed using the encoder–decoder dynamic time features expanding and extracting method (DTFEE) based on the LSTM network [5,6]. The characteristics of the image, together with the characteristics obtained from the time series data information of the process, are used as the input of the encoder–decoder model to train the predicted output of the quality variable. The block diagram of the multi-source data fusion prediction method combined with deep and shallow image features is shown in Figure 15.

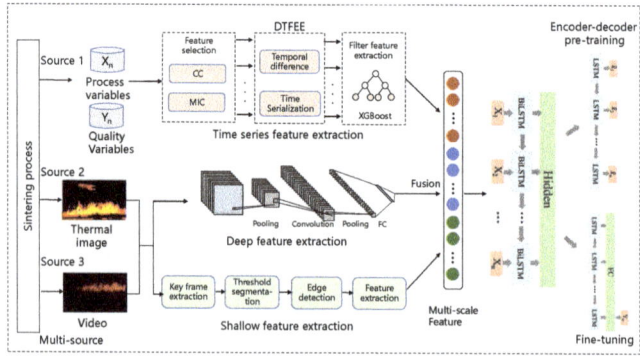

Figure 15. Diagram of Sintering prediction model based on multi-source data fusion.

4. Case Study on Sintering Process

4.1. Introduction to the Multi-Source Dataset of Sintering Process and Settings

The images used for the soft sensor of the sinter are collected via the thermal imager and industrial camera, respectively. Video data were collected from 8 December 2021 to 10 December 2021. The acquisition resolution of the industrial camera is 1920 × 1080 and that of the thermal imager is 640 × 480. Using the feature height method, the keyframes are obtained from the video for expert calibration. The extracted deep and shallow features and process time series data features jointly construct a dataset, with a total of 1319 samples. Each sample has 35 features, including 17 time-series features, 4 shallow features and 14 deep features. There are 1100 sets of samples in the training set and 219 sets of samples in the test set. The model consists of two layers of LSTM, with 50 hidden layer units and an input length of 50. The optimizer uses Adam and the early stop step is set to 20.

4.2. Comparison of Results and Analysis

The effect of shallow feature extraction is shown in Figure 16. The online acquisition of characteristic height, the thickness of the red flame layer, the distribution area and the proportion of four flame layers are presented.

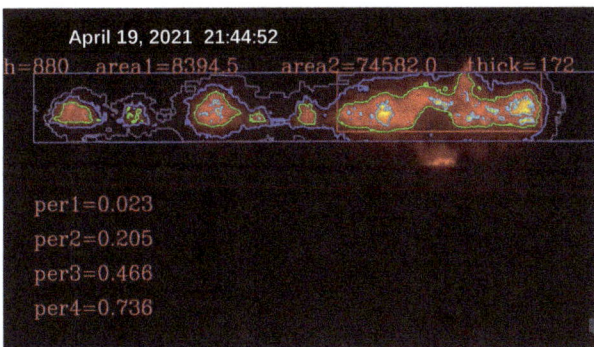

Figure 16. Video feature extraction diagram of the red layer at the end of the sintering machine.

In this experiment, the accuracy of the prediction model was evaluated by mean square error (MSE), mean absolute error (MAE) and hit rate (HR), where y and $\hat{y}$ are the real value and prediction, respectively, and n is the number of test samples. See Table 2 for the average evaluation indexes of the model obtained from the 10 experiments.

$$MSE = \frac{1}{n}\sum_{i=1}^{n}(y_i - \hat{y}_i)^2 \quad (3)$$

$$MAE = \frac{1}{n}\sum_{i=1}^{n}|y_i - \hat{y}_i| \quad (4)$$

$$H_i = \begin{cases} 1, & |y_i - \hat{y}_i|/y_i <= 1.5\% \\ 0, & |y_i - \hat{y}_i|/y_i > 1.5\% \end{cases} \quad (5)$$

$$HR = \frac{1}{n}\sum_{i=1}^{n} H_i \quad (6)$$

As a control group, the model used only time series data from the industrial process and did not use image information fusion. The prediction results are shown in Figure 17 and the decline in the loss function during network training is shown in Figure 18. The second model added shallow image information fused with time series data. The prediction results are shown in Figure 19 and the loss function decline diagram during network training is shown in Figure 20. The prediction results of the model fused with the deep and shallow image information are shown in Figure 21 and the decline in the loss function when training the network is shown in Figure 22.

It can be seen from Table 2 that the prediction model of multi-source data fusion proposed in this paper achieved good results and fast convergence speed. Compared with the method using only time series data and shallow features, the model fusing time series data, deep and shallow features obtains more process information and rich features at different scales, and the prediction effect is improved to some extent.

Figures 10 and 14 show that the correlation of the extracted deep and shallow features is similar to that of the time series data, which has some significance for the prediction model.

Compared with the industrial process time series data model without introducing images, the MSE of the deep and shallow image information model proposed in this paper decreases by about 29% and the hit rate increases from 86.5% to 93.1%. Compared with the temporal data fusion shallow feature model, the MSE of the fusion deep and shallow image information model proposed in this paper decreases by about 24% and the hit rate increases from 89.8% to 93.1%. The actual industrial application verifies the effectiveness of the multi-source data fusion method proposed in this paper.

Table 2. Evaluation index of prediction value of different methods.

Methods	MSE	MAE	HR
Time series data	0.0082	0.072	0.865
Time series data + shallow feature fusion	0.0076	0.069	0.898
Time series data + Deep and shallow feature fusion (ours)	0.0058	0.061	0.931

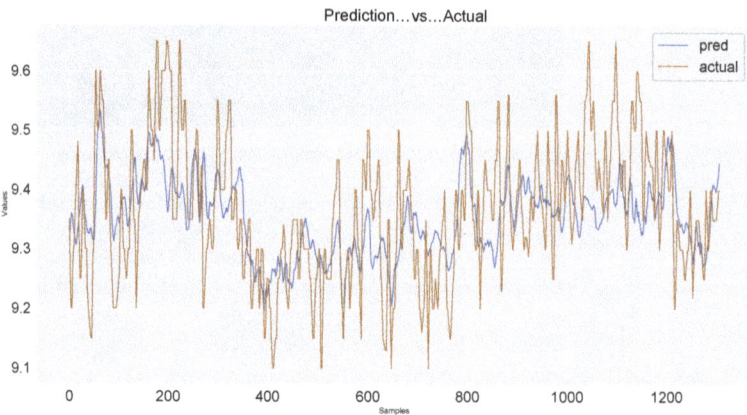

Figure 17. Plot of prediction results using time series data for industrial processes only.

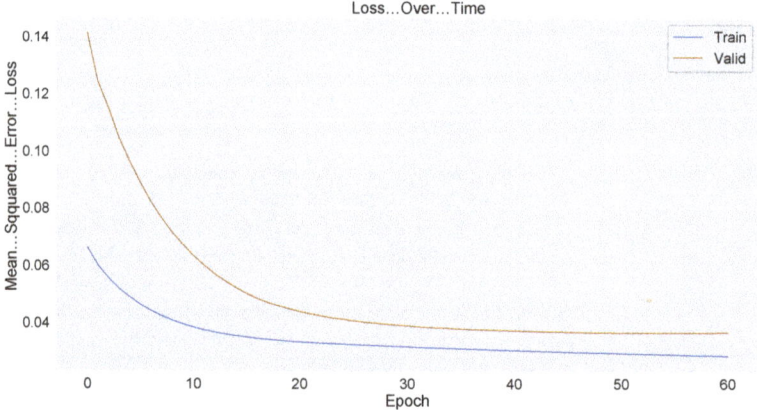

Figure 18. Plot of the loss function of the time series data model during network training.

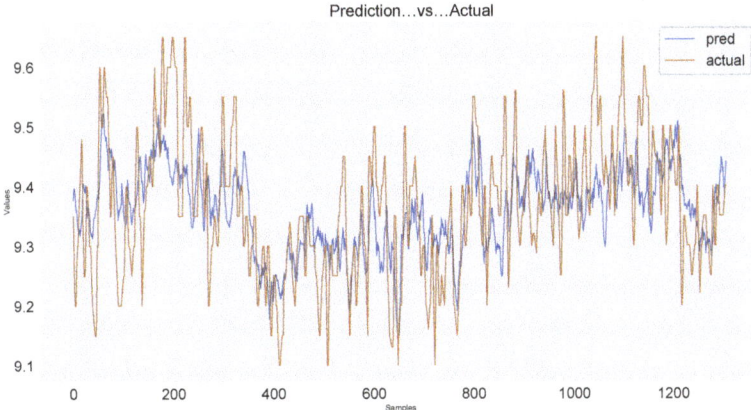

Figure 19. Plot of prediction results using time series data and shallow feature fusion model for industrial processes.

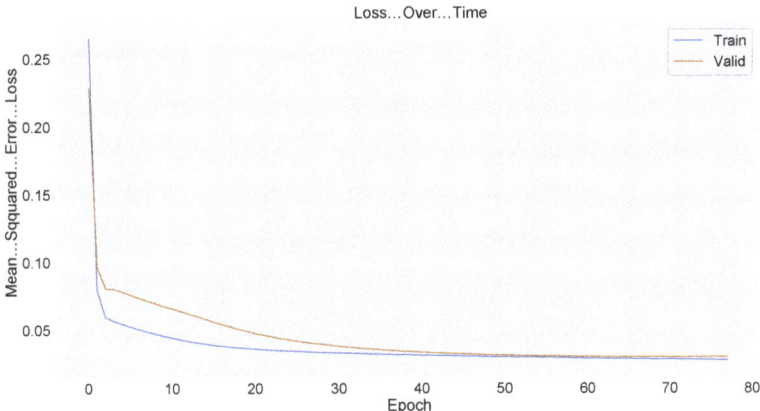

Figure 20. Plot of the loss function of time series data and shallow feature fusion model during network training.

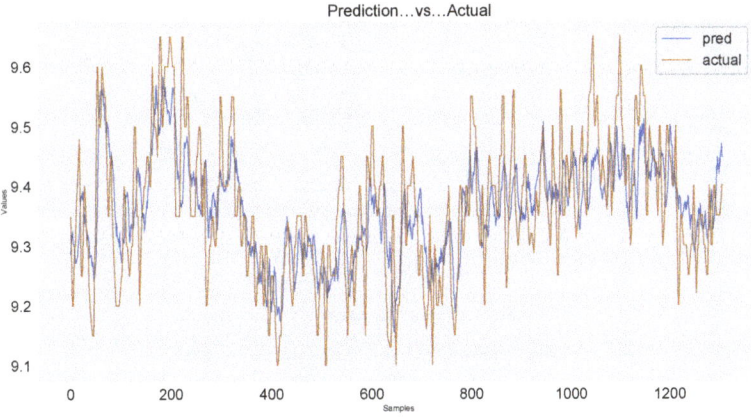

Figure 21. Plot of prediction results using time series data, shallow feature and deep feature fusion model for industrial processes.

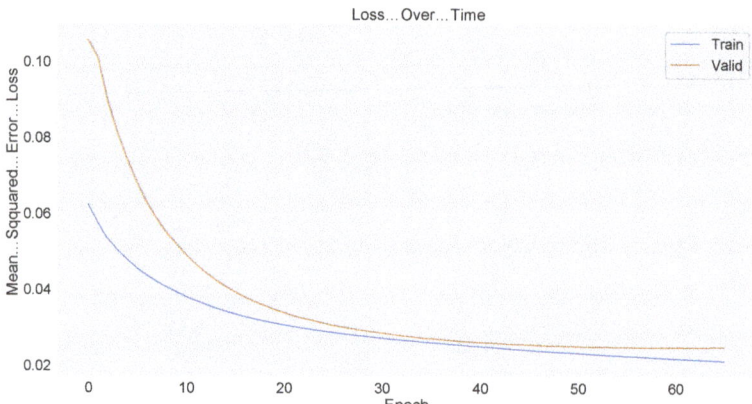

Figure 22. Plot of the loss function of time series data, shallow feature and deep feature fusion model during network training.

5. Conclusions

This paper presents a method to detect FeO content in sinter based on multi-source information fusion. The method first collects video data of the red layer at the end of the sintering machine through an industrial camera. Secondly, the keyframe extraction algorithm based on feature height and the shallow feature construction method based on sinter layering are designed according to the actual process. Then, deep features of sinter tail red layer images are extracted from keyframes by ResNet model. Finally, combined with the process parameters of the production process, an online real-time prediction model of FeO content in sinter is established through the LSTM network.

The model solves the problems of poor time efficiency and high cost of existing technologies by extracting multi-scale information from industrial camera video data and integrating the process parameters. It has practical significance for the guidance of the sinter production process and provides technical support for energy conservation, emission reduction, and quality and efficiency improvement of iron and steel enterprises. There are also quality variables in the sintering process that are relevant to the images of the faults, such as the total iron content, tumbler index, etc. This method can be extended to other variable predictions as long as suitable image labeled data are available. However, the new system requires labeled data before deployment, high quality image labeled data have a direct impact on system accuracy. To reduce manual effort and improve deployment efficiency, a future direction that could be considered is self-supervised learning of images, thus reducing the workload of expert labeling.

Author Contributions: Software, Y.L.; Supervision, W.J.; Writing—original draft, Y.L.; Writing—review and editing, C.Y. and Z.S. All authors have read and agreed to the published version of the manuscript. All authors have read and agreed to the published version of the manuscript.

Funding: Funding was received from the National Natural Science Foundation of China (No. 61933015) and the Fundamental Research Funds for the Central Universities (Zhejiang University NGICS platform).

Institutional Review Board Statement: Not applicable.

Informed Consent Statement: Not applicable.

Data Availability Statement: Not applicable.

Acknowledgments: The authors would like to thank the editors and reviewers for their contribution to the improvement and publication of this article. And we also want to thank Liuzhou Steel Group for its strong support and cooperation.

Conflicts of Interest: The authors declare no conflict of interest.

References

1. Wu, S.-l.; Wang, Q.-F.; Bian, M.-l.; Zhu, J.; Long, F.-Y. Influence of Iron Ore Characteristics on FeO Formation during Sintering. *J. Iron Steel Res. Int.* **2011**, *18*, 5–10. [CrossRef]
2. Yang, S.; Liu, H.; Sun, H.; Zhang, T.; Liu, S. Study on Influencing Factors of High-Temperature Basic Characteristics of Iron Ore Powder and Optimization of Ore Blending. *Materials* **2022**, *15*, 3329. [CrossRef] [PubMed]
3. Yang, S.; Tang, W.; Xue, X. Effect of TiO_2 on the Sintering Behavior of Low-Grade Vanadiferous Titanomagnetite Ore. *Materials* **2021**, *14*, 4376. [CrossRef] [PubMed]
4. Ramelot, D. Systems for the Control of the Sintering Process. *Sinter. Pelletizing* **2010**, *35*, 30–34. [CrossRef]
5. Li, Y.; Yang, C.; Sun, Y. Dynamic Time Features Expanding and Extracting Method for Prediction Model of Sintering Process Quality Index. *IEEE Trans. Ind. Inform.* **2022**, *18*, 1737–1745. [CrossRef]
6. Li, Y.; Yang, C.; Sun, Y. Sintering Quality Prediction Model Based on Semi-Supervised Dynamic Time Feature Extraction Framework. *Sensors* **2022**, *22*, 5861. [CrossRef] [PubMed]
7. Yan, F.; Yang, C.; Zhang, X. DSTED: A Denoising Spatial-Temporal Encoder-Decoder Framework for Multistep Prediction of Burn-Through Point in Sintering Process. *IEEE Trans. Ind. Electron.* **2022**, *69*, 10735–10744. [CrossRef]
8. Yang, C.; Yang, C.; Li, J.; Li, Y.; Yan, F. Forecasting of iron ore sintering quality index: A latent variable method with deep inner structure. *Comput. Ind.* **2022**, *141*, 103713. [CrossRef]
9. Yan, F.; Zhang, X.; Yang, C.; Hu, B.; Qian, W.; Song, Z. Data-driven modeling methods in sintering process: Current research status and perspectives. *Can. J. Chem. Eng.* **2022**, *1*. [CrossRef]
10. Usamentiaga, R.; García, D.F.; Molleda, J.; Bulnes, F.G.; Orgeira, V.G. Temperature Tracking System for Sinter Material in a Rotatory Cooler Based on Infrared Thermography. *IEEE Trans. Ind. Appl.* **2014**, *50*, 3095–3102. [CrossRef]
11. Jiang, Z.; Guo, Y.; Pan, D.; Gui, W.; Maldague, X. Polymorphic Measurement Method of FeO Content of Sinter Based on Heterogeneous Features of Infrared Thermal Images. *IEEE Sens. J.* **2021**, *21*, 12036–12047. [CrossRef]
12. He, K.; Zhang, X.; Ren, S.; Sun, J. Deep Residual Learning for Image Recognition. In Proceedings of the 2016 IEEE Conference on Computer Vision and Pattern Recognition (CVPR), Las Vegas, NV, USA, 27–30 June 2016; pp. 770–778. [CrossRef]
13. Wu, H.; Han, Y.; Zhu, Q.; Geng, Z. Novel Feature-Disentangled Autoencoder integrating Residual Network for Industrial Soft Sensor. *IEEE Trans. Ind. Inform.* **2023**. [CrossRef]
14. Yin, J.; Lei, L.; He, L.; Liu, Q. The infrared moving object detection and security detection related algorithms based on W4 and frame difference. *Infrared Phys. Technol.* **2016**, *77*, 302–315. [CrossRef]
15. Shelhamer, E.; Long, J.; Darrell, T. Fully Convolutional Networks for Semantic Segmentation. *IEEE Trans. Pattern Anal. Mach. Intell.* **2017**, *39*, 640–651. [CrossRef] [PubMed]
16. Kai, Z.; Zuo, W.; Chen, Y.; Meng, D.; Lei, Z. Beyond a Gaussian Denoiser: Residual Learning of Deep CNN for Image Denoising. *IEEE Trans. Image Process.* **2016**, *26*, 3142–3155.

Disclaimer/Publisher's Note: The statements, opinions and data contained in all publications are solely those of the individual author(s) and contributor(s) and not of MDPI and/or the editor(s). MDPI and/or the editor(s) disclaim responsibility for any injury to people or property resulting from any ideas, methods, instructions or products referred to in the content.

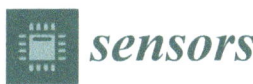

Article

Development and Optimization of a Novel Soft Sensor Modeling Method for Fermentation Process of *Pichia pastoris*

Bo Wang, Jun Liu *, Ameng Yu and Haibo Wang

Key Laboratory of Agricultural Measurement and Control Technology and Equipment for Mechanical Industrial Facilities, School of Electrical and Information Engineering, Jiangsu University, Zhenjiang 212013, China; wangbo@ujs.edu.cn (B.W.); 2222107008@stmail.ujs.edu.cn (A.Y.); 2212107036@stmail.ujs.edu.cn (H.W.)
* Correspondence: liujun4503@126.com

Abstract: This paper introduces a novel soft sensor modeling method based on BDA-IPSO-LSSVM designed to address the issue of model failure caused by varying fermentation data distributions resulting from different operating conditions during the fermentation of different batches of *Pichia pastoris*. First, the problem of significant differences in data distribution among different batches of the fermentation process is addressed by adopting the balanced distribution adaptation (BDA) method from transfer learning. This method reduces the data distribution differences among batches of the fermentation process, while the fuzzy set concept is employed to improve the BDA method by transforming the classification problem into a regression prediction problem for the fermentation process. Second, the soft sensor model for the fermentation process is developed using the least squares support vector machine (LSSVM). The model parameters are optimized by an improved particle swarm optimization (IPSO) algorithm based on individual differences. Finally, the data obtained from the *Pichia pastoris* fermentation experiment are used for simulation, and the developed soft sensor model is applied to predict the cell concentration and product concentration during the fermentation process of *Pichia pastoris*. Simulation results demonstrate that the IPSO algorithm has good convergence performance and optimization performance compared with other algorithms. The improved BDA algorithm can make the soft sensor model adapt to different operating conditions, and the proposed soft sensor method outperforms existing methods, exhibiting higher prediction accuracy and the ability to accurately predict the fermentation process of *Pichia pastoris* under different operating conditions.

Keywords: soft sensor; improved particle swarm algorithm; least squares support vector machine; transfer learning; *Pichia pastoris*

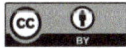

1. Introduction

The *Pichia pastoris* expression system is a eukaryotic expression system that has developed in the past decade and is one of the most successful foreign protein expression systems [1]. Compared with other expression systems, *Pichia pastoris* has significant advantages in processing, secretion, post-translational modifications, and glycosylation of expressed products, and has been widely applied [2]. Over 1,000 proteins have been efficiently expressed using the *Pichia pastoris* expression system. High-density fermentation is an important strategy for improving foreign protein expression levels in *Pichia pastoris* [3]. To effectively increase the expression level of secreted foreign proteins in *Pichia pastoris*, the fermentation process needs to be dynamically regulated and optimized in real-time by changing the fermentation environment and cultivation conditions to find the optimal environmental parameters for improving the secretion effect of foreign proteins [4]. However, *Pichia pastoris* fermentation is a complex, nonlinear, and uncertain process with multiple variables and time-varying properties [5,6]. Due to the actual process technology and cost reasons, key biochemical parameters that directly reflect fermentation process quality, such as cell concentration and product concentration, cannot be directly measured online and can only be estimated roughly through offline sampling and analysis [7]. This not only causes lagging information acquisition but also affects the correct judgment and decision-making of operators on real-time reaction status, while also limiting the implementation of optimization and control strategies. Therefore, there is an urgent need to find a method to achieve optimal estimation and prediction of key biochemical parameters during *Pichia pastoris* fermentation processes.

The soft sensor method is an effective solution to the problem of difficult online measurement of key biochemical parameters in biological fermentation processes. Many scholars worldwide have conducted in-depth research on soft sensor technology and achieved a series of results. Shao et al. [8] proposed a semisupervised Gaussian regression for the ammonia synthesis process, which achieved accurate real-time prediction of ammonia production concentration with fewer labeled samples. However, the accuracy parameter in Bayesian regularization needs to be manually predefined, which greatly reduces the accuracy of the model. Yuan et al. [9] used a supervised long short-term memory network to achieve soft sensor modeling of the penicillin fermentation process, which fully utilized the quality variables in the long short-term memory network and realized nonlinear dynamic modeling of the penicillin fermentation process with a good prediction effect. The limitation of this method is that the amount of computation and training time of the model are greatly increased due to adding the quality variable to each LSTM cell. Zheng et al. [10] proposed a real-time semisupervised extreme learning machine, which integrated semisupervised learning and just-in-time learning strategies into the modeling framework to establish a local prediction model, and fully utilized a large amount of unlabeled data information to achieve fast and accurate measurement of Mooney viscosity in the rubber mixing process. Chang et al. [11] proposed a consistent contrastive network to realize the time awareness and robustness of the soft sensor model, which overcame the limitations of manifold regularization and fully utilized abnormal data and unlabeled data information. The effectiveness of the consistent contrastive network was verified in the soft sensor modeling of ammonia and sulfur removal industrial processes. Fan et al. [12] proposed a soft sensor regression model based on the long short-term memory recurrent neural network in deep learning using the data obtained by the sensor, by designing the relative error loss and the normalized L1 loss function using the time step of the sensor to predict the measured value, to realize the detection of the wafer manufacturing process to reduce the recall rate of the wafer. The experimental results show that the proposed soft sensor model can realize various types of inspection and prediction in complex manufacturing processes. However, the generalization ability of this model is poor, and it can only be used in the manufacturing process of one working condition. Zhang et al. [13] deeply analyzed the relevant factors affecting the formation of glutamate, and proposed a soft sensor model based on fuzzy reasoning based on a support vector machine using the soft sensor method, and used the particle swarm optimization algorithm to optimize the key parameters to realize the control of glutamate concentration. The precise prediction of the model is optimized by using the fuzzy reasoning mechanism and the fuzzy basis function to optimize the kernel function of the support vector machine, which improves the anti-interference ability and adaptability of the model, whose prediction ability is good. However, the generalization ability of the model is insufficient, and the calculation process is relatively complicated, increasing the time cost. Han et al. [14], inspired by the adversarial network, used the adversarial domain adaptation method to improve the performance of the deep migration learning model and realize the accurate diagnosis of mechanical failures with small data volumes in industrial processes. However, this method must have sufficient target domain data. After the migration is completed, the target domain data in the actual industrial process are extremely limited, which affects the predictive performance of the model. Although the soft sensor models established in the above literature achieve accurate online prediction of key biological parameters, they do not consider the problem of model failure and performance degradation caused by the mismatch between modeling data and real-time data under different operating conditions in biological fermentation processes.

Regarding the abovementioned issue, [15] utilized deep transfer learning strategies to reduce the differences in data distribution between the source and target domains, effectively solving the problems of missing data and deterioration of soft sensor model performance in complex industrial processes. However, this method is only suitable for transferring from one working condition to another, which will reduce the ability of the model to fit. Ref. [16] proposed an online transfer learning technique based on slow feature analysis and variational Bayesian inference to improve the predictive performance of the target process, solving the problem of online measurement of water content in crude oil emulsions using steam-assisted gravity drainage technology and greatly improving production efficiency. Two weighting functions related to the transformation and emission equations are introduced and dynamically updated to quantify the transferability from the source domain to the target domain at each moment. Ref. [17] aims at the problem of online detection of key variables in industrial processes, proposes a soft sensor model based on variational mode decomposition, stacked enhanced autoencoder and transfer learning to achieve high-precision regression prediction, and introduces a transfer learning algorithm based on the maximum mean deviation in transfer learning to solve the domain under different operating conditions of the adaptation problem. However, the hyperparameters of the built model need to be manually selected, which greatly increases the prediction error of the model. Ref. [18] implements transfer learning by fine-tuning the weights of the network, freezing inner layers and updating outer layers. The method of transfer learning proposed in the literature realizes the prediction of complex industrial processes with small amounts of data. However, the prediction accuracy of this method is poor, and multiple parameters need to be manually set. Therefore, the application of transfer learning can effectively solve the dilemma of model failure and performance deterioration under different operating conditions. In summary, this paper proposes a multioperating condition transfer learning-based soft sensor modeling method for *Pichia pastoris* fermentation. First, to address the issue of significant data distribution differences between batches in the fermentation process, the BDA method in transfer learning is adopted to reduce the differences [19], and the fuzzy set concept is introduced to improve the BDA method, effectively converting the classification problem into a regression prediction problem of the fermentation process. Then, considering the nonlinearity and small sample characteristics of the *Pichia pastoris* fermentation process, the LSSVM is used as the basic model of the soft sensor process, and the adapted data are used to train the LSSVM model. The model is then optimized using an IPSO based on psychological mechanisms. Finally, the adapted target domain data are used to predict the *Pichia pastoris* cell concentration and product concentration through the constructed soft sensor model. The experimental results demonstrate that this soft sensor method is significantly superior to existing methods, has high prediction accuracy, and can accurately predict the *Pichia pastoris* fermentation process under different operating conditions. This paper makes significant contributions to current research on soft sensors. First, an IPSO algorithm is proposed to optimize the parameters of LSSVM, which greatly improves prediction accuracy. Compared with GWO and ABC optimization algorithms, the proposed IPSO algorithm has good dynamic performance and optimization performance. Second, this paper proposes to use the improved BDA algorithm in transfer learning to adapt the source domain and target domain to reduce the differences between different domains, so that the soft sensor model achieves good performance under multiworking conditions.

2. Methods

2.1. Principle and Solution of Balanced Distribution Adaptation

During the fermentation process of *Pichia pastoris*, the real-time data and modeling data distributions between different fermentation batches do not match due to varying operating conditions [20]. Soft sensor models established based on historical operational data may not be applicable to new batches, leading to model degradation and misalignment issues. Considering that transfer learning can learn useful information from other fermentation batches to assist in completing tasks for the target fermentation batch and does not require training and prediction data to conform to the requirement of independent and identically distributed data [21], it is an effective way to solve the problem of soft sensor modeling for the fermentation process with multiple operating conditions across different batches. Transfer learning has been widely used in medical images, industrial processes, and so on [22,23]. Transfer learning aims to improve the performance of target learners on target domains by transferring knowledge contained in different but related source domains [24]. Therefore, this article introduces a transfer learning strategy to construct a soft sensor model for the fermentation process of *Pichia pastoris*.

Data distribution adaptation is one of the most commonly used feature-based transfer learning methods [25]. The main idea behind this method is to use some transformations to bring the distance between data distributions of different domains closer together [26]. Currently, the most commonly used algorithm for this purpose is BDA, which reduces the joint probability distribution distance between the source and target domains to achieve transfer learning and improve the applicability and predictive accuracy of traditional soft sensor models. However, since the traditional BDA method is only suitable for solving classification problems [27], and soft sensor modeling for the fermentation process of *Pichia pastoris* is a regression problem, this article introduces the concept of fuzzy sets [28] into the BDA method to transform the classification problem into a regression problem and to achieve soft sensor modeling for the fermentation process of *Pichia pastoris*.

For a given labeled source domain data $Q_s = \{x_{s_i}, y_{s_i}\}_{i=1}^{n}$ and unlabeled target domain data $Q_t = \{x_{t_j}, y_{t_j}\}_{j=1}^{m}$ of the *Pichia pastoris* fermentation process, assuming the feature spaces are χ_s and χ_t, respectively, and $\chi_s = \chi_t$, the label spaces are Y_s and Y_t, respectively, and $Y_s = Y_t$, the marginal distributions are $P_s(x_s)$ and $P_t(x_t)$, respectively, and $P_s(x_s) \neq P_t(x_t)$, and the conditional distributions are $P_s(y_s|x_s)$ and $P_s(y_t|x_t)$, respectively, and $P_s(y_s|x_s) \neq P_s(y_t|x_t)$. The goal of BDA is to complete transfer learning by minimizing the marginal and conditional distributions between the source and target domains, which is minimizing the following equation.

$$DIS(Q_s, Q_t) \approx (1-\mu)DIS(P(x_s), P(x_t)) + \mu DIS(P(y_s|x_s), P(y_t|x_t)) \quad (1)$$

where μ is the balance factor to adjust the distance between the two distributions, $\mu \in [0,1]$. When $\mu \to 1$, it indicates that data sets are similar, and the conditional distribution has a greater proportion. When $\mu \to 0$, it indicates that the data sets are dissimilar, and the marginal distribution has a greater proportion.

Since there are no labels in the target domain Q_t, it is impossible to calculate the conditional probability distribution. Therefore, further training of a preclassifier is necessary to obtain soft labels y_{t_j}.

Let $Q_s^c = \{x_i | x_i \in Q_s \wedge y_i = c\}$ be the sample set of class c in the source domain s, and $Q_t^c = \{x_i | x_i \in Q_t \wedge y_i = c\}$ be the sample set of class c in the target domain t.

Using Maximum Mean Discrepancy (MMD) [29] to measure the distance between two neighboring domains, Equation (1) can be expressed as:

$$DIS(Q_s, Q_t) \approx (1-\mu) \left|\left| \frac{1}{n}\sum_{i=1}^{n} x_{s_i} - \frac{1}{m}\sum_{j=1}^{m} x_{t_j} \right|\right|_H^2 + \mu \sum_{c=1}^{C} \left|\left| \frac{1}{n_c}\sum_{x_{s_i} \in Q_s^c} x_{s_i} - \frac{1}{m_c}\sum_{x_{t_j} \in Q_t^c} x_{t_j} \right|\right|_H^2 \quad (2)$$

where H is the Reproducing Kernel Hilbert Space [30], c denotes different class labels, and $c \in \{1, 2, \cdots, C\}$, n and m represent the number of samples in the source and target domains, respectively. Q_s^c and Q_t^c refer to class c samples in the source and target domains, respectively. n_c and m_c, respectively, represent the number of samples in Q_s^c and Q_t^c. The first term in Equation (2) computes the distance between the marginal probability distributions of the source and target domains, and the second term calculates the distance between the conditional probability distributions.

Considering that the soft sensor problem of *Pichia pastoris* fermentation process studied in this paper is a regression problem, while the BDA method is only applicable to classification problems, this paper introduces the fuzzy set method to improve the BDA method and make it applicable to regression problems.

In traditional classification problems, a sample can only belong to one class, while using the fuzzy set method allows a sample to belong to multiple classes to varying degrees, therefore, for the output $\{y_i^z\}_{i=1,\cdots,n}$ of the z-th source domain, the 5th, 50th, and 95th percentile values are found and denoted as $p_5^z, p_{50}^z, p_{95}^z$. Three fuzzy sets denoted as $small^z$, $medium^z$, $large^z$ are defined based on these percentiles, as shown in Figure 1.

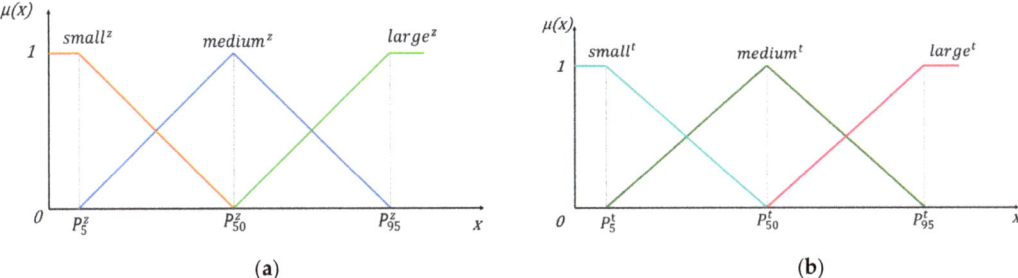

Figure 1. Percentage based fuzzy set division (**a**) Fuzzy sets in the source domain; (**b**) Fuzzy sets in the target domain.

Let the membership degree of y_i^z in class p in the source domain be denoted as α_{ip}^z, and the membership degree of y_i^t in class q in the target domain be denoted as α_{iq}^t, and normalize α_{ip}^z and α_{iq}^t, as shown in Equations (3) and (4):

$$\overline{\alpha}_{ip}^z = \frac{\alpha_{ip}^z}{\sum_{i=1}^{n} \alpha_{ip}^z} \quad p=1,2,3; i=1,2,\cdots,n \tag{3}$$

$$\overline{\alpha}_{iq}^t = \frac{\alpha_{iq}^t}{\sum_{i=1}^{n} \alpha_{iq}^t} \quad q=1,2,3; i=1,2,\cdots,n \tag{4}$$

Based on Equations (3) and (4), Equation (2) can be represented as:

$$DIS(Q_s, Q_t) \approx (1-\mu)||\frac{1}{n}\sum_{i=1}^{n} x_{s_i} - \frac{1}{m}\sum_{j=1}^{m} x_{t_j}||_H^2 + \mu \sum_{c=1}^{3} || \sum_{x_{s_i} \in D_s^{(c)}} \overline{\alpha}_{ic}^z x_{s_i} - \sum_{x_{t_j} \in D_t^{(c)}} \overline{\alpha}_{ic}^t x_{t_j} ||_H^2 \tag{5}$$

Using matrix techniques, Equation (5) can be written in the following form:

$$DIS(Q_s, Q_t) \approx A^T X(1-\mu) M_0 X^T A + A^T X \mu \sum_{c=1}^{3} M_c X^T A$$
$$= A^T X[(1-\mu) M_0 + \mu M_R] X^T A \tag{6}$$

where $M_R = M_1 + M_2 + M_3$, M_1, M_2 and M_3 are matrices for maximum mean discrepancy, defined as follows:

$$(M_c)_{ij} = \begin{cases} \overline{\alpha}_{ic}^z \overline{\alpha}_{jc}^z & x_i, x_j \in Q_s^c \\ \overline{\alpha}_{ic}^t \overline{\alpha}_{jc}^t & x_i, x_j \in Q_t^c \\ -\overline{\alpha}_{ic}^z \overline{\alpha}_{jc}^z & x_i \in Q_s^c, x_j \in Q_t^c \\ -\overline{\alpha}_{ic}^t \overline{\alpha}_{jc}^t & x_i \in Q_s^c, x_j \in Q_t^c \\ 0 & \text{other} \end{cases} \quad (7)$$

The calculation formula of M_0 is as follows:

$$(M_0)_{ij} = \begin{cases} \frac{1}{n^2} & x_i, x_j \in Q_s \\ \frac{1}{m^2} & x_i, x_j \in Q_t \\ \frac{-1}{mn} & \text{other} \end{cases} \quad (8)$$

The objective function Equation (2) can be represented as:

$$\begin{array}{c} \min tr(A^T X[(1-\mu)M_0 + \mu M_R]X^T A) + \lambda ||A||_F^2 \\ s.t. \ A^T X H X^T A = I, 0 \le \mu \le 1 \end{array} \quad (9)$$

where λ is the regularization parameter, A is the transformation matrix, X is the input matrix composed of x_{s_i} and x_{t_j}, $||\bullet||_F^2$ is the Hilbert-Schmidt norm, I is the identity matrix, $I \in \mathbb{R}^{(n+m)*(n+m)}$, and $H = I - (1/n)E$, E is the identity matrix. By using the Lagrange multiplier method, the Lagrange function for Equation (9) is:

$$L = tr(A^T X[(1-\mu)M_0 + \mu M_R]X^T A) + \lambda ||A||_F^2 + tr([I - A^T X H X^T A]\phi) \quad (10)$$

where the Lagrange multiplier $\phi = (\phi_1, \phi_2, \cdots, \phi_d)$, set derivative $\partial L/\partial A = 0$, then the optimization problem can be transformed into a generalized eigenvalue decomposition problem, which can be expressed as:

$$(X[(1-\mu)M_0 + \mu M_R]X^T + \lambda I)A = XHX^T A\phi \quad (11)$$

The optimal transformation matrix A can be obtained by solving Equation (11).

By using the optimal transformation matrix A, the distributions of the source domain data and the target domain data can be adapted, thereby improving the applicability and prediction accuracy of the soft sensor model.

2.2. Improving Particle Swarm—Least Squares Support Vector Machine Algorithm

2.2.1. Least Squares Support Vector Machine

The key biochemical parameters reflecting the real-time fermentation status and fermentation quality of *Pichia pastoris* (such as cell concentration and product concentration) are currently mainly obtained through offline sampling and laboratory analysis methods. However, this method is cumbersome and leads to long intervals between data collection for the same batch of fermentation, resulting in a limited number of actual collected data samples. In addition, the fermentation process has strong nonlinear characteristics. In light of the favorable performance of LSSVM in solving small sample, nonlinear, and high-dimensional regression tasks [31] and its fast solution speed and robust fitting ability, this paper applied LSSVM to soft sensor modeling of *Pichia pastoris* fermentation.

Suykens et al. [32] proposed the least LSSVM as a variant of the support vector machine (SVM). This method greatly reduces the complexity of the algorithm by using the sum of squared errors as the loss function. Given a dataset $\{x_i, y_i\}_{i=1}^l$ with the input data $x_i \in R^n$

and the output data $y_i \in R^n$, the optimization objective of LSSVM can be represented as follows:

$$\min_{\omega,e} J(\omega,e) = \frac{1}{2}\omega^T\omega + \frac{\gamma}{2}\sum_{i=1}^{l} e_i^2 \quad (12)$$

Subject to:

$$y_i[\omega^T \varphi(x_i) + b] = 1 - e_i \ i = 1, 2, \cdots, l \quad (13)$$

where ω represents the weight vector, $\varphi(i)$ is a nonlinear function that maps the data to a high-dimensional space, γ is the regularization parameter, e_i is the error introduced by the samples, and b is the constant bias. The optimization objective can be converted into a dual variable optimization problem using the Lagrange duality, which can be expressed as follows:

$$\begin{aligned} L(\omega,b,e,\alpha) &= J(\omega,e) - \sum_{i=1}^{l} \alpha_i(\omega^T \varphi(x_i) + b + e_i - y_i) \\ &= \tfrac{1}{2}\omega^T\omega + \tfrac{\gamma}{2}\sum_{i=1}^{l} e_i^2 - \sum_{i=1}^{l} \alpha_i\{[\omega^T \varphi(x_i) + b] + e_i - y_i\} \end{aligned} \quad (14)$$

where α_i is the Lagrange multiplier for the i-th constraint, according to the Karush–Kuhn–Tucker (KKT) conditions:

$$\begin{aligned} \tfrac{\partial L}{\partial \omega} &= 0 \to \sum_{i=1}^{l} \alpha_i \varphi(x_i) = \omega \\ \tfrac{\partial L}{\partial b} &= 0 \to -\sum_{i=1}^{l} \alpha_i y_i = 0 \\ \tfrac{\partial L}{\partial e_i} &= 0 \to \alpha_i = \gamma e_i \\ \tfrac{\partial L}{\partial \alpha_i} &= 0 \to \omega^T \varphi(x_i) + b + e_i - y_i = 0 \end{aligned} \quad (15)$$

After eliminating ω, e, Equation (16) is obtained as follows:

$$\begin{bmatrix} 0 & E^T \\ E & \Omega + \gamma^{-1} I_l \end{bmatrix} \begin{bmatrix} b \\ \alpha \end{bmatrix} = \begin{bmatrix} 0 \\ y \end{bmatrix} \quad (16)$$

where $E = [1, \ldots, 1]^T$, I_l is an $l \times l$ identity matrix, $\alpha = [\alpha_1, \ldots, \alpha_l]^T$, and Ω is the kernel matrix, $\Omega \in \mathbb{R}^{N \times N}$, and $\Omega_{ij} = \varphi(x_i)^T \varphi(x_j) = K(x_i, x_j)$ for a given RBF kernel function:

$$K(x_i, x_j) = \exp(\frac{-\|(x_i - x_j)\|^2}{2\sigma^2}) \quad (17)$$

Thus, the objective function can be derived as follows:

$$f(x) = \sum_{i=1}^{l} \alpha_i K(x, x_i) + b \quad (18)$$

where α, b are the solutions to Equation (16).

The predictive performance of LSSVM mainly depends on the regularization parameter γ and the kernel width σ, where γ balances the trade-off between fitting accuracy and model generalization ability, and σ affects the complexity of the distribution of the sample data in the mapped space. Traditional methods for parameter selection are often based on experience and trial, which may not guarantee regression accuracy and computational efficiency. To improve the LSSVM model, the IPSO algorithm is used to optimize the parameters (σ, γ) of LSSVM.

2.2.2. Improved Particle Swarm Optimization

Particle swarm optimization (PSO) is an evolutionary algorithm used to solve global optimization problems [33]. However, PSO has certain limitations such as a lack of dynamic adaptability, which can result in local optima trapping and slow convergence speed [34]. Researchers have proposed improved PSO algorithms to address these limitations, including dynamic PSO and adaptive PSO [35]. These algorithms have shown promising results in enhancing PSO's performance.

Yang Ge et al. [36] introduced a psychological model into PSO and proposed Emotional PSO (EPSO) to enhance the search ability of particles and accelerate the convergence speed of PSO. However, the algorithm lacks dynamic adaptability and is prone to getting trapped in local optima [37]. Therefore, this paper proposes an improved PSO algorithm based on EPSO to optimize the regularization parameter and kernel width of the LSSVM. The improved PSO algorithm is expected to overcome the limitations of EPSO and enhance the performance of PSO in solving optimization problems.

Assuming that each particle possesses emotional states and perception abilities, the Weber–Fechner law [38] has been utilized to enhance the performance of PSO. Specifically, particles utilize their emotional states to determine their next actions, and they can perceive stimuli by evaluating the difference between their current position and the historical best position. When the stimulus exceeds the perception threshold, the particle's emotional state changes, resulting in a stronger response to the stimulus. Three emotional states have been defined for the particles, namely happy, normal, and sad, which correspond to different particle reactions. The emotional state of each particle is updated in each iteration. If the particle's fitness is higher than that of the previous iteration, its emotional state increases; otherwise, its emotional state decreases. The emotional state of the i-th particle in the t-th iteration is represented by eX_i^t, and its initial emotional state is a random number. The formula for eX_i^0 can be expressed as:

$$eX_i^0 = rand[-0.1, 0.1] \quad (19)$$

The emotional state of the particle is adjusted according to its fitness. If the particle's fitness is better than the previous iteration, its emotional state increases; otherwise, its emotional state decreases. The increase and decrease of emotional state can be represented as:

$$\Delta^+ = \frac{(f(X_i^{t-1}) - f(X_i^t)) \cdot (f(X_i^t) - f(gb^t))}{(f(g\omega^t) - f(gb^t))^2} \quad (20)$$

$$\Delta^- = \frac{(f(X_i^t) - f(X_i^{t-1})) \cdot (f(g\omega^t) - f(X_i^t))}{(f(g\omega^t) - f(gb^t))^2} \quad (21)$$

where X_i^t represents the position of the i-th particle during the t-th iteration, gb^t represents the global best position at the t-th iteration, and $g\omega^t$ represents the global worst position at the t-th iteration.

Regarding particle swarm $pX = \{pX_i; i = 1, 2, \cdots, n\}$, its emotional state is sorted, and all particles are divided into three different emotional states based on the average value of their emotional state, as shown in Figure 2.

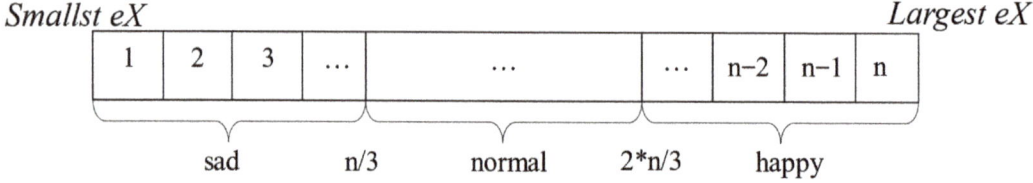

Figure 2. Particle swarm emotional state eX sorting.

Subsequently, the particle's behavior is determined based on its emotional state. The Weber–Fechner law is employed to describe the particle's perception ability, which can be expressed as:

$$r_g = -k \ln \frac{S(f(gBest) - f(pX_i))}{S_0} \qquad (22)$$

$$r_h = -k \ln \frac{S(f(pBest_i) - f(pX_i))}{S_0} \qquad (23)$$

where r_g represents global perception, r_h represents historical perception, k is a constant factor, $S(\cdot)$ is the stimulus function, S_0 is the stimulus threshold, $gBest$ is the historical best position of the particle swarm, and $pBest_i$ is the historical position of the i-th particle. According to the paper [35], the velocity and position update formulas for a particle in a normal emotional state are:

$$V_i^{t+1} = \zeta \cdot V_i^t + c_1 \cdot r_1 \cdot (pBest_i^t - pX_i^t) + c_2 \cdot r_2 \cdot (gBest^t - pX_i^t) \qquad (24)$$

$$pX_i^t = pX_i^{t-1} + V_i^t \qquad (25)$$

When the particle is in the happy state, it will be more energetic in the current position. The update formula of the particle speed and position in the happy state is:

$$V_i^{t+1} = \zeta \cdot V_i^t + c_1 \cdot r_1 \cdot r_g \cdot (pBest_i^t - X_i^t) + c_2 \cdot r_2 \cdot r_h \cdot (gBest^t - X_i^t) \qquad (26)$$

$$pX_i^t = pX_i^{t-1} + V_i^t \qquad (27)$$

When a particle is in a sad emotional state, it primarily focuses on its historical best position and contracts towards it from its current position. However, due to the decreasing fitness over iterations, the particle may become trapped in a local optimum. Based on the psychological model, a particle in a sad emotional state is on the verge of collapse and requires assistance from particles with better emotional states in the swarm to improve its condition. To address this issue, this paper proposes a restart strategy for updating the velocity of sad particles. The restart strategy is as follows:

$$V_i^t = c_1 \cdot (u - l) \cdot rand[-1, 1] \qquad (28)$$

where c_1 is a constant, u represents the upper limit of the particle search range, l represents the lower limit of the particle search range, and rand $[-1, 1]$ denotes a random number within the range of $[-1, 1]$. To maintain both convergence performance and diversity in the particle swarm, a combination of random initialization and the global best position is employed for updating the position of sad particles, which can be expressed as follows.

$$pX_i^t = \begin{cases} gb^{t-1} & r < 0.5 \\ l + (u - l) \cdot rand[-1, 1] & r \geq 0.5 \end{cases} \qquad (29)$$

The IPSO algorithm workflow is illustrated in Figure 3.

According to the analysis presented above, the improved PSO algorithm that utilizes the psychological mechanism demonstrates desirable dynamic and convergence performance, as well as enhanced search ability of particles when compared to traditional PSO algorithms. As a result, this study employed the improved PSO algorithm based on the psychological mechanism to optimize the key parameters (γ, σ) of the LSSVM.

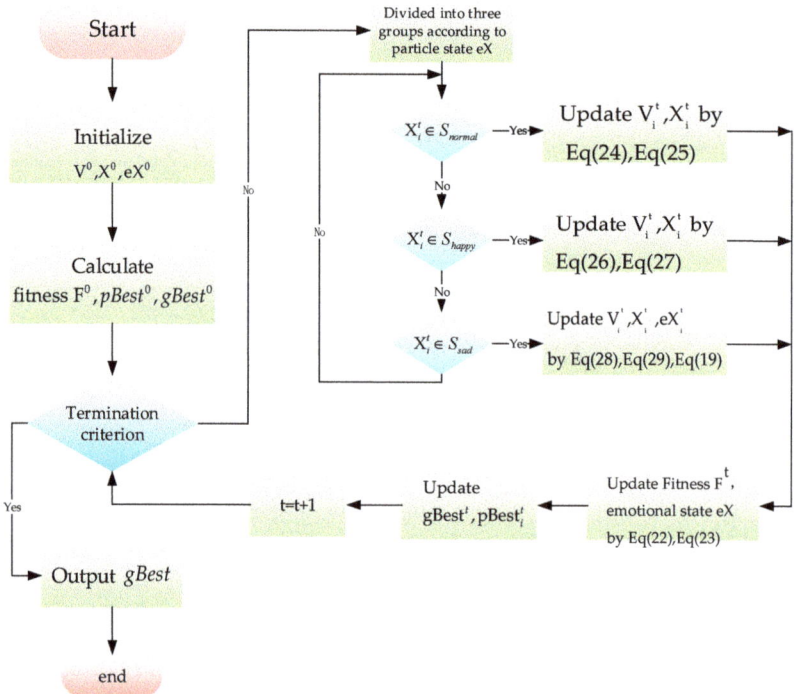

Figure 3. The framework of the IPSO algorithm.

2.3. Soft Sensor Modeling Based on BDA-IPSO-LSSVM

In this study, a soft sensor modeling strategy based on BDA-IPSO-LSSVM is proposed to address the issue of soft sensor model failure caused by the mismatch between training data and actual operating condition data in the fermentation process of *Pichia pastoris*. The proposed strategy utilizes the idea of transfer learning and employs the improved BDA method to match the training data and operating condition data, thereby enhancing the generalization ability and prediction accuracy of the established soft sensor model. Additionally, an improved PSO algorithm is proposed to optimize the established LSSVM-based soft sensor model and overcome the problem of arbitrary local optima in the PSO algorithm. To illustrate the proposed soft sensor modeling strategy based on BDA-IPSO-LSSVM, Figure 4 is provided, which presents a graphical representation of the strategy.

2.4. Introduction of the Pichia pastoris Experimental Work

The focus of this study is on *Pichia pastoris*, and *Pichia pastoris* GS115, MutsHis+ strain was selected as the strain. The RTY-C-100L fermenter was used as the fermentation equipment. The input variables for the soft sensor model were chosen based on the analysis of the fermentation process of *Pichia pastoris* using the absolute relation degree method. The stirring speed v, temperature T, airflow q, pH of the fermentation liquid, dissolved oxygen Do, and fermenter pressure p were selected as input variables, and the concentrations of production P and cell concentration C were selected as output variables. The fermentation process is shown in Figure 5.

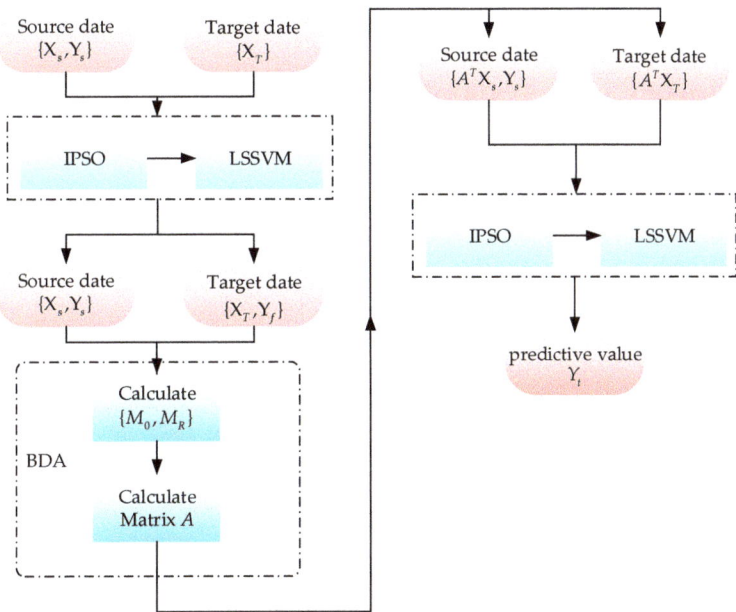

Figure 4. The framework of the BDA-IPSO-LSSVM.

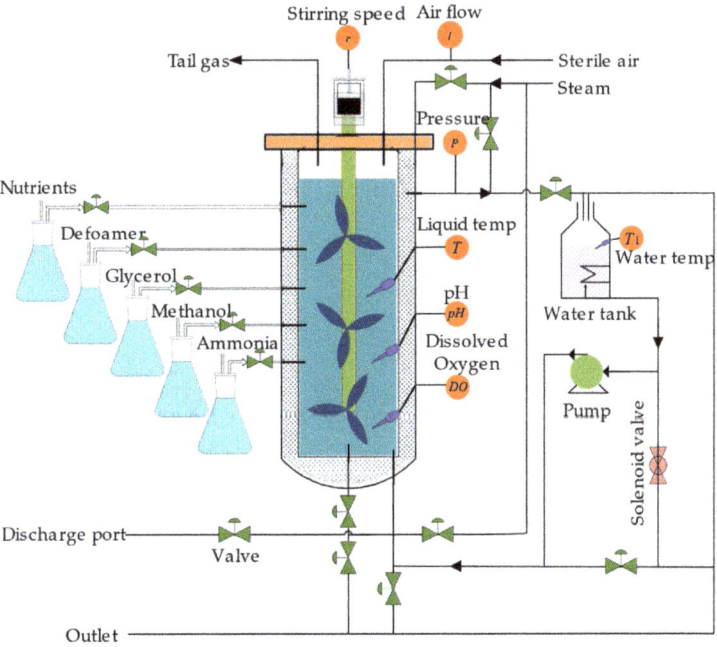

Figure 5. Structure of *Pichia pastoris* fermentation process.

The specific steps for modeling the *Pichia pastoris* fermentation soft sensor model based on BDA method are as follows, where the source domain data and the target domain data are represented by $Q_s = \{x_{s_i}, y_{s_i}\}_{i=1}^n$ and $Q_t = \{x_{t_l}, y_{t_l}\}_{l=1}^m$, respectively:

Step 1: Carry out *Pichia pastoris* fermentation experiments, build the datasets, and normalize the dataset.

Step 2: Establish the IPSO-LSSVM model: the first step is to determine the parameters of the LSSVM model, including regularization parameter γ and kernel width σ. IPSO-LSSVM is an optimization method based on the improved particle swarm algorithm, which automatically selects the optimal model parameters. The IPSO-LSSVM uses the IPSO algorithm proposed in this paper to automatically obtain regularization parameter γ and kernel width σ.

Step 3: Train the IPSO-LSSVM model using labeled source domain data $Q_s = \{x_{s_i}, y_{s_i}\}_{i=1}^n$: labeled source domain data can be used to train the initial IPSO-LSSVM model, which can serve as the starting point for the iterative process, helping to improve the subsequent optimization results.

Step 4: Obtain soft label y_f for target domain data x_t by iteratively inputting unlabeled data into the IPSO-LSSVM model: Since the target domain data are unlabeled, the unlabeled target domain data x_t are input into the IPSO-LSSVM model obtained in step 3 to generate predicted values y_t, which are then used as soft labels. The soft labels y_f are then combined with the target domain data x_t.

Step 5: Compute the transformation matrix A using the source domain data, target domain data, and soft labels as inputs for the improved BDA algorithm: the improved BDA algorithm utilizes the source domain data Q_s, target domain data x_t, and target domain data soft labels y_f to compute a transformation matrix A that matches the source domain data and the target domain data, facilitating the transfer of knowledge from the source domain to the target domain.

Step 6: Input the matched source domain $\{A^T x_s, y_s\}$ and target domain $\{A^T x_t\}$ into the IPSO-LSSVM model to obtain the actual predicted key parameters y_t in the fermentation process of *Pichia pastoris*.

The specific steps of the *Pichia pastoris* fermentation experiment are as follows:

1. The fermentation system was sterilized and the bacterial strain was cultured according to the requirements of the *Pichia pastoris* fermentation process. The medium was sterilized at 130 °C for 30 min, and the bacterial strain was inoculated by flame when the temperature dropped to 30 °C. The initial fermentation conditions were set: initial tank pressure control at 0.02~0.05 MPa; pH control at 5.0; temperature control at 28 °C; speed set at 300~400 rpm; and airflow velocity control at 150~300 L/M.

2. We selected the stirring speed v, temperature T, airflow q, pH of the fermentation liquid, dissolved oxygen Do, and fermenter pressure P as auxiliary variables by the absolute relation degree method. All auxiliary variables were transmitted to the database through the distributed control system. The auxiliary variables in this experiment were sampled every 0.5 h.

3. We selected different batches of *Pichia pastoris* fermentation data as data samples. Since the fermentation cycle of *Pichia pastoris* is 90 h, each batch contained 180 data samples. We used auxiliary variables as input variables, cell density and product concentration as output variables, and input the data into the established *Pichia pastoris* fermentation soft sensor model to complete the establishment of the soft sensor model of the *Pichia pastoris* fermentation process and realize real-time prediction of key biological parameters. The root mean square error ($RMSE$), coefficient of determination (R^2), and mean absolute error (MAE) and floating point operations ($GFLOPs$) were used as performance evaluation indicators for the soft sensor model. The calculation formulas are as follows:

$$RMSE = \sqrt{\frac{1}{n}\sum_{i=1}^{n}(y_{pre}^{(i)} - \hat{y}_{real}^{(i)})^2} \tag{30}$$

$$R^2 = 1 - \frac{\sum_{i=1}^{n}(y_{pre}^{(i)} - y_{real}^{(i)})^2}{\sum_{i=1}^{n}(y_{real}^{(i)} - \hat{y}_{real})^2} \tag{31}$$

$$MAE = \frac{1}{n}\sum_{i=0}^{n}|y_{pre}^{(i)} - y_{real}^{(i)}| \tag{32}$$

3. Result and Discussion

3.1. Result

To better demonstrate the effectiveness of the proposed method in this article, simulations were conducted for the LSSVM soft sensor model, the PSO-LSSVM soft sensor model, the IPSO-LSSVM soft sensor model, and the BDA-IPSO-LSSVM soft sensor model, respectively, to achieve real-time prediction of cell concentration C and product concentration P of *Pichia pastoris*. The simulation results for cell concentration C are shown in Figure 6, where Figure 6a represents the simulation result for LSSVM, using the RBF function as the kernel function, the regularization parameter set to 125, and the RBF kernel width set to 10. PSO and IPSO were introduced to optimize the LSSVM model, with the regularization parameter lower bound set to zero, the upper bound set to 300, the initialization set to 100, the kernel width lower bound set to zero, the upper bound set to 50, the particle swarm size set to 100, and c_1 set to 0.35, when the number of iterations reaches 200 or the global optimal position is less than 110, it is used as the termination condition of the IPSO algorithm. Finally, the IPSO algorithm was used to obtain the optimized LSSVM regularization parameter of 132.4 and kernel width of 16.4, resulting in the simulation results shown in Figure 6b,c, respectively. The "actual value" in the figures represents the real value measured during the fermentation experiment of *Pichia pastoris*. In order to further illustrate the effectiveness of the proposed IPSO algorithm, Figure 7 shows the fitness curves of the PSO algorithm and the IPSO algorithm. It can be seen that the fitness of the IPSO algorithm is significantly better than that of the PSO algorithm. To further demonstrate the favorable convergence performance and optimization capability of the IPSO algorithm, a comparative analysis was conducted by the IPSO with two classical optimization algorithms, namely Grey Wolf Optimization [39] (GWO) and Artificial Bee Colony [40] (ABC), under identical input conditions. Figure 7 presents the fitness curves of the IPSO, PSO, GWO, and ABC optimization algorithms. It is evident that the IPSO algorithm exhibits a significantly accelerated optimization speed in comparison to the other algorithms. Concerning the prediction results for the cell concentration of *Pichia pastoris*, Figure 8 shows the prediction result of the IPSO-LSSVM, WOLF-LSSVM and ABC-LSSVM. The figure distinctly illustrates that IPSO-LSSVM produces markedly smaller prediction errors compared to the other two algorithms. The results provide substantial evidence that the IPSO algorithm demonstrates pronounced superiority in terms of parameter optimization effectiveness, surpassing both GWO and ABC algorithms.

The improved BDA algorithm was used to further improve the prediction accuracy by adapting the source domain data and target domain data. In the BDA algorithm, the balancing factor μ approaches one as the conditional probability distribution becomes more important and approaches zero as the marginal probability distribution becomes more important. In this simulation, the balancing factor was set to 0.62 to achieve optimal prediction performance. The final simulation result for the BDA-IPSO-LSSVM soft sensor model is shown in Figure 6d.

By comparing Figure 6a,b, it can be observed that the PSO algorithm can enhance the prediction accuracy of the LSSVM model. However, the prediction effect of the LSSVM model is not ideal and cannot meet the needs of the fermentation industry, significant errors remain present in the model by comparing the predicted value with the actual value. A further comparison of Figure 6b,c indicates that the IPSO algorithm can effectively enhance the prediction accuracy of the model by improving the dynamic performance of the PSO algorithm, and the IPSO algorithm reduces the prediction error of the model. The result presented in Figure 6d demonstrates that the proposed IBDA algorithm is effective in reducing the distribution distance between the source domain and the target domain and makes the predicted value of the model meet the actual fermentation production needs.

It can be seen that the proposed BDA-IPSO-LSSVM model has good prediction accuracy in Figure 6e.

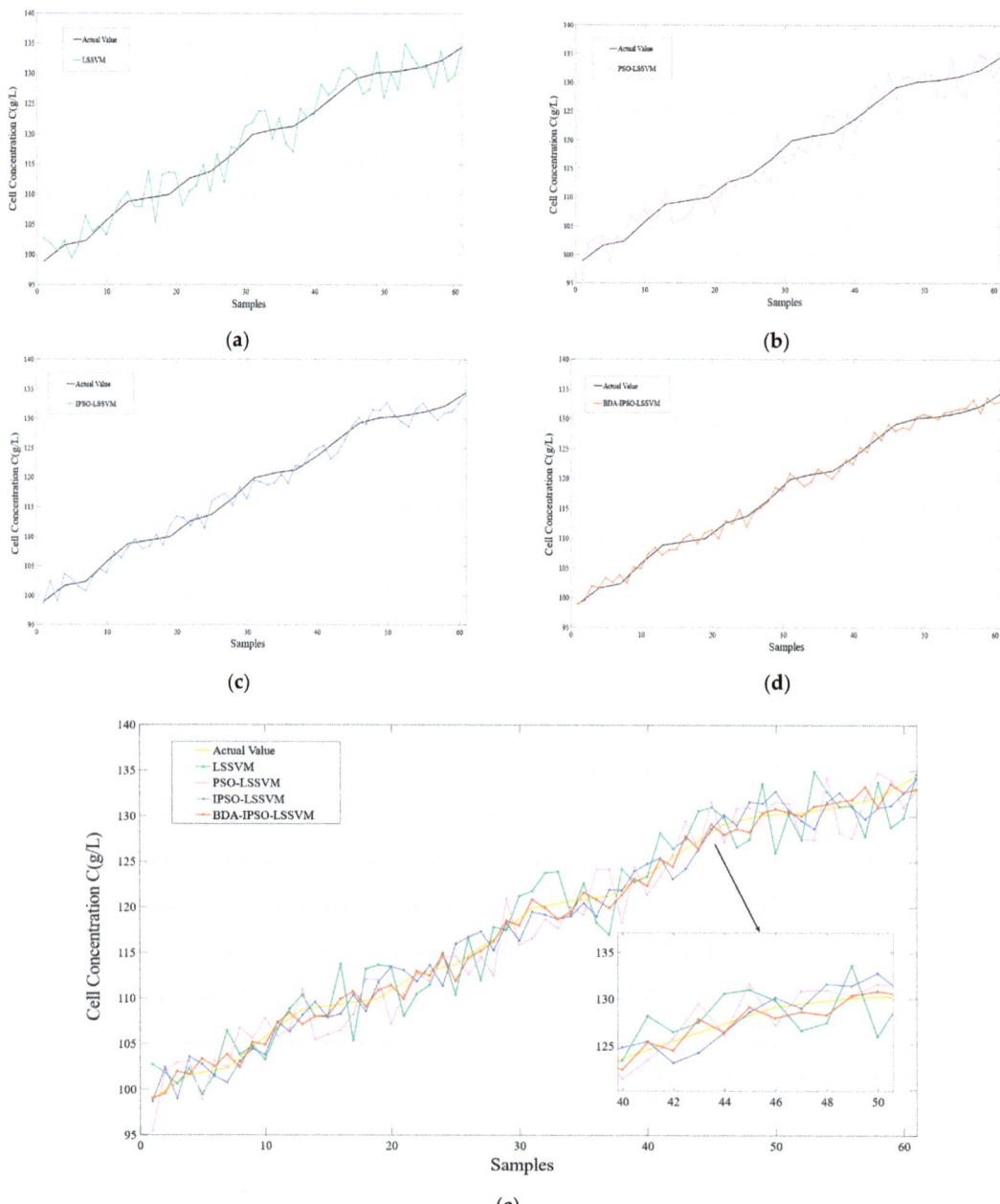

Figure 6. Prediction results of different models for cell concentration: (**a**) LSSVM; (**b**) PSO-LSSVM; (**c**) IPSO-LSSVM; (**d**) BDA-IPSO-LSSVM; (**e**) Combination of the four models.

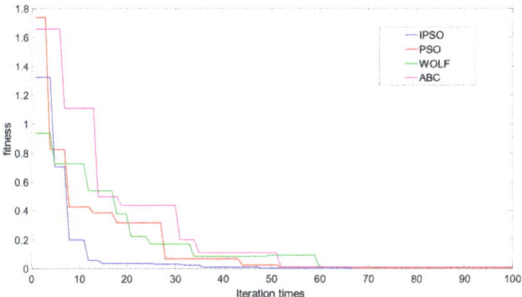

Figure 7. The fitness curve of the IPSO, PSO, WOLF and ABC optimization algorithms.

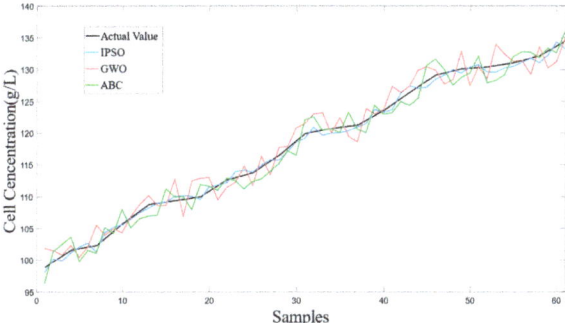

Figure 8. The prediction result of the IPSO-LSSVM, WOLF-LSSVM and ABC-LSSVM.

Figure 9 shows the residuals of the different soft sensor models in predicting the cell concentration of *Pichia pastoris*. The prediction performance of the soft sensor models is shown in Table 1. It can be intuitively seen in Figure 8 and Table 1 that the BDA-IPSO-LSSVM residual is relatively small compared to other models, and it performs well in the *RMSE*, R^2, and *MAE* performance metrics. GFLOPs reflects the complexity of the model. From the value of GFLOPs of each model in Table 1, it can be seen that the proposed hybrid model does not increase the complexity of the model.

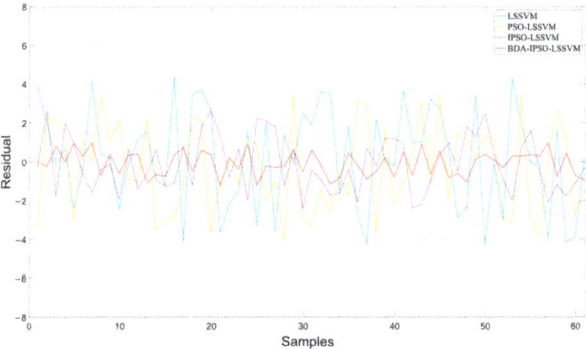

Figure 9. The residuals of the different soft sensor models in predicting the cell concentration of *Pichia pastoris*.

To further illustrate the effectiveness of the proposed BDA-IPSO-LSSVM model, similar to Figure 6, Figure 10 illustrates the predicted values of the Pichia pastoris product concentration. Specifically, Figure 10 presents the results of the four different soft sensor models, while Figure 10a–d show the prediction results of the LSSVM model, PSO-LSSVM model, IPSO-LSSVM model, and BDA-IPSO-LSSVM model for product concentration during the fermentation process of *Pichia pastoris*. As evidenced by Figure 10e, the BDA-IPSO-LSSVM model proposed in this paper exhibits strong predictive performance in regard to the key parameters during the fermentation process of *Pichia pastoris*. Figure 11 displays the residuals of the different soft sensor models, and Table 2 presents the performance metrics of the prediction results. By means of comparison, it can be concluded that the proposed BDA-IPSO-LSSVM soft sensor model exhibits superior prediction accuracy compared to the other models.

Table 1. Prediction performance indexes of different soft sensor models in predicting cell concentration.

	RMSE	R^2	MAE	GFLOPs
LSSVM	2.3356	0.9425	2.1929	0.0014
PSO-LSSVM	2.1830	0.9572	1.9425	0.0016
IPSO-LSSVM	1.5902	0.9779	1.4154	0.0016
BDA-IPSO-LSSVM	1.0485	0.9912	0.8554	0.0016

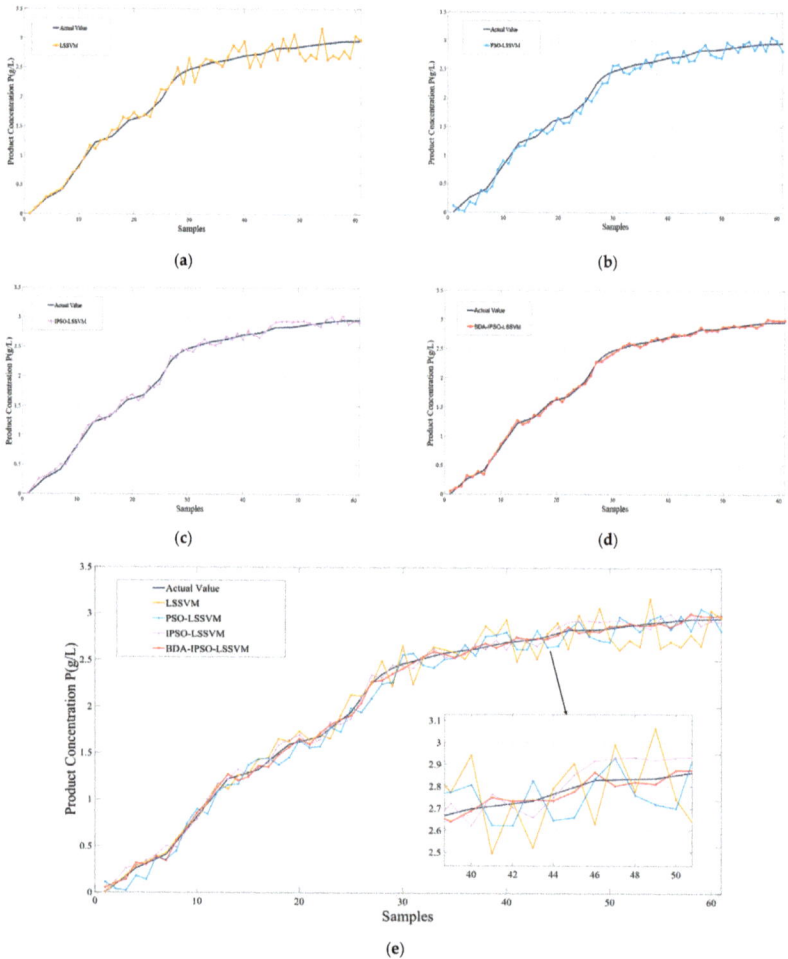

Figure 10. Prediction results of different models for product concentration: (**a**) LSSVM; (**b**) PSO-LSSVM; (**c**) IPSO-LSSVM; (**d**) BDA-IPSO-LSSVM; (**e**) Combination of the four models.

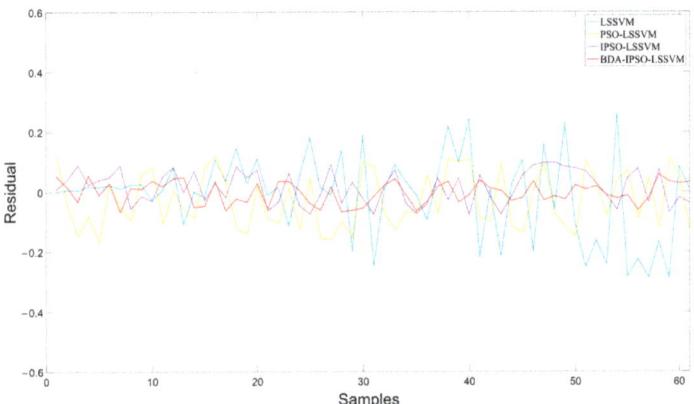

Figure 11. The residuals of the different soft sensor models in predicting the product concentration of *Pichia pastoris*.

Table 2. Prediction performance indexes of different soft sensor models in predicting product concentration.

	RMSE	R^2	MAE	FLOPs
LSSVM	0.1397	0.9773	0.1046	0.0013
PSO-LSSVM	0.0973	0.9890	0.0887	0.0015
IPSO-LSSVM	0.0569	0.9962	0.0508	0.0015
BDA-IPSO-LSSVM	0.0368	0.9984	0.0322	0.0015

3.2. Discussion

This paper proposes a soft sensor model of *Pichia pastoris* based on LSSVM. Through Figures 6 and 10, it can be seen that the proposed soft sensor model has good predictive performance and can better realize the real-time monitoring of the fermentation process of *Pichia pastoris*. This paper first proposes an IPSO algorithm to optimize the parameters of LLSVM to achieve good prediction performance of LSSVM. Figures 7 and 8 show that compared with the GWO and ABC optimization algorithms, the IPSO algorithm proposed in this paper has good dynamic performance and convergence performance: it better solves the optimization problem of LSSVM parameters and realizes an accurate prediction of the LSSVM model. Second, this paper uses the BDA method in transfer learning to match the source domain data and target domain data, and realizes the accurate prediction of the *Pichia pastoris* soft sensor model under different working conditions. In Figures 9 and 11, it can be seen that, compared with the model without transfer, the proposed hybrid model reduces the prediction error of the model to a large extent and solves the problem of model failure under different working conditions. It can be seen from Tables 1 and 2 that the hybrid model proposed in this paper has good performance in various evaluation indicators. Moreover, the simulation results show that the hybrid model proposed in this paper has good predictive performance and can realize the real-time and accurate prediction of the cell concentration and product concentration in the fermentation process of *Pichia pastoris*, which greatly improves the production efficiency of *Pichia pastoris* fermentation products.

4. Conclusions

This study has proposed a novel soft sensor modeling strategy based on BDA-IPSO-LSSVM to address the issue of data distribution differences resulting from different operating conditions during the fermentation process of *Pichia pastoris*. The proposed strategy employs the BDA method and a fuzzy set-based improvement to reduce the distribution differences and improve the generalization ability of the traditional soft sensor model. Additionally, an improved PSO algorithm is proposed to optimize the established LSSVM-based soft sensor model, which addresses the issue of PSO algorithms becoming trapped in local optima and results in a significant improvement in the prediction accuracy of the soft sensor model. The experimental results demonstrate that the proposed BDA-IPSO-LSSVM soft sensor model exhibits strong performance in terms of the *RMSE*, R^2, and *MAE* prediction performance indicators. The soft sensor model can effectively predict the key parameters of *Pichia pastoris* fermentation in real-time, including cell concentration and product concentration. The proposed strategy offers a promising solution to the issue of soft sensor model failure caused by the mismatch between training data and actual operating condition data and has potential applications in the fermentation industry. Future studies may explore the generalization of the proposed strategy to other fermentation processes or even other fields. The main limitation at present is that only one source domain and one target domain can be adapted, and the IPSO can be optimized for a single objective. In the future, we aim to research the transfer learning from the data of multiple historical operating conditions to further reduce the difference between data, and generalization of IPSO to multiobjective optimization problems.

Author Contributions: Conceptualization, B.W. and J.L.; methodology, B.W.; software, J.L.; validation, J.L., A.Y. and H.W.; formal analysis, J.L.; investigation, J.L.; resources, J.L.; data curation, H.W.; writing—original draft preparation, H.W.; writing—review and editing, A.Y.; visualization, J.L.; supervision, B.W.; project administration, B.W.; funding acquisition, B.W. All authors have read and agreed to the published version of the manuscript.

Funding: This research was funded by Natural Science Foundation of China (No. 61705093) and the Wuxi Science and Technology Plan Project—Basic Research: No. K20221054.

Institutional Review Board Statement: Not applicable.

Informed Consent Statement: Not applicable.

Data Availability Statement: The dataset in this article is unavailable because it involves privacy.

Conflicts of Interest: The authors declare no conflict of interest.

Abbreviations

BDA	balanced distribution adaptation
LSSVM	least squares support vector machine
IPSO	improved particle swarm optimization
LSTM	Long Short Term Memory
GWO	Grey Wolf Optimization
ABC	Artificial Bee Colony
MMD	Maximum Mean Discrepancy
H	Reproducing Kernel Hilbert Space
KKT	Karush–Kuhn–Tucker
PSO	Particle Swarm Optimization
EPSO	Emotional Particle Swarm Optimization
RMSE	Root Mean Square Error
R^2	R-Square
FLOPs	Floating Point Operations
MAE	Mean Absolute Error

Nomenclature

Q_s	the source domain data
x_{s_i}	*i*-th input source domain data
y_{s_i}	*i*-th output source domain data
n	the amount of data in the source domain
Q_t	target domain data
x_{t_j}	*j*-th input source domain data
y_{t_j}	*j*-th output source domain data

m	the amount of data in the target domain
χ_s	the source domain future space
χ_t	the target domain future space
γ_s	the source domain label space
γ_t	the target domain label space
$P_s(x_s)$	the source domain marginal distribution
$P_t(x_t)$	the target domain marginal distribution
$P_s(y_s|x_s)$	the source domain conditional distribution
$P_t(y_t|x_t)$	the target domain conditional distribution
μ	the balance factor
Q_s^c	the sample set of class c in the source domain
Q_t^c	the sample set of class c in the target domain
C	the number of classes
c	the c-th classes
n_c	the number of samples in $Q_s{}^c$
m_c	the number of samples in $Q_t{}^c$
y_i^z	the z-th source domain i-th data
P_5^z	the z-th source domain 5-th percentile values
P_{50}^z	the z-th source domain 50-th percentile values
P_{95}^z	the z-th source domain 95-th percentile values
α_{ip}^z	the membership degree of y_i^z in class p in the source domain
α_{iq}^t	the membership degree of y_i^t in class q in the target domain
M_c	the matrices for maximum mean discrepancy
λ	the regularization parameter
A	the transformation matrix
X	the input matrix composed of x_{s_i} and x_{t_j}
$\|\bullet\|_F^2$	the Hilbert–Schmidt norm
E	the identity matrix
ϕ	the Lagrange multiplier
ω	the weight vector
$\varphi(i)$	a nonlinear function that maps the data to a high-dimensional space
γ	the regularization parameter
e_i	the error introduced by the samples
b	the constant bias
$L(\omega, b, e, \alpha)$	the LSSVM optimization objective
α_i	the Lagrange multiplier for the i-th constraint
I_l	an $l*l$ identity matrix
Ω	the kernel matrix
σ	the kernel width
$K(x_i, x_j)$	the RBF kernel
eX_i^t	The emotional state of the i-th particle in the t-th iteration
Δ^+	the increase of emotional state
Δ^-	the increase of emotional state
X_i^t	the position of the i-th particle during the t-th iteration
gb^t	the global best position at the t-th iteration
gw^t	the lobal worst position at the t-th iteration
pX	the particle swarm
pX_i	the i-th particle position
r_g	the global perception
r_h	The historical perception
k	a constant factor
$S(\cdot)$	the stimulus function
S_0	the stimulus threshold
$gBest$	the historical best position of the particle swarm
$pBest_i$	the historical position of the i-th particle
μ	the upper limit of the particle search range
l	the lower limit of the particle search range

v	The stirring speed
T	temperature
q	airflow
Do	dissolved oxygen
C	cell concentration
p	fermenter pressure
P	the concentrations of production
$y_{pre}^{(i)}$	the model i-th prediction data
$y_{real}^{(i)}$	i-th real data

References

1. Karbalaei, M.; Rezaee, S.A.; Farsiani, H. *Pichia pastoris*: A Highly Successful Expression System for Optimal Synthesis of Heterologous Proteins. *J. Cell. Physiol.* **2020**, *235*, 5867–5881. [CrossRef] [PubMed]
2. Yang, Y.; Madden, K.; Sha, M. Human IgG Fc Production Through Methanol-Free *Pichia pastoris* Fermentation. *BioProcess. J.* **2022**, *21*, 1–10.
3. Wu, J.; Zhang, X.; Yu, H.; Li, W.; Jia, Y.; Guo, J.; Zhang, L.; Song, X. Research Progress of High Density Fermentation Process of *Pichia pastoris*. *China Biotechnol.* **2016**, *36*, 108–114. [CrossRef]
4. Zhu, X.; Rehman, K.U.; Wang, B.; Shahzad, M. Modern Soft-Sensing Modeling Methods for Fermentation Processes. *Sensors* **2020**, *20*, 1771. [CrossRef]
5. Mohanty, S.; Khasa, Y.P. Nitrogen Supplementation Ameliorates Product Quality and Quantity during High Cell Density Bioreactor Studies of *Pichia pastoris*: A Case Study with Proteolysis Prone Streptokinase. *Int. J. Biol. Macromol.* **2021**, *180*, 760–770. [CrossRef]
6. Chai, W.Y.; Teo, K.T.K.; Tan, M.K.; Tham, H.J. Fermentation Process Control and Optimization. *Chem. Eng. Technol.* **2022**, *45*, 1731–1747. [CrossRef]
7. Wang, B.; Wang, X.; He, M.; Zhu, X. Study on Multi-Model Soft Sensor Modeling Method and Its Model Optimization for the Fermentation Process of *Pichia pastoris*. *Sensors* **2021**, *21*, 7635. [CrossRef] [PubMed]
8. Shao, W.; Ge, Z.; Song, Z. Soft-Sensor Development for Processes With Multiple Operating Modes Based on Semisupervised Gaussian Mixture Regression. *IEEE Trans. Control Syst. Technol.* **2019**, *27*, 2169–2181. [CrossRef]
9. Yuan, X.; Li, L.; Wang, Y. Nonlinear Dynamic Soft Sensor Modeling With Supervised Long Short-Term Memory Network. *IEEE Trans. Ind. Inform.* **2020**, *16*, 3168–3176. [CrossRef]
10. Zheng, W.; Liu, Y.; Gao, Z.; Yang, J. Just-in-Time Semi-Supervised Soft Sensor for Quality Prediction in Industrial Rubber Mixers. *Chemom. Intell. Lab. Syst.* **2018**, *180*, 36–41. [CrossRef]
11. Chang, S.; Zhao, C.; Li, K. Consistent-Contrastive Network With Temporality-Awareness for Robust-to-Anomaly Industrial Soft Sensor. *IEEE Trans. Instrum. Meas.* **2022**, *71*, 1–12. [CrossRef]
12. Fan, A.; Huang, Y.; Xu, F.; Bom, S. Soft Sensing Regression Model: From Sensor to Wafer Metrology Forecasting. *arXiv* **2023**, arXiv:2301.08974.
13. Zhang, C.; Li, Z.; Sun, Y. Study on Soft Sensing of Glutamic Acid Fermentation Process Based on LS-SVM. In Proceedings of the 2022 IEEE International Conference on Artificial Intelligence and Computer Applications (ICAICA), Dalian, China, 24–26 June 2022; pp. 354–360.
14. Han, T.; Liu, C.; Wu, R.; Jiang, D. Deep Transfer Learning with Limited Data for Machinery Fault Diagnosis. *Appl. Soft Comput.* **2021**, *103*, 107150. [CrossRef]
15. Chai, Z.; Zhao, C.; Huang, B.; Chen, H. A Deep Probabilistic Transfer Learning Framework for Soft Sensor Modeling With Missing Data. *IEEE Trans. Neural Netw. Learn. Syst.* **2021**, *33*, 7598–7609. [CrossRef]
16. Xie, J.; Huang, B.; Dubljevic, S. Transfer Learning for Dynamic Feature Extraction Using Variational Bayesian Inference. *IEEE Trans. Knowl. Data Eng.* **2022**, *34*, 5524–5535. [CrossRef]
17. Ren, J.-C.; Liu, D.; Wan, Y. VMD-SEAE-TL-Based Data-Driven Soft Sensor Modeling for a Complex Industrial Batch Processes. *Measurement* **2022**, *198*, 111439. [CrossRef]
18. Hsiao, Y.-D.; Kang, J.-L.; Wong, D.S.-H. Development of Robust and Physically Interpretable Soft Sensor for Industrial Distillation Column Using Transfer Learning with Small Datasets. *Processes* **2021**, *9*, 667. [CrossRef]
19. Wang, J.; Chen, Y.; Hao, S.; Feng, W.; Shen, Z. Balanced Distribution Adaptation for Transfer Learning. *arXiv* **2018**, arXiv:1807.00516.
20. Zhu, X.; Liu, W.; Wang, B.; Wang, W. A Soft Sensor Model of *Pichia pastoris* Cell Concentration Based on IBDA-RELM. *Prep. Biochem. Biotechnol.* **2022**, *52*, 618–626. [CrossRef]
21. Tang, Y.; Rahmani Dehaghani, M.; Wang, G.G. Review of Transfer Learning in Modeling Additive Manufacturing Processes. *Addit. Manuf.* **2023**, *61*, 103357. [CrossRef]
22. Kora, P.; Ooi, C.P.; Faust, O.; Raghavendra, U.; Gudigar, A.; Chan, W.Y.; Meenakshi, K.; Swaraja, K.; Plawiak, P.; Rajendra Acharya, U. Transfer Learning Techniques for Medical Image Analysis: A Review. *Biocybern. Biomed. Eng.* **2022**, *42*, 79–107. [CrossRef]
23. Curreri, F.; Patanè, L.; Xibilia, M.G. RNN- and LSTM-Based Soft Sensors Transferability for an Industrial Process. *Sensors* **2021**, *21*, 823. [CrossRef]

24. Zhuang, F.; Qi, Z.; Duan, K.; Xi, D.; Zhu, Y.; Zhu, H.; Xiong, H.; He, Q. A Comprehensive Survey on Transfer Learning. *Proc. IEEE* **2021**, *109*, 43–76. [CrossRef]
25. Weiss, K.; Khoshgoftaar, T.M.; Wang, D. A Survey of Transfer Learning. *J. Big Data* **2016**, *3*, 9. [CrossRef]
26. Pan, S.J.; Tsang, I.W.; Kwok, J.T.; Yang, Q. Domain Adaptation via Transfer Component Analysis. *IEEE Trans. Neural Netw.* **2011**, *22*, 199–210. [CrossRef]
27. Zhou, X.; Sbarufatti, C.; Giglio, M.; Dong, L. A Fuzzy-Set-Based Joint Distribution Adaptation Method for Regression and Its Application to Online Damage Quantification for Structural Digital Twin. *Mech. Syst. Signal Process.* **2023**, *191*, 110164. [CrossRef]
28. Wu, D.; Lawhern, V.J.; Gordon, S.; Lance, B.J.; Lin, C.-T. Driver Drowsiness Estimation From EEG Signals Using Online Weighted Adaptation Regularization for Regression (OwARR). *IEEE Trans. Fuzzy Syst.* **2017**, *25*, 1522–1535. [CrossRef]
29. Alon, I.; Globerson, A.; Wiesel, A. On the Optimization Landscape of Maximum Mean Discrepancy. *arXiv* **2021**, arXiv:2110.13452.
30. Berlinet, A.; Thomas-Agnan, C. *Reproducing Kernel Hilbert Spaces in Probability and Statistics*; Springer Science & Business Media: Berlin/Heidelberg, Germany, 2011; ISBN 978-1-4419-9096-9.
31. Guo, H.; Cui, M.; Feng, Z.; Zhang, D.; Zhang, D. Classification of Aviation Alloys Using Laser-Induced Breakdown Spectroscopy Based on a WT-PSO-LSSVM Model. *Chemosensors* **2022**, *10*, 220. [CrossRef]
32. Suykens, J.A.K.; Vandewalle, J. Least Squares Support Vector Machine Classifiers. *Neural Process. Lett.* **1999**, *9*, 293–300. [CrossRef]
33. Jain, M.; Saihjpal, V.; Singh, N.; Singh, S.B. An Overview of Variants and Advancements of PSO Algorithm. *Appl. Sci.* **2022**, *12*, 8392. [CrossRef]
34. Tao, X.; Li, X.; Chen, W.; Liang, T.; Li, Y.; Guo, J.; Qi, L. Self-Adaptive Two Roles Hybrid Learning Strategies-Based Particle Swarm Optimization. *Inf. Sci.* **2021**, *578*, 457–481. [CrossRef]
35. Shami, T.M.; El-Saleh, A.A.; Alswaitti, M.; Al-Tashi, Q.; Summakieh, M.A.; Mirjalili, S. Particle Swarm Optimization: A Comprehensive Survey. *IEEE Access* **2022**, *10*, 10031–10061. [CrossRef]
36. Ge, Y.; Rubo, Z. An Emotional Particle Swarm Optimization Algorithm. In Proceedings of the Advances in Natural Computation; Wang, L., Chen, K., Ong, Y.S., Eds.; Springer: Berlin/Heidelberg, Germany, 2005; pp. 553–561.
37. Gou, J.; Lei, Y.-X.; Guo, W.-P.; Wang, C.; Cai, Y.-Q.; Luo, W. A Novel Improved Particle Swarm Optimization Algorithm Based on Individual Difference Evolution. *Appl. Soft Comput.* **2017**, *57*, 468–481. [CrossRef]
38. Kausik, B.N. Accelerating Machine Learning via the Weber-Fechner Law. *arXiv* **2022**, arXiv:2204.11834.
39. Mirjalili, S.; Mirjalili, S.M.; Lewis, A. Grey Wolf Optimizer. *Adv. Eng. Softw.* **2014**, *69*, 46–61. [CrossRef]
40. Sharma, A.; Sharma, A.; Choudhary, S.; Pachauri, R.; Shrivastava, A.; Kumar, D. A review on artificial bee colony and it's engineering applications. *J. Crit. Rev.* **2020**, *7*, 4097–4107. [CrossRef]

Disclaimer/Publisher's Note: The statements, opinions and data contained in all publications are solely those of the individual author(s) and contributor(s) and not of MDPI and/or the editor(s). MDPI and/or the editor(s) disclaim responsibility for any injury to people or property resulting from any ideas, methods, instructions or products referred to in the content.

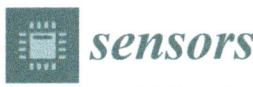

Article

Halfway to Automated Feeding of Chinese Hamster Ovary Cells

Simon Tomažič *,† and Igor Škrjanc †

Faculty of Electrical Engineering, University of Ljubljana, 1000 Ljubljana, Slovenia; igor.skrjanc@fe.uni-lj.si
* Correspondence: simon.tomazic@fe.uni-lj.si; Tel.: +386-1-4768-760
† These authors contributed equally to this work.

Abstract: This paper presents a comprehensive study on the development of models and soft sensors required for the implementation of the automated bioreactor feeding of Chinese hamster ovary (CHO) cells using Raman spectroscopy and chemometric methods. This study integrates various methods, such as partial least squares regression and variable importance in projection and competitive adaptive reweighted sampling, and highlights their effectiveness in overcoming challenges such as high dimensionality, multicollinearity and outlier detection in Raman spectra. This paper emphasizes the importance of data preprocessing and the relationship between independent and dependent variables in model construction. It also describes the development of a simulation environment whose core is a model of CHO cell kinetics. The latter allows the development of advanced control algorithms for nutrient dosing and the observation of the effects of different parameters on the growth and productivity of CHO cells. All developed models were validated and demonstrated to have a high robustness and predictive accuracy, which were reflected in a 40% reduction in the root mean square error compared to established methods. The results of this study provide valuable insights into the practical application of these methods in the field of monitoring and automated cell feeding and make an important contribution to the further development of process analytical technology in the bioprocess industry.

Keywords: spectroscopy; Raman; modelling; soft sensor; variable selection; outliers; simulator; kinetic model

---

Citation: Tomažič, S.; Škrjanc, I. Halfway to Automated Feeding of Chinese Hamster Ovary Cells. *Sensors* **2023**, *23*, 6618. https://doi.org/10.3390/s23146618

Academic Editor: Yuan Yao

Received: 26 June 2023
Revised: 14 July 2023
Accepted: 21 July 2023
Published: 23 July 2023

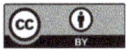

Copyright: © 2023 by the authors. Licensee MDPI, Basel, Switzerland. This article is an open access article distributed under the terms and conditions of the Creative Commons Attribution (CC BY) license (https://creativecommons.org/licenses/by/4.0/).

1. Introduction

Chemometrics, which deals with the application of various mathematical and statistical methods, could be described by a broad definition in which the most important part is the application of a multivariate data analysis to data relevant to chemistry [1]. The multivariate statistical data analysis is a powerful tool for analysing and structuring data sets obtained from different measurement systems and for building empirical mathematical models that can predict, for example, the values of important properties that cannot be measured directly [2,3]. Multivariate calibration is often used in the industry for the rapid online determination of important process parameters and critical quality characteristics and enables non-destructive measurements, online monitoring and process control.

In analytical chemistry, molecular spectroscopic methods, including infrared, near-infrared and Raman spectroscopy, are widely used to determine the molecular structure of various substances [4–6]. These methods work by assessing the radiant energy that is either absorbed or scattered when excited by a high intensity monochromatic beam that induces a transient energy state in the molecule. The process of Raman scattering occurs when the material under investigation is exposed to monochromatic light, causing a tiny percentage of the light to be inelastically scattered at wavelengths other than the incident light.

Raman spectroscopy is an optical method that enables the non-destructive investigation of molecular structures and chemical compositions. However, due to its low intensity, the study of Raman scattering requires the use of sophisticated instruments [7]. The data obtained from spectroscopy contain thousands of wavenumbers (variables) and measurements (observations), which requires multivariate analysis to determine the relationship between these variables [8,9]. Modern Raman instruments usually use a laser as the illumination source because of its high-intensity monochromatic properties. The wavelength of this laser can range from the UV ($\lambda = 200$ nm) to the near-infrared ($\lambda = 1064$ nm), but for pharmaceutical or biological applications, near-infrared wavelengths ($\lambda = 785$ or $\lambda = 830$ nm) are usually preferred to minimise fluorescence interference.

In bioprocess literature, spectroscopic sensors are sometimes referred to as soft sensors [10] because the spectroscopic data are modelled in software programmes that provide information analogous to that of hardware sensors. It is critical that data analysis models are used to extract the optimal amount of information from Raman spectra, an area that has received much attention in research [11]. The complexity and difficulties associated with interpreting results from Raman and IR spectroscopy can be mitigated by applying various data mining methods required for a more comprehensive understanding. These methods must be able to manage large multidimensional data sets while exploring the totality of spectral information [12].

Chemometric techniques, including the commonly used Partial Least Squares (PLS) [13,14] method, exploit the transformation capabilities of the principal component analysis (PCA). In this technique, the attributes of a data set are transformed into uncorrelated principal components, which allows a reduction in data dimensions with minimal loss of information. PCA-based techniques complemented by machine learning methods such as decision trees [15], Support Vector Machine (SVM) [16] and artificial neural networks (ANN) [17,18] allow for an even finer analysis. Additional preprocessing steps can be implemented, including normalisation and smoothing via k-th order Savitzky–Golay derivative [19], while model accuracy can be assessed by the standard error of calibration, factors used and coefficient of determination (R^2).

The inherent complexity of spectral data derived from vibrational spectroscopic techniques, including IR, NIR and Raman, has sparked debates on the topic of variable selection in PLS regression models [20,21]. This complexity arises from the interference caused by the scattering of diffuse light, instrumental noise and overlapping absorption bands. Given this complexity, variable selection strategies focus either on single wavelengths (e.g., variable importance in projection [22]) or on informative spectral intervals (such as interval PLS [23]). These methods help to eliminate superfluous information, a concept introduced by Spiegelman et al. [24]. More recently, the technique of the Competitive Adaptive Reweighted Sampling (CARS) has proven its effectiveness in processing NIR and RAMAN spectra [25,26].

Certain Raman spectra obtained from the same sample may differ from the group due to factors such as instrumental artefacts and variations in the sample. These spectra are often referred to as unwanted spectra or outliers. Omitting these spectra is considered crucial before applying multivariate techniques to obtain the desired results.

Raman spectroscopy, known for its precise spectral features that correlate with the molecular structure of a sample, has demonstrated its strengths in a non-destructive analysis and its ability to work with aqueous systems. These properties make it particularly suitable for the study of cell cultures and tissues [27]. It is widely used for the study of polysaccharides, amino acids, alcohols and metabolites and has secured its position as an important process analytical technology (PAT) in the bioprocess industry [18,28,29]. The ability of inline Raman spectroscopy to monitor and adjust critical parameters in real time ensures consistent drug production.

Although mammalian cell cultures are widely used in the pharmaceutical industry to produce biological products such as antibodies and growth factors, the full potential of advances in process monitoring and control has not yet been realised [10,27]. Conventional methods, often based on offline sampling and manual calculations, are still widely used. In particular, mammalian cells are mainly used for the production of protein therapeutics, which account for 60–70% of biopharmaceuticals. These processes usually involve the delivery of glucose to CHO cells [30–33].

By using non-invasive real-time measurements PAT in conjunction with closed-loop feedback control, feeding strategies can be optimised to improve yield [29,34,35]. Raman spectroscopy plays an important role in this, as it enables in-situ measurements and process control in real time. In situ Raman measurements, first presented by [36], allow the simultaneous measurement of total cell density (TCD), viable cell density (VCD) and concentrations of glucose, glutamate, lactate and ammonia. This method has proven successful in monitoring mammalian cell cultures in bioreactors. Several successful examples can be found in recent literature [18,34,36]. Subsequent studies have extended this application from developmental scales of 3 to 15 L [27,34] to clinical production scales of 2000 L [37], demonstrating the scaling potential of this approach.

This manuscript represents a significant advance in the field of bioprocess technology by providing a comprehensive PLS model construction procedure for Raman spectroscopy that incorporates data preprocessing and outlier removal, thereby improving the understanding and control of bioprocess behaviour. In addition, the development of a simulator that incorporates CHO cell kinetics is an important contribution to the field. It paves the way for the development of a model predictive control system for the automated feeding of CHO cells, revolutionising the way we approach the automation and control of bioprocesses.

The paper is organized as follows. Sections 2 and 2.1 describe the process of data acquisition and introduce the process of spectra processing, which is the initial step of data analysis. Section 2.2 explains the development of the PLS models for soft sensor design and different methods for variable selection in spectroscopic multivariate calibration. This subsection also discusses the process of identifying and removing outlier spectra to improve the robustness and accuracy of the PLS model. Section 3 discusses the CHO cell kinetics model required to develop an advanced simulation environment. Section 4 presents the results of the model construction and simulator implementation. Sections 5 and 6 provide the discussion and concluding remarks.

2. Materials and Methods

2.1. Spectra Processing

The extensive research began with the systematic compilation of measurements and data obtained from the cultivation of CHO cells in a stainless steel bioreactor. The local pharmaceutical company, which was in charge of designing the experiment, played an important role. Our task, on the other hand, was to analyse the collected data, create the necessary models and establish a suitable simulation environment, which is described in this paper.

The cultivation of the CHO cells took place in a bioreactor with a volume of 10 L. To collect measurements (Raman spectra), the probe of a Kaiser RamanRXN2 spectrometer was inserted into the bioreactor. The RamanRXN2 spectrometer is a sophisticated analytical device that uses laser light with a wavelength of 532 nm. The resulting Raman spectrum is collected over a period of at least 30 min, a measure that improves the signal-to-noise ratio. It is important to note that Raman scattering, which is essentially inelastic photon scattering, is a rather small fraction compared to its elastic counterpart.

For data storage, a desktop computer with a Windows operating system was used, which was directly connected to the Raman spectrometer. Four different experiments were performed to grow the cells in the bioreactor, with each batch lasting about two weeks. The bioreactor contained CHO-S cell lines. This cell line is a sub-line of the original CHO-K1, with adaptations for suspension culture. CHO-S cells are commonly used in the industrial production of therapeutic proteins.

To maintain the optimal environment of the bioreactor, the pH and temperature were strictly controlled and nutrient dosing (glucose and glutamine) was conducted manually on a daily basis using reference measurements. A Roche Cedex Bio Analyzer, known for its reliability and precision, was used to record these reference measurements daily. This allowed for the accurate monitoring of parameters such as glucose and glutamine concentration, viable cell count and others.

The development of useful models depends on appropriate methods, but even more important is the selection of appropriate data. In our case, the raw data consist of the Raman spectra shown in Figure 1. For a first experiment, the choice between regression methods such as principal component regression, partial least squares or an artificial neural network may not be so important [27]. However, it is important that the selected independent variables (x-data) have a strong relationship with the dependent variables (y-data) to be modelled [38]. The choice of method then depends on the type and amount of data available.

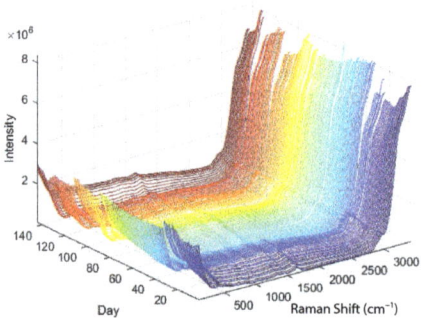

Figure 1. Spectra obtained with Raman spectroscopy (from four different batches where only spectra, which are used for training and validation, are shown).

In cases where the x-data for objects represent time series or digitised data from a continuous spectrum (e.g., Raman spectra, see Figure 1), possible pre-processing strategies could include smoothing or a transition to a first or second derivative. Smoothing attempts to reduce random noise by eliminating sharp peaks in the spectrum, while differencing brings relevant data to light despite noise amplification. The first derivative achieves alignment of spectra with different absorbance values that are shifted in parallel by cancelling out an additive baseline. A second derivative removes a constant and linear baseline. Each object vector, referred to as x_i, undergoes separate processes of smoothing and differentiation.

For both differentiation and smoothing, the Savitzky–Golay method is used. This is a method widely used in chemistry. This technique, a local polynomial regression using the method of least linear squares, requires x-values that are both exact and uniformly distributed. For each point, symbolised as j with value x_j, a linear combination is used to calculate the weighted sum of the neighbouring values. These weights determine whether smoothing or a derivative calculation is performed. Factors such as the number of neighbours and the polynomial order determine the strength of the smoothing. Choosing the right polynomial order is crucial, as incorrectly chosen higher order polynomials could misinterpret significant Raman bands as mere background. In the Savitzky–Golay method, a vector component x_j is transformed by

$$x_j^* = \frac{1}{N} \sum_{h=-k}^{k} c_h x_{j+h}, \qquad (1)$$

where x_j^* is the new value (of a smoothed curve or a derivative), N is the normalisation constant, k is the number of neighbouring values (determining the size of the moving window) on each side of j and c_h are the coefficients, which depend on the degree of the polynomial used and the objective (smoothing, first or second derivative). For example, if a second order polynomial is fitted through a window of five points ($k = 2$), the following coefficients c_{-2}, c_{-1}, c_0, c_1, c_2 can be used for smoothing: $-3, 12, 17, 12, -3$, the first derivative: $-2, -1, 0, 1, 2$, and the second derivative: $2, -1, -2, -1, 2$ [19]. Figure 2 shows the Raman spectra to which the Savitzky–Golay filtering was applied.

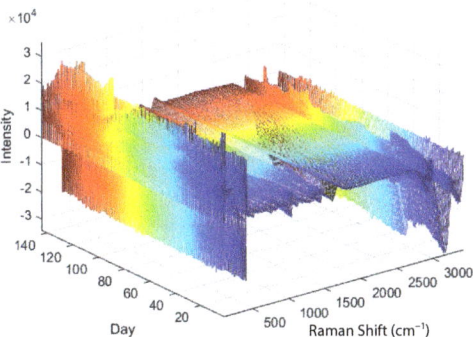

Figure 2. Raman spectra to which Savitzky–Golay filtering has been applied.

The process of pre-processing includes both filtering and normalisation, with the latter playing an important role. The reason for this is that even spectra recorded for the same material may demonstrate differences due to different recording times or unequal instrument conditions such as laser power and alignment. These variations can lead to different intensity values for spectra of the same material.

To compensate for these intensity differences, normalisation comes into play. This process ensures a maximum similarity of the intensity of a given Raman band of a given material when the spectra were taken under the same experimental parameters; however, some conditions are slightly different. Various normalisation methods are explored in the literature, including min-max normalisation, vector normalisation and Standard Normal Variate (SNV) normalisation. Of these methods, SNV normalisation is the most commonly used [39,40]. SNV normalisation works on the basis of the Equation (2), which can be outlined as follows:

$$\hat{x}_j^* = \frac{x_j^* - \bar{x}^*}{\sigma} \text{ where } \sigma = \sqrt{\frac{1}{N}\sum_{j=1}^{N}(x_j^* - \bar{x}^*)^2} \text{ and } j = 1, 2, ..., N. \qquad (2)$$

Figure 3 shows the Raman spectra for which SNV normalisation was performed in addition to Savitzky–Golay filtering.

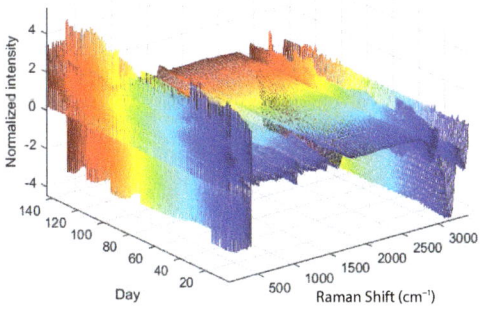

Figure 3. Raman spectra to which Savitzky–Golay filtering and SNV normalization are applied.

2.2. Model Construction

The construction of predictive models for bioprocesses, particularly for the cultivation of CHO cells in bioreactors, has made significant progress through the application of chemometric methods to Raman spectroscopic data [38]. These models can predict several key variables such as the concentrations of glucose, glutamine, lactate and other biochemical parameters, as well as cell growth metrics such as total cell count (TCC) and viable cell count (VCC). Raman spectroscopy, a non-invasive, label-free technique, provides detailed chemical information about the bioprocess by recording the molecular vibrations of the components. The resulting Raman spectra serve as input data for the prediction model and provide a comprehensive, high-dimensional data set.

Model construction begins with a calibration phase in which known samples are analysed using Raman spectroscopy and appropriate laboratory tests. This process generates a set of reference data that includes Raman spectra and associated concentrations of glucose, glutamine, lactate and cell counts. Another way to collect reference measurements is to use a device such as Roche's Cedex Analyzer. Once the reference data are prepared, multivariate analysis techniques such as Partial Least Squares Regression (PLSR) are used to build the predictive model. These methods work by identifying correlation patterns within the Raman spectra and relating them to the biochemical parameters of interest.

For more complex data sets or non-linear relationships, machine learning techniques such as Random Forest or SVM can be used. Advanced deep learning techniques such as Convolutional Neural Networks (CNN) are particularly effective for processing high-dimensional spectral data, as they can automatically extract meaningful features and improve prediction accuracy [18]. However, one must be aware that such a method of creating a model requires a large database, which is not always available.

This approach not only improves our understanding of the bioprocess, but also our control over it. The real-time predictive capability of the model leads to optimised and consistent bioproduction outcomes by enabling rapid, data-driven decision-making and process adjustments, thereby increasing bioprocess performance, reducing costs and improving product quality. The model is continuously refined as more data become available, improving its predictive power over time.

2.2.1. Partial Least Squares

Partial Least Squares (PLS) is a statistical method that finds a linear regression model by projecting the predicted variables and the observable variables onto a new space. The method was first developed by Swedish statistician Herman Wold and has since been widely used in fields such as chemometrics, neuroimaging, bioinformatics and social sciences [41,42].

PLS simultaneously accounts for the covariance of both the independent variables (predictors) and the dependent variables (responses). This approach is advantageous when dealing with complex, multivariate data sets where the predictors are highly collinear or where there are more predictors than observations. The method can handle noisy and missing data, which makes it robust and flexible.

Partial Least Squares (PLS) regression is a multivariate technique that combines features of principal component analysis (PCA) and multiple linear regression. Although PCA is not explicitly used in the PLS method, the concept of extracting principal components or latent variables is central to both methods. In PCA, the goal is to find a small number of uncorrelated variables, called principal components, that explain most of the variation in the data. Each principal component is a linear combination of the original variables and is orthogonal to all other components. PLS works in a similar way, but instead of trying to explain as much of the variance in the predictor variables as possible, PLS tries to extract components that explain as much of the covariance between the predictor and response variables as possible. Essentially, PLS looks for directions in which the predictors not only explain a large part of their own variance (as in PCA), but are also highly correlated with the response. PLS regression can be summarised in the following steps:

- Standardisation of data: The first step in PLS regression is to standardise the predictor and response matrices. This ensures that the model is not overly influenced by variables that have large values or a large range of values.
- Extraction of PLS components: PLS decomposes the predictor and response matrices into a set of orthogonal components. These are linear combinations of the original variables that explain the maximum covariance between the predictors and the responses. The number of PLS components is chosen to optimise the predictive power of the model.
- Estimation of the PLS model: The PLS regression coefficients are estimated by relating the PLS components to the responses. These coefficients show the relationship between the changes in the predictor variables and the changes in the response variables.
- Prediction and validation: The PLS model can then be used to predict responses for new data. Cross-validation is often used to assess the predictive performance of the model and to determine the optimal number of PLS components.

In terms of its statistical properties, PLS is a form of regularised regression. Like other forms of regularisation, it can prevent overfitting by introducing some bias into the model, but it reduces the variance of the model and thus improves its predictive performance.

PLS has been extended to handle different types of data and different modelling scenarios. The most popular versions of PLS include PLS-DA (PLS Discriminant Analysis) [43] for classification problems and PLS-PM (PLS Path Modelling) [44] for structural equation modelling. These extensions have made PLS a versatile and powerful tool for multivariate analysis. When considering the use of PLS, it is important to understand its assumptions and limitations. Although PLS does not assume that predictors are independent or normally distributed, it does assume a linear relationship between predictors and responses. In addition, PLS may not work well with unrelated predictors because it attempts to use all predictors in the model, which can lead to overfitting. It is recommended to evaluate the performance of PLS against other multivariate methods such as principal component regression (PCR) or ridge regression to ensure that it is appropriate for a particular data set and research question.

The Nonlinear Iterative Partial Least Squares (NIPALS) algorithm is a common method for calculating PLS components. The goal is to find a set of components (also called latent vectors) that capture the covariance between the predictors and the responses. The algorithm of the simplified NIPALS method can be summarised in the following five points:

- Initialization:

$$\mathbf{X} \in \mathbb{R}^{n \times m}, \mathbf{Y} \in \mathbb{R}^{n \times p}, \qquad (3)$$

where X is a predictor matrix and Y is a response matrix.
- Selection of an initial column vector. Typically, the first column of the Y matrix represents the vector u:

$$\mathbf{u} = \mathbf{Y}[:, 1] \qquad (4)$$

- Iteratively compute the weights w and t until convergence:

$$\mathbf{w} = \frac{\mathbf{X}^T \mathbf{u}}{\mathbf{u}^T \mathbf{u}} \qquad (5)$$

Normalize the weights:

$$\mathbf{w} = \frac{\mathbf{w}}{\|\mathbf{w}\|} \qquad (6)$$

Compute the score vector:

$$\mathbf{t} = \mathbf{X}\mathbf{w} \qquad (7)$$

Reassign u as:

$$u = Y^T t / t^T t \qquad (8)$$

The iteration continues until the difference between the new and old score vectors falls below a certain threshold, indicating convergence.
- Deflate X and Y:
Calculate the outer product of t and p (the loading vector for the X), then subtract it from X. Do the same for Y with t and q (the loading vector for the Y):

$$p = \frac{X^T t}{t^T t}, \quad q = \frac{Y^T t}{t^T t} \qquad (9)$$

$$X = X - t p^T, \quad Y = Y - t q^T \qquad (10)$$

The iterations end when X (or Y) can no longer be deflated or when the number of extracted latent variables is enough to describe the data according to some criterion.
- Calculate the regression coefficients. Once all the latent vectors are extracted, the regression coefficients B can be calculated as:

$$B = W(P^T W)^{-1} Q^T, \qquad (11)$$

where W is the matrix of weight vectors, P is the loading matrix of X.

The Root Mean Square Error of Cross-Validation (RMSECV), which is calculated during the creation of the PLS model, can be used as a criterion to find the right number of latent variables and prevent overfitting. For example, Figure 4 shows that in the case of a PLS model for glucose concentration, the most appropriate number of latent variables is four, as the RMSECV does not drop drastically after that.

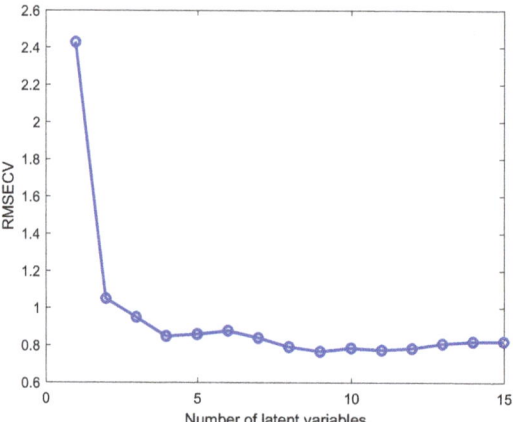

Figure 4. Finding the most appropriate number of latent variables in a PLS model.

2.2.2. Selection of Key Variables

To further improve the PLS models and reduce the possibility of overfitting, the Variable Importance in Projection (VIP) and Competitive Adaptive Reweighted Sampling—Partial Least Squares (CARS-PLS) methods were used.

Variable Importance in the Projection is a popular method for assessing the importance of variables in a Partial Least Squares (PLS) regression model. PLS is a statistical approach used in predictive modelling where the prediction of a set of dependent variables from a set of independent variables is conducted through latent variable regression.

The VIP score for a variable is a measure of that variable's contribution to the model, taking into account both its contribution to explaining the dependent variable and its contribution to explaining the independent variable. A high VIP score indicates that the variable is highly significant in the model (Figure 5 shows an example of selecting key variables in a PLS model of glucose concentration). However, the VIP method also has some disadvantages:

- Overemphasis on highly collinear variables: If variables are highly collinear, the VIP score can overestimate the importance of those variables and result in a model that may not be as accurate as possible. This can be problematic in areas where variables may be highly correlated, such as genomics or metabolomics.
- Unreliable with small data sets: The VIP method can be unreliable with small data sets because it depends on having enough data to estimate the PLS model accurately.

On the other hand, Competitive Adaptive Reweighted Sampling—Partial Least Squares is a more recent technique used for variable selection in spectroscopic multivariate calibration. It has gained considerable attention in the field of chemometrics. CARS-PLS was developed to overcome two major challenges in the analysis of spectroscopic data: high dimensionality and multicollinearity. These problems can lead to overfitting of the model, poor generalisation ability and difficulties in interpretation. The method CARS-PLS consists of two main stages:

- Competitive Adaptive Reweighted Sampling: This is a Monte Carlo-based sampling technique that helps identify relevant variables (wavelengths) for building the model. Initially, CARS assigns equal weights to all variables. Then, a set of subsets of variables is generated, each subset containing each variable with a probability proportional to its weight. A PLS model is created for each subset and its performance is evaluated. Based on the evaluation, the weights of the variables are updated—variables that frequently contribute to good models are given higher weights, while those that contribute to poor models are given lower weights. This process is repeated many times (usually thousands of iterations) until the best subset of variables is found.
- Partial Least Squares (PLS): After identifying the best subset of variables with CARS, a PLS model is built using only these selected variables (Figure 5). This model is simpler and less prone to overfitting than a model built with all variables. Moreover, because only relevant variables are included, the model is often easier to interpret.

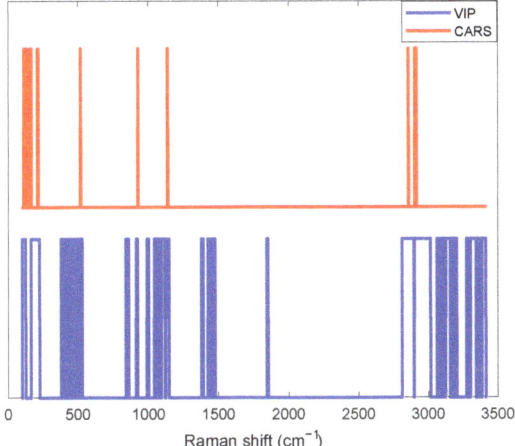

Figure 5. Key variables determined with the methods VIP and CARS for the PLS model of glucose concentration.

The CARS-PLS method has been used successfully in many areas where spectroscopic data are used, such as pharmaceutical analysis, food quality control and environmental monitoring. However, like all methods, it has its limitations and assumptions. It assumes that there is a linear relationship between predictors and responses, and it may not work well if this assumption is not met. In addition, the performance of CARS-PLS may depend on the initial weights of the variables and the number of Monte Carlo iterations. Therefore, it is often advisable to make several runs of CARS-PLS with different initial settings and determine the consensus of the results.

Compared to VIP, CARS offers the following advantages:

- Better handling of collinearity: In contrast to the method VIP, CARS can better handle the problem of collinearity between variables.
- Simplicity and interpretability: CARS tends to lead to simpler and more interpretable models, which is of great importance in practical applications.
- Better performance on small data sets: CARS is not as reliant on large data sets as VIP and is therefore a more reliable method for variable selection on small data sets.
- More robustness: CARS is less prone to overfitting because it focuses on a subset of particularly relevant variables instead of considering all variables in the model.
- Adaptive: CARS is an adaptive method, able to adjust its selection as more data becomes available or the nature of the data changes.

2.2.3. Removal of Outlier Spectra

The PLS model can be further improved by searching for spectra representing outliers. Therefore, a resampling method commonly used in statistics and machine learning was used, which can also be referred to as Monte Carlo cross-validation or repeated random sub-sampling validation. The outlier detection method consists of the following five steps:

- Partitioning: first, the original training dataset is randomly partitioned into a training dataset and a test dataset. For example, the partitioning could be 4:1, i.e., 80% of the data are used for training and 20% for testing. This partitioning is conducted many times, which is characteristic of a Monte Carlo approach.
- PLS modelling and prediction: A Partial Least Squares (PLS) regression model is built using the training data. This model is then used to make predictions for the test subset.
- Error calculation: The prediction errors for each spectrum in the test set are then calculated. Each spectrum will occur multiple times in different test sets; thus, an average error and standard deviation can be calculated for each spectrum across all iterations.
- Identification of outliers: Spectra that consistently produce high prediction errors (based on their average error or a combination of average error and standard deviation) can be considered outliers. These outliers represent spectra that are not well modelled by the PLS and thus affect the accuracy of the model. In Figure 6, for example, it can quickly be observed that the 25th and 58th spectra are outliers.
- Removal of outliers: The identified outlier spectra are removed from the original dataset, hopefully improving the robustness and accuracy of the model.
- Iterating: This entire process can be repeated as needed, each time recalculating the errors for each spectrum and identifying and removing outliers.

The advantage of this method is that it can help to increase the robustness of the PLS models by removing outliers that would otherwise distort the model parameters. It is a relatively simple and intuitive approach that combines the robustness of resampling with the ability to identify and remove problematic data points. This method helps to further reduce the Root Mean Square Error of Prediction (RMSEP) and thus improve the overall performance of the model.

However, as with any method, it should be used judiciously. Removing outliers too aggressively can lead to over-fitting, where the model becomes over-fitted to the "typical" data points and performs poorly on new, unknown data. This method is most useful if you have a large enough dataset so that removing some data points does not significantly reduce the overall size of the dataset.

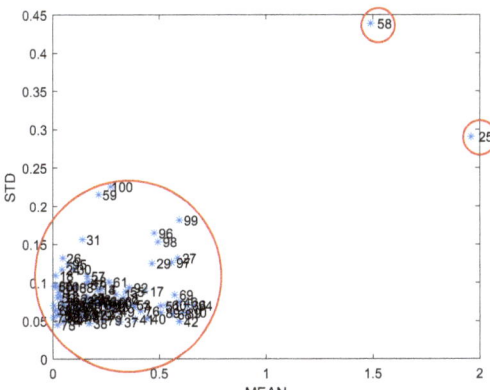

Figure 6. The mean error and standard deviation for all spectra.

3. Simulator Construction

In order to develop a predictive control algorithm for automated nutrient feeding in a bioreactor, a simulation environment based on a dynamic model was implemented. The latter describes the kinetics of the growth of a CHO cell culture in a fed-batch bioreactor. It is well known that the process parameters (temperature, pH, feeding, ammonia removal, etc.) have a significant impact on cell growth and especially on the quality of the monoclonal antibodies (mAbs) produced [45]. Therefore, the model is important not only for the development of management algorithms, but also for the observation and identification of the key factors (variables and parameters) that have the greatest influence on cell productivity. This is particularly important from the point of view of optimising protein production in a mammalian cell line.

3.1. Modelling CHO Cell Culture Kinetics

Chinese Hamster Ovary cells are the most commonly used mammalian hosts for the industrial production of therapeutic proteins, due to their capacity to perform human-like post-translational modifications. The growth kinetics of CHO cells can be studied using a mechanistic model [32]. A mechanistic model is a type of model used to describe biological processes based on underlying physiological mechanisms. These models allow us to interpret, predict and simulate biological phenomena by using mathematical equations to represent the interactions and transformations that occur in a system. In the context of CHO cell growth kinetics, a mechanistic model would include at least the following components. One of the most important mechanisms determining the growth kinetics of CHO cells is cell division. The rate at which cells grow and divide depends on various influencing factors such as the availability of nutrients, the accumulation of waste products and the passage of time. Mathematical models such as the Gompertz model or the logistic growth model are often used to represent these complicated dynamics of cell growth. Another crucial determinant of cell growth is the assimilation and utilisation of nutrients such as glucose and glutamine. The rate at which these nutrients are consumed can have a significant impact on cell growth and is usually modelled using Monod or Michaelis–Menten kinetics, which provides essential insights into cell metabolism and growth patterns. As cells grow and metabolise nutrients, they inevitably generate waste products such as lactate or ammonia. The accumulation of these waste products can have a suppressive effect on cell growth. To quantify this inhibitory effect, mathematical models are used to provide detailed insight into the relationship between the accumulation of waste products and cell proliferation. The loss of cells through mechanisms such as apoptosis, nutrient deprivation or the toxic effect of accumulated by-products is an inevitable aspect of cell culture. Mathematical models are used to express the rate of cell death as a function of various parameters, providing valuable insights into the factors that influence cell viability over time. Finally, the growth kinetics of CHO cells are significantly influenced by external environmental factors such as temperature, pH and osmolality. These factors must be carefully incorporated into the mechanistic model to ensure its relevance and accuracy. These environmental influences represent an additional layer of complexity and require a comprehensive understanding of their effects on cell growth and survival. Each of these components is interconnected and forms a complex network of interactions that determine the growth kinetics of CHO cells. Together, they form a robust mechanistic model that allows the prediction, interpretation and simulation of the behaviour of CHO cells under different conditions. A mechanistic model of CHO cell growth kinetics would typically be a system of differential equations, where each equation represents a particular biological process (such as cell growth, nutrient consumption, production of waste products, etc.). These models can be quite complex and usually require a large amount of experimental data for their parameterisation.

However, despite their complexity, mechanistic models can provide valuable insights into the cell growth process and can be helpful in optimising cell culture conditions for maximum productivity. Many authors [45–48] who have worked on modelling the kinetics of CHO cell cultures have set up various dynamic models in the form of differential equations based on steady-state analysis. In most cases, these simple models only describe the variation of extracellular metabolite concentrations and the number of live/dead cells during the cell cycle. The models differ in the number of factors considered (number of variables and parameters), which are more or less relevant to describe what actually happens in a mammalian cell line (in a bioreactor). However, in order to have a practical and universally applicable simulator, a model was needed that took all the important variables into account. An example of such a model was also developed by M. Ivarsson [48] in her PhD thesis, as it takes into account the four phases of the cell cycle, temperature, glutamine concentration, number of dead cells, etc., in addition to the number of living cells and the concentrations of glucose, lactate and ammonia. For the development of a predictive controller for automated feeding, only a model prediction of glucose concentration would be required at this stage. However, as glucose concentration variations are also highly dependent on other variables, these should also be considered in the model. As mentioned above, the chosen dynamic model [48] describes four phases of the cell cycle: G_0, G_1, S and G_2/M and the number of cells per phase: X_{G0}, X_{G1}, X_S and $X_{G2/M}$:

G_1 phase:

$$\frac{d(X_{G1}V)}{dt} = 2k_{G2/M-G1}X_{G2/M}V - k_{G1-S}X_{G1}V - k_{G1-G0}X_{G1}V - k_d X_{G1}V - F_{OUT}X_{G1} \quad (12)$$

S phase:

$$\frac{d(X_S V)}{dt} = k_{G1-S}m_{stress}X_{G1}V - k_{S-G2/M}X_S V - k_d X_S V - F_{OUT}X_S \quad (13)$$

G_2/M phase:

$$\frac{d(X_{G2/M}V)}{dt} = k_{S-G2/M}X_S V - k_{G2/M-G1}X_{G2/M}V - k_d X_{G2/M}V - F_{OUT}X_{G2/M} \quad (14)$$

G_0 phase:

$$\frac{d(X_{G0}V)}{dt} = k_{G1-S}(1 - m_{stress})X_{G1}V + k_{G1-G0}X_{G1}V - k_d X_{G0}V - F_{OUT}X_{G0} \quad (15)$$

The equations include transition factors k, where, e.g., k_{G1-S} represents the transition from the G_1 phase to the S phase. The transition factors between subpopulations depend mainly on the growth rate, which in turn is determined by the times (t_{G1}, t_S and $t_{G2/M}$) required for the completion of each cellular phase:

$$\mu = \frac{\ln(2)}{t_{G1} + t_S + t_{G2/M}} \quad (16)$$

The transition from the G_1 to the G_0 phase is determined by the transition factor k_{G1-G0}, which represents the temperature stress. However, the transition to phase G_0 may also cause metabolic stress m_{stress}. The number of viable cells is calculated as the sum of the cells from each phase, where V represents the current volume of material in the bioreactor:

$$\frac{d(X_V V)}{dt} = \frac{d(X_{G0} V)}{dt} + \frac{d(X_{G1} V)}{dt} + \frac{d(X_S V)}{dt} + \frac{d(X_{G2/M} V)}{dt} \tag{17}$$

The volume varies depending on the nutrient dosage (F_{Glc} and F_{Gln}) and the potential sampling F_{OUT}:

$$\frac{dV}{dt} = F_{Glc} + F_{Gln} - F_{OUT} \tag{18}$$

Glutamine concentration varies according to consumption factor Q_{Gln} and degradation to ammonia K_{deg} and potential dose F_{Gln}. Glutamine consumption depends on the cell growth factor, the specific yield Y_{Gln} and the limiting function f_{upt}:

$$\frac{d(GlnV)}{dt} = -Q_{Gln} X_V V - K_{deg} GlnV + F_{Gln} Gln_{Feed} - F_{OUT} Gln \tag{19}$$

The ammonia concentration depends largely on changes in the glutamine concentration, since the ammonia concentration increases with glutamine consumption (factors Y_{Amn} and K_{deg}):

$$\frac{d(A_{mn} V)}{dt} = Q_{Gln} Y_{Amn} X_V V + K_{deg} GlnV - F_{OUT} Amn \tag{20}$$

The glucose concentration varies according to the consumption factor Q_{Glc} and the minimum consumption to keep the cells alive m_{Glc}, and the amount of glucose added F_{Glc}. The consumption factor Q_{Glc} is influenced by temperature and lactate as an inhibitor:

$$\frac{d(GlcV)}{dt} = -Q_{Glc} X_V (1 - f_{G0}) V - m_{Glc} X_V f_{G0} V + F_{Glc} Glc_{Feed} - F_{OUT} Glc \tag{21}$$

The lactate concentration depends on the glucose consumption (Q_{Glc} and m_{Glc}):

$$\frac{d(LacV)}{dt} = Y_{Lac} Q_{Glc} X_V (1 - f_{G0}) V - Y_{Lac} m_{Glc} X_V f_{G0} V - F_{OUT} Lac \tag{22}$$

The change in monoclonal antibody concentration is determined by factors representing the productivity level ($q_{G1/G0}$, q_S and $q_{G2/M}$) per cell phase:

$$\frac{d(mAbV)}{dt} = \mu [q_{\frac{G1}{G0}} (X_{G1} + X_{G0}) + q_S X_S + q_{\frac{G2}{M}} X_{\frac{G2}{M}}] - F_{OUT} mAb \tag{23}$$

4. Results

In order to be able to monitor the process in the bioreactor in detail during the entire batch, which usually takes about 14 days, seven PLS models were developed in the Matlab environment. The latter models, which represent soft sensors, allow the monitoring of the most important process variables in CHO cell cultivation. These variables are: Glucose concentration, viable cell concentration (VCC), total cell count (TCC), glutamine, glutamate, lactate and ammonium.

Data from four different batches were available to us for the development of PLS models. Raman spectra were collected every half hour and reference measurements (offline) were performed once or twice a day with Cedex Analyzer. Thus, the first step was to find the pairs of spectra and reference measurements that matched best in terms of acquisition time. The Raman measurement takes about half an hour to obtain a good signal-to-noise ratio and to remove fluorescence interference.

As described in Section 2.1, two key initial steps in the development of PLS models are the preprocessing of the Raman spectra with the Savitzky–Golay filter and the normalisation with the Standard Normal Variate method (see Figures 2 and 3). Savitzky–Golay low-pass filtering was performed for all independent variables (Raman shift (cm^{-1})) of each spectrum, with a quadratic function chosen for smoothing with the Savitzky–Golay filter and the window length (smoothing) set to 15 samples. In addition, a normalisation or Standard Normal Variate function is applied to the independent variables for all spectra, resulting in spectra with a mean of zero and a standard deviation of one.

As described in Section 2.2 and illustrated in Figure 2, careful consideration is also required in the selection of the parameter that determines the number of latent variables. For each PLS model, the optimal number of latent variables is determined based on cross-validation, aiming for the smallest RMSECV error. In general, it is preferred to keep the number of latent variables as small as possible.

Characteristic independent variables of the spectrum (i.e., energy shifts) at which a spike occurs can be extracted from the literature for individual observed variables. Taking these characteristic energy shifts into account when calculating PLS models is therefore considered useful as it further weighs the individual independent variables of the spectrum and improves the model in this way. If these characteristic energy shifts are not known, various methods are available to identify the more important independent variables and take them into account to a greater extent.

The Variable Importance in the Projection method, described in Section 2.2.2, was tested first. However, the prediction results were not improved by this simple method; thus, alternative approaches to selecting key variables were investigated. Attempts to select "key" intervals or several independent variables of the spectrum together also did not lead to better results.

It turned out that the Competitive Adaptive Reweighted Sampling method, which is also discussed in Section 2.2.2, gave the best results for selecting key variables when building PLS models. As can be observed in Figure 5, the method CARS identifies fewer key variables than the method VIP. Nevertheless, the validation results of the PLS model (using glucose concentration as an example) were better when the method CARS was used, as evidenced by the smaller Root Mean Square Error (see Figure 7 and Table 1).

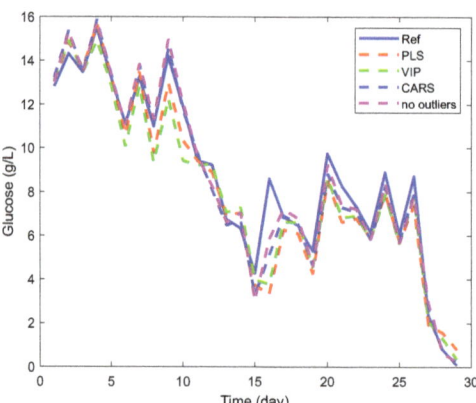

Figure 7. Validation of the PLS glucose model using VIP, CARS and outlier removal methods.

Table 1. Root Mean Square Error of glucose concentration prediction and the coefficient of determination (R^2).

	RMSE (g/L)	R^2
PLS	1.25	0.92
VIP	1.26	0.92
CARS	0.84	0.96
No outliers	0.75	0.97

The reference values in Figure 7 represent offline measurements performed with the Cedex Analyzer. In some cases of glucose measurement, the VIP method even leads to worse results than not using a method, as shown in Table 1 (see RMSE).

Assuming that Cedex's offline measurements are reliable, the training set was examined for spectra representing outliers that could affect the parameters of the PLS model during the learning phase and consequently affect the prediction accuracy. Applying the Monte Carlo sampling method and calculating the mean error and standard deviation for each PLS model led to the identification of spectra within the dataset that represent outliers, as shown in Figure 6 and discussed in Section 2.2.3. This process allowed a further increase in the accuracy and robustness of the PLS models, as can be observed in Figure 7 and Table 1. In this case, the coefficient of determination for the PLS model for glucose is $R^2 = 0.97$, which means that the PLS model has been further improved compared to the method CARS (where $R^2 = 0.96$). An accurate prediction of glucose concentration can also be observed in Figure 8, which shows a comparison of experimental and predicted values using CARS and methods to remove outliers. Ideally, all points should lie on a straight line.

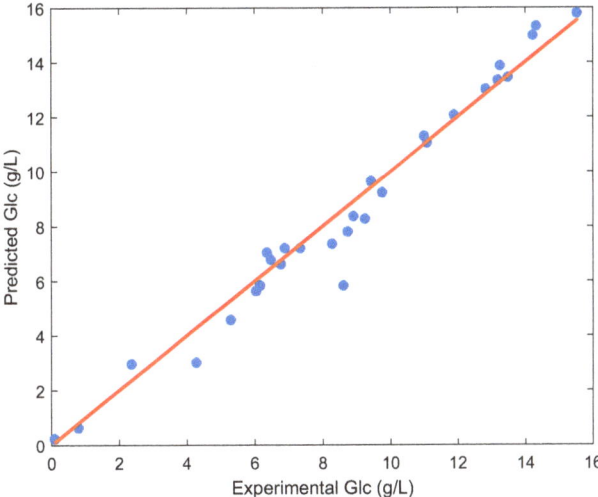

Figure 8. Validation of the PLS glucose model: comparison of experimental and predicted values using CARS and outlier removal methods.

Table 2 shows the RMSE and coefficient of determination (R^2) for the following constructed PLS models in addition to the glucose PLS model. VCC, TCC, glutamine, glutamate, lactate and ammonium. The results demonstrate that all PLS models developed provide an accurate prediction of the main process variables ($R^2 > 0.8$), and only the PLS model for glutamine has a slightly worse prediction ($R^2 = 0.33$). The reason for this lies in the following fact. In Raman spectroscopy, glutamine and glutamate are related because they have a similar molecular structure and similar active Raman vibrational modes that produce similar spectral features. Glutamine and glutamate are structurally similar amino acids, both containing a carboxyl group (-COOH) and an amine group (-NH2). The main structural difference between them is that glutamate has an additional carboxyl group, while glutamine has an amide group (-CONH2) instead. It is important to note that while Raman spectroscopy is a powerful technique for identifying molecules, its resolution is often insufficient to distinguish between similar molecules in a mixture. In such cases, additional techniques, such as chromatographic separation or more sophisticated spectral analysis methods, are required.

Table 2. Root Mean Square Error and the coefficient of determination (R^2) for all other constructed PLS models.

	RMSE	R^2
VCC	0.86 (10^6 cells/mL)	0.93
TCC	1.06 (10^6 cells/mL)	0.91
Glutamine	1.60 (g/L)	0.33
Glutamate	0.26 (g/L)	0.95
Lactate	0.10 (g/L)	0.99
Ammonium	1.16 (mmol/L)	0.83

Table 3 shows the best RMSE results for PLS models according to the existing literature [11,37]. A comparison with the data in Tables 1 and 2 shows that our method for building PLS models excels at accurately predicting key variables from Raman spectra. This comparison essentially underlines the effectiveness of our approach. It is particularly noteworthy that our PLS models have an RMSE that is on average three times smaller than the RMSE published in recent research [11,37].

Table 3. The best RMSE results for PLS models found in the literature [11,37].

	RMSE
VCC	4.87 (10^6 cells/mL)
TCC	3.68 (10^6 cells/mL)
Glucose	1.13 (g/L)
Glutamate	1.18 (g/L)
Lactate	0.19 (g/L)
Ammonium	1.21 (mmol/L)

The learning process for the PLS models depended on a single offline measurement (Cedex) of each variable (e.g., glucose) per day. Therefore, only the Raman spectroscopy spectra that matched the offline measurements in time could be used. However, once the PLS models were built, all spectra collected every half hour could be used, giving an informative representation of the time course of each variable (see Figure 9). These data are then used in the optimisation to determine the parameters of the dynamic model for the CHO cell kinetics, as described in the Section 3.1. Careful examination of the time series signal for glucose and glutamine concentrations in Figure 9 reveals a sawtooth pattern due to the daily manual dosing of nutrients. This pattern is not conducive to the optimal growth of the CHO cells.

The problem can be solved by implementing an automated feeding system that continuously doses the nutrients according to a predefined reference signal. However, such a system requires not only the application of the previously developed soft sensors (PLS models), but also a simulation environment. In this environment, a control algorithm can be developed and different scenarios such as different feeding regimes, the removal of inhibitors and the observation of important process variables can be investigated. The heart of the simulator, represented by the Simulink schema in Figure 10, is a dynamic model of CHO cell kinetics, which is explained in the Section 3.1. Figure 10 also shows the controller and optimisation blocks, the details of which will be explained in more detail in forthcoming scientific publications.

Based on known process parameters (temperature and pH) and time series signals of the main process variables (VCC, glucose, glutamine, etc.), it is possible to perform the optimisation of the parameters of the dynamic model of CHO cell kinetics (presented in the Section 3.1). This optimisation aims at aligning the model results as much as possible with the measurements of previous batches.

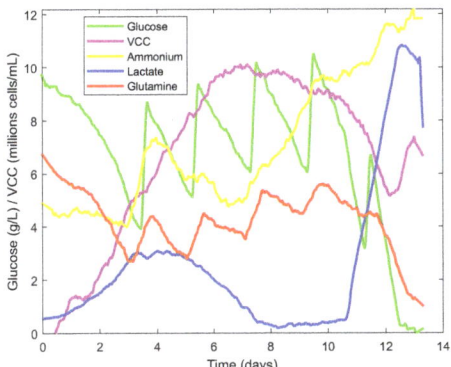

Figure 9. Signal reconstruction of key process variables via PLS models.

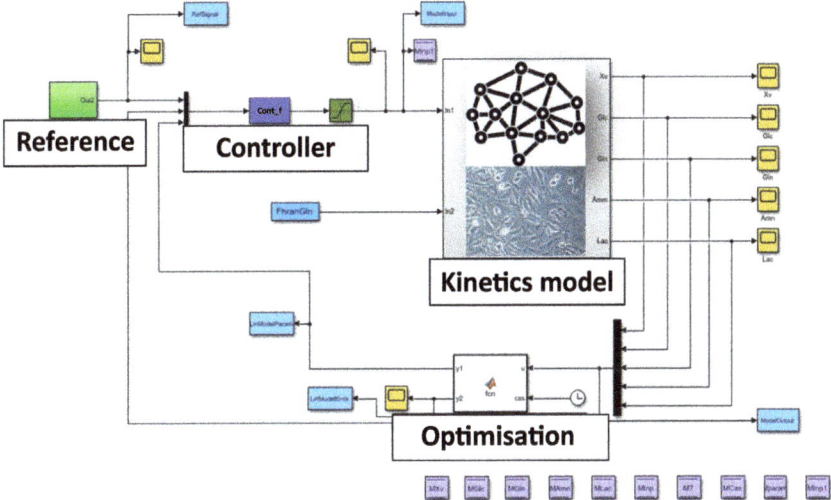

Figure 10. Implementation of a simulator within the Simulink environment based on the CHO cell kinetics model.

For the parameter optimisation, the particle swarm optimisation (PSO) method was used, which makes it possible to find the global minimum of the chosen criterion function while optimising a large number of parameters. In this case, the criterion function was given as RMSE, with the final values presented in the Table 4.

Table 4. Root Mean Square Error and the coefficient of determination (R^2) in the case of predicting all important process variables using the CHO cell kinetics model.

	RMSE	R^2
VCC	0.15 (10^6 cells/mL)	0.99
Glucose	0.18 (g/L)	0.99
Glutamine	0.20 (g/L)	0.98
Lactate	0.14 (g/L)	0.99
Ammonium	0.10 (mmol/L)	0.99

A comparison of glucose concentration measurements from one of the batches with a glucose concentration prediction derived from a mechanistic model of CHO cell kinetics is shown in Figure 11. The results of the agreement were excellent in this case, with an RMSE of 0.18 g/L and $R^2 = 0.99$.

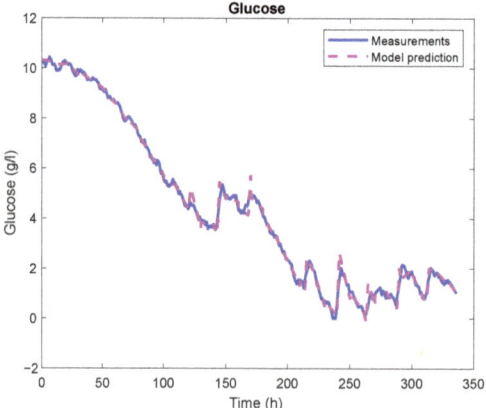

Figure 11. Validation of the CHO cell kinetics model in the case of glucose concentration prediction for the entire batch run.

Furthermore, Figure 12 shows the remarkable matching between the measurements and the predicted values; ideally, all points should lie on a straight line. However, it is important to note that the available data were limited to only four batches. If a larger number of batches are included in the optimisation process, a slight deviation between the individual batches and the process variables is to be expected. In the future, it would be beneficial to combine the data from the individual batches based on the criterion of mutual similarity and then determine the model parameters for the individual clusters.

The predictions for the other process variables, as shown in Table 4, prove satisfactory when the CHO cell kinetics model is used. Only in the case of glutamine concentration does a somewhat larger error occur, which has already been pointed out. The reason for this is that when the PLS model predicts the time series signal for glutamine with less accuracy, the variance of the "measurements" (derived from the soft sensor) increases. Consequently, the time series signal of glutamine is predicted with lower accuracy by the mechanistic model.

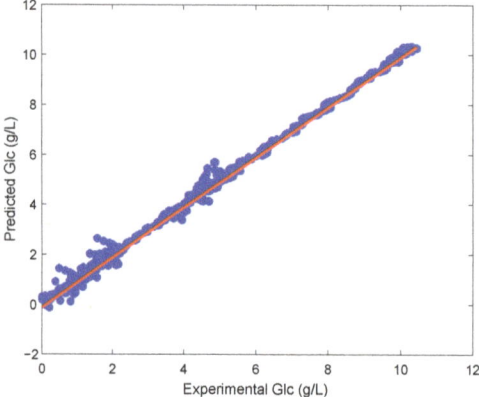

Figure 12. Validation of the CHO cell kinetics model: comparison of experimental and predicted glucose concentrations.

5. Discussion

In developing models that allow the use of soft sensors to monitor key process variables (VCC, TCC, glucose, glutamine, glutamate, lactate and ammonium) in the bioreactor, it was found that using the PLS method alone did not provide the required accuracy and robustness of the models. In particular, with a limited data set (a few batches), the model can be overfitted, leading to a sharp drop in predictive performance compared to what the validation with limited data promises.

Since in our work only about 100 spectra with reference measurements were available during the learning phase and Raman spectra contain more than 3000 components, the phase of selecting key variables became crucial for model construction. By using the CARS method, better handling of collinearity between variables was observed, as well as better performance on small data sets and higher robustness compared to the VIP method. As a result, the RMSE was reduced by up to 30%.

It was found that the VIP method further impaired the predictive ability of the models in certain cases, indicating an overfitting problem, as the number of key variables selected was significantly larger than required by the CARS method. The VIP method also had stability problems, as the results may have become unstable with small samples. Minor variations in the data can lead to significant shifts in the scores, making it difficult to extrapolate the results to other data sets. When calculating the VIP scores based on the weighted sum of squares of the PLS loadings, high variability was found in small data sets.

In Raman spectroscopy, it is important to understand that outlier spectra can occur, influenced by various factors. For example, if the sample in the bioreactor is not evenly mixed, this can lead to deviations in the spectra obtained. Raman spectroscopy derives its readings from the average properties of the area illuminated by the laser. Therefore, a lack of homogeneity in the sample can lead to inconsistent measurements.

Moreover, the components of the sample can play an important role. If components fluoresce under the laser light of the Raman spectrometer, the resulting fluorescence could overshadow the Raman signal and distort the spectra. Additionally, bubbles or particles in the bioreactor can cause scattering or absorption of the laser light, resulting in unpredictable spectra.

Given these potential sources of error, it is important to carefully identify and remove outlier spectra during the modelling phase, as described in Section 2.2.3. This step reduced the root mean square error (RMSE) by 10% (in addition to 30% reduction with the method CARS).

The efficient growth and production of desired products by CHO cells requires specific, strictly controlled conditions in the bioreactor. These conditions include the regulation of pH and temperature, which affect cell metabolic rate, protein folding and expression levels. Equally important is the careful control of nutrient content, especially glucose and glutamine, according to a predetermined profile for the duration of the batch.

Another critical factor is the control of inhibitor concentrations. Metabolic by-products such as ammonia and lactate can potentially inhibit cell growth and protein production if they reach high concentrations. Since glucose is the primary source of energy, its concentration directly affects cell metabolism. Too little glucose can starve cells and inhibit growth, while too much glucose can cause osmotic stress or trigger overproduction of waste products such as lactate.

Given these complexities, the use of an automated bioreactor control system is essential for CHO cell cultivation. Such a system offers several advantages, including maintaining consistent conditions, real-time monitoring, reducing human error and improving efficiency and scalability. Given the significant costs associated with realistic bioreactor experiments, the development of a simulation environment is essential. This environment enables the creation of control algorithms and the evaluation of the effects of different parameters on cell growth and productivity.

The main reason for the lack of advanced automated control techniques in cell culture bioprocesses and bioreactor operations is that these techniques require robust and reliable measurement methods that are available on site. Concentrations of nutrients and metabolites, cell densities and viability are not measured and are uncontrolled or are only controlled manually with long sampling times (12–24 h, as shown in Figure 9). As a result, possible process disturbances may only be detected after long delays, making it difficult to take corrective action and increasing the risk of batch losses.

For the development of an advanced simulation environment, the choice of a CHO kinetic model is also crucial. The chosen model should represent the complex kinetics of CHO cells in sufficient detail. Simpler models based on the Monod equation, for example, are often inadequate in this respect. More complex models, however, pose the challenge of determining numerous parameters that can only be accurately determined with a suitable optimisation method and sufficiently heterogeneous data. In our study, the parameters of a dynamic model of CHO cell kinetics were successfully determined using the PSO method.

To enable the development of a predictive control algorithm, the complex kinetics model will be simplified and linearised, and online adjustment of the (adaptive) model parameters will be facilitated. This adjustment is made possible by an optimisation method that uses the measurements of the current batch to facilitate the online parameterisation.

Future efforts include the development of a model predictive control algorithm based on the simplified model of CHO cell kinetics. Subsequently, the monitoring and control system will be integrated into a real bioreactor. Finally, a practical test of the implemented system will be carried out.

6. Conclusions

This study demonstrates the significant advances in fully automated feeding of CHO cells achieved through the development of advanced models, soft sensors and a novel simulation environment. The research has required a thorough understanding of various chemometric methods and demonstrated their context-specific application in combination with Raman spectroscopy. It has demonstrated the effectiveness of CARS-PLS and an outlier removal method in overcoming difficult challenges such as high dimensionality, multicollinearity and outlier detection. The models created are versatile and scalable and can be applied to a wide range of products, media and cell lines based on CHO host cells. They can be conveniently scaled up for use in large pilot studies and extensive manufacturing processes. However, the success of these methods depends not only on the right choice of techniques, but also crucially on the quality of the input data. Therefore, the preprocessing of the data to remove interfering signals is of the utmost importance. Raman spectra have no inherent value, but when integrated with the appropriate models, they allow for the creation of a sophisticated measurement system. This system, which consists of soft sensors, is used for real-time monitoring and control of important process variables. The measurements reconstructed with these soft sensors play a crucial role in the design of the simulation environment, which significantly speeds up and cheapens the development of control algorithms and thus the automated nutrient dosing system. In essence, this study provides essential insights into the pragmatic application of Raman spectroscopy and innovative methods that form a solid foundation for further research and development in the field of automated cell feeding.

Author Contributions: Methodology, S.T. and I.Š.; Software, S.T.; Validation, S.T. and I.Š.; Formal analysis, S.T.; Investigation, S.T.; Data curation, S.T.; Writing—original draft, S.T. and I.Š.; Writing—review & editing, I.Š.; Supervision, I.Š.; Project administration, I.Š. All authors have read and agreed to the published version of the manuscript.

Funding: This research received no external funding.

Institutional Review Board Statement: Not applicable.

Informed Consent Statement: Not applicable.

Data Availability Statement: The data presented in this study are available on request from the corresponding author. The data is not publicly available due to trade secrets.

Conflicts of Interest: The authors declare no conflict of interest.

References

1. Vital-López, L.; Mercader-Trejo, F.; Rodríguez-Reséndiz, J.; Zamora-Antuñano, M.A.; Rodríguez-López, A.; Esquerre-Verastegui, J.E.; Farrera Vázquez, N.; García-García, R. Electrochemical Characterization of Biodiesel from Sunflower Oil Produced by Homogeneous Catalysis and Ultrasound. *Processes* **2023**, *11*, 94. [CrossRef]
2. Filzmoser, P.; Varmuza, K.; Filzmoser, M.P. *Introduction to Multivariate Statistical Analysis in Chemometrics*; CRC Press: Boca Raton, FL, USA, 2009.
3. García-García, R.; Bocanegra-García, V.; Vital-López, L.; García-Mena, J.; Zamora-Antuñano, M.A.; Cruz-Hernández, M.A.; Rodríguez-Reséndiz, J.; Mendoza-Herrera, A. Assessment of the Microbial Communities in Soil Contaminated with Petroleum Using Next-Generation Sequencing Tools. *Appl. Sci.* **2023**, *13*, 6922. [CrossRef]
4. Reddy, R.K.; Bhargava, R. Chemometric methods for biomedical Raman spectroscopy and imaging. In *Emerging Raman Applications and Techniques in Biomedical and Pharmaceutical Fields*; Springer: Berlin/Heidelberg, Germany, 2010; pp. 179–213.
5. Ferraro, J.R.; Nakamoto, K.; Brown, C.W. Chapter 1—Basic theory. In *Introductory Raman Spectroscopy*, 2nd ed.; Ferraro, J.R., Nakamoto, K., Brown, C.W., Eds.; Academic Press: San Diego, CA, USA, 2003; pp. 1–94. [CrossRef]
6. Kudelski, A. Analytical applications of Raman spectroscopy. *Talanta* **2008**, *76*, 1–8. [CrossRef]
7. Hof, M.; Macháň, R. Chapter 3—Basics of optical spectroscopy. In *Handbook of Spectroscopy*; John Wiley & Sons, Ltd.: Hoboken, NJ, USA, 2014; pp. 31–38. [CrossRef]
8. Horton, R.B.; Duranty, E.; McConico, M.; Vogt, F. Fourier Transform Infrared (FT-IR) Spectroscopy and Improved Principal Component Regression (PCR) for Quantification of Solid Analytes in Microalgae and Bacteria. *Appl. Spectrosc.* **2011**, *65*, 442–453. [CrossRef]
9. O'Connell, M.L.; Ryder, A.G.; Leger, M.N.; Howley, T. Qualitative Analysis Using Raman Spectroscopy and Chemometrics: A Comprehensive Model System for Narcotics Analysis. *Appl. Spectrosc.* **2010**, *64*, 1109–1121. [CrossRef]
10. Mehdizadeh, H.; Lauri, D.; Karry, K.M.; Moshgbar, M.; Procopio-Melino, R.; Drapeau, D. Generic Raman-based calibration models enabling real-time monitoring of cell culture bioreactors. *Biotechnol. Prog.* **2015**, *31*, 1004–1013. [CrossRef] [PubMed]
11. Yousefi-Darani, A.; Paquet-Durand, O.; von Wrochem, A.; Classen, J.; Tränkle, J.; Mertens, M.; Snelders, J.; Chotteau, V.; Mäkinen, M.; Handl, A.; et al. Generic Chemometric Models for Metabolite Concentration Prediction Based on Raman Spectra. *Sensors* **2022**, *22*, 5581. [CrossRef] [PubMed]
12. Goldrick, S.; Umprecht, A.; Tang, A.; Zakrzewski, R.; Cheeks, M.; Turner, R.; Charles, A.; Les, K.; Hulley, M.; Spencer, C.; et al. High-Throughput Raman Spectroscopy Combined with Innovate Data Analysis Workflow to Enhance Biopharmaceutical Process Development. *Processes* **2020**, *8*, 1179. [CrossRef]
13. Geladi, P.; Kowalski, B.R. Partial least-squares regression: A tutorial. *Anal. Chim. Acta* **1986**, *185*, 1–17. [CrossRef]
14. Lourenço, N.D.; Lopes, J.A.; Almeida, C.F.; Sarraguça, M.C.; Pinheiro, H.M. Bioreactor monitoring with spectroscopy and chemometrics: A review. *Anal. Bioanal. Chem.* **2012**, *404*, 1211–1237. [CrossRef]
15. Markey, M.K.; Tourassi, G.D.; Floyd, C.E., Jr. Decision tree classification of proteins identified by mass spectrometry of blood serum samples from people with and without lung cancer. *Proteomics* **2003**, *3*, 1678–1679. [CrossRef]
16. Zou, T.; Dou, Y.; Mi, H.; Zou, J.; Ren, Y. Support vector regression for determination of component of compound oxytetracycline powder on near-infrared spectroscopy. *Anal. Biochem.* **2006**, *355*, 1–7. [CrossRef]
17. Yang, H.; Griffiths, P.R.; Tate, J. Comparison of partial least squares regression and multi-layer neural networks for quantification of nonlinear systems and application to gas phase Fourier transform infrared spectra. *Anal. Chim. Acta* **2003**, *489*, 125–136. [CrossRef]
18. Guardalini, L.G.O.; Dias, V.A.T.; Leme, J.; Bernardino, T.C.; Astray, R.M.; da Silveira, S.R.; Ho, P.L.; Tonso, A.; Jorge, S.A.C.; Núñez, E.G.F. Comparison of Chemometric Models Using Raman Spectroscopy for Offline Biochemical Monitoring Throughout the VLP-making Upstream Process. *Biochem. Eng. J.* **2023**, *198*, 109013. [CrossRef]
19. Savitzky, A.; Golay, M.J.E. Smoothing and Differentiation of Data by Simplified Least Squares Procedures. *Anal. Chem.* **1964**, *36*, 1627–1639. [CrossRef]
20. Cai, W.; Li, Y.; Shao, X. A variable selection method based on uninformative variable elimination for multivariate calibration of near-infrared spectra. *Chemom. Intell. Lab. Syst.* **2008**, *90*, 188–194. [CrossRef]
21. Gosselin, R.; Rodrigue, D.; Duchesne, C. A Bootstrap VIP approach for selecting wavelength intervals in spectral imaging applications. *Chemom. Intell. Lab. Syst.* **2010**, *100*, 12–21. [CrossRef]
22. Performance of some variable selection methods when multicollinearity is present. *Chemom. Intell. Lab. Syst.* **2005**, *78*, 103–112. [CrossRef]
23. Nørgaard, L.; Saudland, A.; Wagner, J.; Nielsen, J.P.; Munck, L.; Engelsen, S.B. Interval Partial Least-Squares Regression (iPLS): A Comparative Chemometric Study with an Example from Near-Infrared Spectroscopy. *Appl. Spectrosc.* **2000**, *54*, 413–419. [CrossRef]
24. Spiegelman, C.H.; McShane, M.J.; Goetz, M.J.; Motamedi, M.; Yue, Q.L.; Coté, G.L. Theoretical Justification of Wavelength Selection in PLS Calibration: Development of a New Algorithm. *Anal. Chem.* **1998**, *70*, 35–44. [CrossRef]
25. Li, H.; Liang, Y.; Xu, Q.; Cao, D. Key wavelengths screening using competitive adaptive reweighted sampling method for multivariate calibration. *Anal. Chim. Acta* **2009**, *648*, 77–84. [CrossRef]

26. Tang, G.; Huang, Y.; Tian, K.; Song, X.; Yan, H.; Hu, J.; Xiong, Y.; Min, S. A new spectral variable selection pattern using competitive adaptive reweighted sampling combined with successive projections algorithm. *Analyst* **2014**, *139*, 4894–4902. [CrossRef] [PubMed]
27. Graf, A.; Woodhams, A.; Nelson, M.; Richardson, D.D.; Short, S.M.; Brower, M.; Hoehse, M. Automated Data Generation for Raman Spectroscopy Calibrations in Multi-Parallel Mini Bioreactors. *Sensors* **2022**, *22*, 3397. [CrossRef] [PubMed]
28. Miller, C.E. Chapter 8—Chemometrics in process analytical chemistry. In *Process Analytical Technology*; John Wiley & Sons, Ltd.: Hoboken, NJ, USA, 2007; pp. 226–328. [CrossRef]
29. Esmonde-White, K.A.; Cuellar, M.; Uerpmann, C.; Lenain, B.; Lewis, I.R. Raman spectroscopy as a process analytical technology for pharmaceutical manufacturing and bioprocessing. *Anal. Bioanal. Chem.* **2017**, *409*, 637–649. [CrossRef] [PubMed]
30. Wurm, F.M. Production of recombinant protein therapeutics in cultivated mammalian cells. *Nat. Biotechnol.* **2004**, *22*, 1393–1398. [CrossRef] [PubMed]
31. Lim, Y.; Wong, N.S.C.; Lee, Y.Y.; Ku, S.C.Y.; Wong, D.C.F.; Yap, M.G.S. Engineering mammalian cells in bioprocessing—Current achievements and future perspectives. *Biotechnol. Appl. Biochem.* **2010**, *55*, 175–189. [CrossRef]
32. Okamura, K.; Badr, S.; Murakami, S.; Sugiyama, H. Hybrid Modeling of CHO Cell Cultivation in Monoclonal Antibody Production with an Impurity Generation Module. *Ind. Eng. Chem. Res.* **2022**, *61*, 14898–14909. [CrossRef]
33. Berry, B.N.; Dobrowsky, T.M.; Timson, R.C.; Kshirsagar, R.; Ryll, T.; Wiltberger, K. Quick generation of Raman spectroscopy based in-process glucose control to influence biopharmaceutical protein product quality during mammalian cell culture. *Biotechnol. Prog.* **2016**, *32*, 224–234. [CrossRef]
34. Whelan, J.; Craven, S.; Glennon, B. In situ Raman spectroscopy for simultaneous monitoring of multiple process parameters in mammalian cell culture bioreactors. *Biotechnol. Prog.* **2012**, *28*, 1355–1362. [CrossRef]
35. Matthews, T.E.; Berry, B.N.; Smelko, J.; Moretto, J.; Moore, B.; Wiltberger, K. Closed loop control of lactate concentration in mammalian cell culture by Raman spectroscopy leads to improved cell density, viability, and biopharmaceutical protein production. *Biotechnol. Bioeng.* **2016**, *113*, 2416–2424. [CrossRef]
36. Abu-Absi, N.R.; Kenty, B.M.; Cuellar, M.E.; Borys, M.C.; Sakhamuri, S.; Strachan, D.J.; Hausladen, M.C.; Li, Z.J. Real time monitoring of multiple parameters in mammalian cell culture bioreactors using an in-line Raman spectroscopy probe. *Biotechnol. Bioeng.* **2011**, *108*, 1215–1221. [CrossRef] [PubMed]
37. Berry, B.; Moretto, J.; Matthews, T.; Smelko, J.; Wiltberger, K. Cross-scale predictive modeling of CHO cell culture growth and metabolites using Raman spectroscopy and multivariate analysis. *Biotechnol. Prog.* **2015**, *31*, 566–577. [CrossRef] [PubMed]
38. Xu, W.J.; Lin, Y.; Mi, C.L.; Pang, J.Y.; Wang, T.Y. Progress in fed-batch culture for recombinant protein production in CHO cells. *Appl. Microbiol. Biotechnol.* **2023**, *107*, 1063–1075. [CrossRef] [PubMed]
39. Bocklitz, T.; Walter, A.; Hartmann, K.; Rösch, P.; Popp, J. How to pre-process Raman spectra for reliable and stable models? *Anal. Chim. Acta* **2011**, *704*, 47–56. [CrossRef] [PubMed]
40. Gautam, R.; Vanga, S.; Ariese, F.; Umapathy, S. Review of multidimensional data processing approaches for Raman and infrared spectroscopy. *EPJ Tech. Instrum.* **2015**, *2*, 8. [CrossRef]
41. Rosipal, R.; Krämer, N. Overview and recent advances in partial least squares. In *International Statistical and Optimization Perspectives Workshop "Subspace, Latent Structure and Feature Selection"*; Saunders, C., Grobelnik, M., Gunn, S., Shawe-Taylor, J., Eds.; Springer: Berlin/Heidelberg, Germany, 2006; pp. 34–51.
42. Madden, M.G.; Howley, T. A Machine Learning Application for Classification of Chemical Spectra. In *Applications and Innovations in Intelligent Systems XVI*; Allen, T., Ellis, R., Petridis, M., Eds.; Springer: London, UK, 2009; pp. 77–90.
43. Brereton, R.G.; Lloyd, G.R. Partial least squares discriminant analysis: taking the magic away. *J. Chemom.* **2014**, *28*, 213–225. [CrossRef]
44. Tenenhaus, M.; Vinzi, V.E.; Chatelin, Y.M.; Lauro, C. PLS path modeling. *Comput. Stat. Data Anal.* **2005**, *48*, 159–205. [CrossRef]
45. Robitaille, J.; Chen, J.; Jolicoeur, M. A Single Dynamic Metabolic Model Can Describe mAb Producing CHO Cell Batch and Fed-Batch Cultures on Different Culture Media. *PLoS ONE* **2015**, *10*, e0136815. [CrossRef]
46. Galleguillos, S.N.; Ruckerbauer, D.; Gerstl, M.P.; Borth, N.; Hanscho, M.; Zanghellini, J. What can mathematical modelling say about CHO metabolism and protein glycosylation? *Comput. Struct. Biotechnol. J.* **2017**, *15*, 212–221. [CrossRef]
47. López-Meza, J.; Araíz-Hernández, D.; Carrillo-Cocom, L.M.; López-Pacheco, F.; Rocha-Pizaña, M.d.R.; Alvarez, M.M. Using simple models to describe the kinetics of growth, glucose consumption, and monoclonal antibody formation in naive and infliximab producer CHO cells. *Cytotechnology* **2016**, *68*, 1287–1300. [CrossRef]
48. Ivarsson, M. Impact of Process Parameters on Cell Growth, Metabolism and Antibody Glycosylation. Ph.D. Thesis, ETH Zurich, Zürich, Switzerland, 2014.

Disclaimer/Publisher's Note: The statements, opinions and data contained in all publications are solely those of the individual author(s) and contributor(s) and not of MDPI and/or the editor(s). MDPI and/or the editor(s) disclaim responsibility for any injury to people or property resulting from any ideas, methods, instructions or products referred to in the content.

MDPI

St. Alban-Anlage 66

4052 Basel

Switzerland

www.mdpi.com

Sensors Editorial Office

E-mail: sensors@mdpi.com

www.mdpi.com/journal/sensors

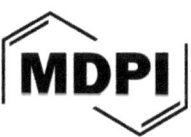

Disclaimer/Publisher's Note: The statements, opinions and data contained in all publications are solely those of the individual author(s) and contributor(s) and not of MDPI and/or the editor(s). MDPI and/or the editor(s) disclaim responsibility for any injury to people or property resulting from any ideas, methods, instructions or products referred to in the content.

www.ingramcontent.com/pod-product-compliance
Lightning Source LLC
LaVergne TN
LVHW070415100526
838202LV00014B/1462